CARIBBEAN HEALING TRADITIONS

As Caribbean communities become more international, clinicians and scholars must develop new paradigms for understanding treatment preferences and perceptions of illness. Despite evidence supporting the need for culturally appropriate care and the integration of traditional healing practices into conventional health and mental health care systems, it is unclear how such integration would function since little is known about the therapeutic interventions of Caribbean healing traditions.

Caribbean Healing Traditions: Implications for Health and Mental Health fills this gap. Drawing on the knowledge of prominent clinicians, scholars, and researchers of the Caribbean and the diaspora, these healing traditions are explored in the context of health and mental health for the first time, making *Caribbean Healing Traditions* an invaluable resource for students, researchers, faculty, and practitioners in the fields of nursing, counseling, psychotherapy, psychiatry, social work, youth and community development, and medicine.

Patsy Sutherland, MEd, is a psychotherapist and PhD candidate in counseling psychology at the University of Toronto. She has authored or coauthored over 15 peer-reviewed papers and book chapters and served as a reviewer for the *Counseling Psychology Quarterly*. Patsy cofounded the Society for Integrating Traditional Healing into Counseling, Psychology, Psychotherapy, and Psychiatry.

Roy Moodley, PhD, is associate professor of counseling psychology at the University of Toronto. He is the director for the Centre for Diversity in Counselling and Psychotherapy. He has authored or edited several journal articles, book chapters and books, including *Outside the Sentence* and Handbook of Counseling and Psychotherapy in an International Context.

Barry Chevannes, PhD, was emeritus professor of social anthropology at the University of the West Indies, Mona. He authored three books, one edited collection, and scores of articles on the Rastafari and Revival religions, male socialization, and culture. A public scholar, he served as chair of the Institute of Jamaica, the National Ganja Commission, and the Jamaica Justice System Reform Task Force.

CARIBBEAN HEALING TRADITIONS

Implications for Health and Mental Health

Edited by
Patsy Sutherland, Roy Moodley,
and Barry Chevannes

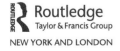

Routledge
Taylor & Francis Group
NEW YORK AND LONDON

First published 2014
by Routledge
711 Third Avenue, New York, NY 10017

Simultaneously published in the UK
by Routledge
27 Church Road, Hove, East Sussex BN3 2FA

Library of Congress Cataloging in Publication Data
Caribbean healing traditions : implications for health and mental health /
edited by Patsy Sutherland, Roy Moodley, and Barry Chevannes.
    pages cm
    Includes bibliographical references and index.
 1. Traditional medicine–Caribbean Area–History. 2. Healing–Caribbean
Area–History. 3. Medicine, Magic, mystic, and spagiric–Caribbean area.
 I. Sutherland, Patsy, 1965– II. Moodley, Roy. III. Chevannes, Barry.
 GR120.C38 2014
 610.9729–dc23   2012051145

ISBN: 978–0–415–88339–9 (hbk)
ISBN: 978–0–415–84233–4 (pbk)
ISBN: 978–0–203–84450–2 (ebk)

Typeset in Bembo
by Swales & Willis Ltd, Exeter, Devon

In loving memory of Kennedy Salim
– PS

CONTENTS

ACKNOWLEDGMENTS

We extend our sincerest appreciation to all of the contributors in this book for sharing their expertise in the way that the book necessitated. Thank you for your patience and understanding in configuring your chapters in accordance with our specifications.

Our deepest gratitude to family and several colleagues for their unwavering support throughout this project; they are Clarence St. Louis, Melina Sutherland, Natasha Sutherland, Diana Cassie, Anissa Talahite, Zina Claude, Tara Isabelle, Maya Florence, Roisin Anna, Daniel McGrath, and Uwe Gielen.

We would also like to acknowledge the help and support of the editors, copy editors and staff at Routledge, Dana Bliss, Christopher Tominich, Anna Moore, and Sam Rosenthal.

It is with profound sadness that we remember the death of our colleague and co-editor Dr. Barry Chevannes who died during the preliminary stages of this book.

We would like to thank the Caribbean healers (in Toronto and Grenada) who in many ways contributed directly and indirectly to this book and to our understanding of Caribbean healing traditions.

– Patsy Sutherland and Roy Moodley

CONTRIBUTORS

Jicinta M. Alexis, BA, obtained her degree from St. George's University. Her interest is in community health with special focus on gender and traditional medicine.

E. Anthony Allen, MDiv, MRC Psych, is a psychiatrist and a consultant with Wholistic Health Ministries. He has pioneered community-based whole person healing ministries in local congregations. He has also authored the books *Caring for the Whole Person* and *Simple Steps to Wellness*.

Omowale Amuleru-Marshall, PhD, MPH, is a counseling and public health psychologist. He is originally from Guyana and is currently the director of Community Health and Outreach in the office of the Provost at St. George's University in Grenada.

Claudette A. Anderson, PhD, obtained her degree from the Graduate Institute of the Liberal Arts at Emory University. Her research and scholarship focuses on Jamaican Ethno-medicine and Africa-derived religions with a specialization in Revival and Obeah.

Michel'e Bertrand, MEd, is an EdD candidate in counseling psychology at the University of Toronto and a psychotherapist in private practice in Toronto.

Yuri Clement, PhD, holds the post of senior lecturer in pharmacology at the University of the West Indies, Trinidad and Tobago. His laboratory research includes evaluation of medicinal plant extracts for anticancer and hepatoprotective properties using in vitro and in vivo techniques.

Wendy Crawford-Daniel, PhD, is a research sociologist, assistant professor, and acting chair of the department of liberal studies at St. Georges University in Grenada. Her areas of interest include cultural competency in working with diverse populations and international organizations.

Jesus Soto Espinosa, PhD, is a clinical psychologist who has carried out research into asthma as a member of a team from the University of Puerto Rico Medical Sciences Campus. Dr. Soto is a co-investigator on a research project that studies spirituality and Spiritism among Puerto Rican doctors.

Stephen D. Glazier, PhD, is professor of anthropology and a graduate faculty fellow at the University of Nebraska-Lincoln. He is author and/or editor of seven books, including *Marchin' the Pilgrims Home* and *The Encyclopedia of African and African American Religions*.

Angela Gomez, PhD, is an applied anthropologist. Her research interests are on human vulnerability with an emphasis on poverty and the impact of social policies and programs aimed at its alleviation in Latin America, the Caribbean, and developing countries.

Camille Hernandez-Ramdwar, PhD, is an associate professor in the department of sociology at Ryerson University in Toronto, Canada, who also teaches in Caribbean studies. Her areas of research include Caribbean cultures and identities and African traditional religions in the Caribbean.

Gerard Hutchinson, MD, is currently the head of the department of clinical medical sciences and unit lead in psychiatry at the school of medicine at the University of the West Indies, St Augustine. His research interests are in migration-related issues in mental health and suicidal behaviour in the Caribbean.

Abrahim H. Khan, PhD, is professor in the faculty of divinity at Trinity College in the University of Toronto and director of its advanced degree studies program. His publications are in the areas of Kierkegaard studies, religion and international diplomacy, and comparative studies in religion.

Joan D. Koss-Chioino, PhD, is professor emerita of anthropology at Arizona State University and research professor of psychology at George Washington University. Her primary interest is the etiology and treatment of illness and emotional problems.

Kumar Mahabir, PhD, is an assistant professor in the Centre for Education Programmes at the University of Trinidad and Tobago. His most recent books are *Indian Caribbean Folklore Spirits*, *The Indian Diaspora in the Caribbean*, and *Traditional Medicine and Women Healers in Trinidad*.

Keith E. McNeal, PhD, is an anthropologist and assistant professor of comparative cultural studies at the University of Houston. He is the author of *Trance and Modernity in the Southern Caribbean: African and Hindu Popular Religions in Trinidad and Tobago.*

Ghislène Méance, PsyD, is a licensed psychologist. She is the founder of the Multicultural Counseling and Testing Center which provides culturally sensitive psychological evaluation, individual, group, and family therapy to individuals from all cultures.

Kai A. D. Morgan, PsyD, has been lecturing in clinical psychology at the University of the West Indies, Mona, Jamaica for the past 12 years and serves as the consultant psychologist in the department of psychiatry.

Nathaniel Samuel Murrell, PhD, is associate professor of philosophy and religion at the University of North Carolina, Wilmington. His book publications include *Chanting Down Babylon* and, most recently, *Afro-Caribbean Religions: An Introduction to their Historical, Cultural, and Sacred Traditions.*

Kristyn O'Rita Neckles, MA, MS, is a doctoral student in clinical psychology at Carlos Albizu University in Miami, Florida. Her current research interest is in exploring the influences of culture and spirituality on the behaviors of Caribbean people.

Arvilla Payne-Jackson, PhD, is a professor at Howard University. Her primary areas of research are in the fields of medical anthropology, sociolinguistics, ethnographic evaluation, and service learning.

Anahí Viladrich, PhD, originally from Argentina, is an associate professor in the departments of sociology and anthropology at Queens College and in the public health program at the graduate center of the City University of New York. She has published more than 50 articles and book chapters on immigrants and folk healing traditions, and on gender and culture.

William Wedenoja, PhD, is professor of anthropology and head of the department of sociology and anthropology at Missouri State University, where he also serves as director of the master's in applied anthropology program. Dr. Wedenoja has published on Revival Zion, trance, healing, Pentecostalism, cultural psychiatry, heritage conservation, and multicultural education.

Paul Younger, PhD, professor emeritus, McMaster University, is the author of 8 books and 40 book chapters. His most recent book is: *New Homelands: Hindu Communities in Mauritius, Guyana, Trinidad, South Africa, Fiji and East Africa.*

Wallace W. Zane, PhD, is an anthropologist, teaching at California State University, Northridge, at Santa Monica College, and Art Center College of Design. He studies religion and culture. His book about the Spiritual Baptists is *Journeys to the Spiritual Lands: The Natural History of a West Indian Religion.*

FOREWORD

Biomedical psychiatry and Western psychology incorporating west-European post-Enlightenment ideologies of the human condition—its division into mind and body, its dependence on individual striving as opposed to communal harmony and so on—has dominated mental health systems in Europe and North America. However, the meaning of "mental health" and illness—both "psychological" and "somatic" if we think in those reductionist terms—are culturally determined. As a result of colonialism and postcolonial Westernization the Euro-American system of mental health has been promoted to a greater or lesser extent in the rest of world, the Global South. As Western psychiatry and psychology come to dominate mental health systems in countries with predominantly non-Western cultural backgrounds, the loss to cultural diversity (which I think most of us value in all things and makes for a truly human world rather than one of machines) is obvious. But what is less evident but equally true is that the alleviation of human suffering, which is an inevitable part of our existence, is ill-served by such a loss.

Healing traditions have been there in all human societies from time immemorial—they may well be a *sine qua non* of the very existence of human beings as social beings—in other words we would not be here if not for such traditions. But cultural traditions never stand still; they are dynamic and alive, changing according to the social and political forces that impinge on the societies that they underpin and sustain. The Caribbean is a place where people from many different cultural traditions have come together—sometimes by forcible transportation—and survived, fought, and suffered together. Out of all this have emerged what are called "new ethnicities" with hybrid (creolized) cultural forms—except of course that all people everywhere are culturally "hybrid" in one way or another. The editors of this book have got together an impressive collection of contributions to present us with a vivid picture of the healing traditions that are alive and well in the Caribbean. This is particularly welcome at a time when Caribbean diasporas in other parts of the Western world—especially in the UK and Canada—are concerned by the inadequacy of the mental health systems they encounter. They are being over-diagnosed as "schizophrenic" clearly because of the limitations of the psychiatric system to properly understand the nature of their cultural backgrounds and the problems they face in living and thriving in an environment that is institutionally racist. But even more importantly, what Caribbean users of mental health services complain about is the lack of spirituality in the types of "treatment" offered to them in the systems of psychiatry and psychology that they encounter. But of course white British and North American people, too, often complain of this; so there is obvious need for statutory services to take heed and take some lessons, at least from healing traditions that may well show us alternative approaches that we should all have access to—and perhaps a knowledge of these traditions would result in fundamental changes to the way mental health services are delivered.

Today there is much discussion around the concept of a "global" mental health—the implication being that what Western psychiatry and psychology have developed in Europe and North America should be actively exported to the Global South—the countries of the "third world." Fortunately this so-called "global mental health movement" has stimulated a countermovement proposing that mental health is a *local* matter—and that systems for promoting mental health must take on board the traditions of local communities and what they want from "health." In this context there is a rising demand for knowledge and understanding of local customs, local ways of seeing health and illness, and, above all, of local healing systems. Healing traditions coexist and overlap with medical traditions the world over and so in planning mental health services, there is an imperative to take on board both local medical traditions *and* local healing traditions. And what is even more important, is the need for knowledge about ways of healing that are currently being used and nurtured by people—currently active systems of healing. The more we know about systems of healing that are serving people in different parts of the world, the better prepared are we to think about and plan services that are culturally consistent with the needs and wishes of communities the world over. We know something about healing systems in Asia and Africa but we have very little knowledge in this respect about the Caribbean region. This book is then a valuable resource at this point of the "global" debate.

So for all these reasons, it is my pleasure to welcome this book.

Dr. Suman Fernando
Honorary Professor, Faculty of Social Sciences & Humanities,
London Metropolitan University; Formerly Senior Lecturer in Mental Health,
European Centre for Migration & Social Care (MASC) University of Kent;
Consultant Psychiatrist, Chase Farm Hospital, Enfield, Middlesex

INTRODUCTION

Traditional, cultural, and indigenous healing practices have been a part of the sociocultural and geopolitical landscape of the Caribbean since the time of slavery, and possibly before, since the Amerindians would have had a form of health care system in place. In the colonial period very little attention was paid to the health of enslaved Africans and indentured Indians; they had to rely on the knowledge, skills, and expertise that came with them from West Africa and India. Most, if not all, of these individuals used religion, knowledge of herbs, and folk medicine to manage their health and mental health (see Handler & Jacoby, 1993, for discussion). This practice of traditional medicine was made possible through its integration with Christianity which in turn resulted in the formation of new forms of religion, spirituality, and healing, such as Shango, Vodou, Spiritual Baptists, Santeria, Obeah, and Spiritism to name a few; practices which are currently in place in the Caribbean. Despite the hegemonic influences of colonialism these religions and their healing practices have remained strong and are continuing to grow (Gibson, Morgado, Brosyle, Mesa, & Sanchez, 2010).

Any critical and reflective view of Caribbean healing traditions must take into account the complex and traumatic experience of slavery, the racism of colonialism, and the postcolonial need for social stability and economic development. Against this background, globalization and neoliberal policies of health care practices often dictated by capitalist multinational pharmaceutical companies appear to influence how individuals and communities understand their health and mental health. In this environment of constant change the medical model and Western psychological sciences are seemingly failing to address the complex needs of the Caribbean people. Critics assert that this can be attributed to the imposition of Western medical and psychological theories and methods that have hindered a holistic and accurate understanding of the health and mental health needs of

Caribbean and other non-Western individuals and groups (Poortinga, 1999). The result, according to a Baptist leader, Reverend Simpson (as cited in Rahming, 2001) is a zombification or colonization of the consciousness and "theft of spirit" of the Caribbean people.

In the Caribbean context, the colonial past is not simply a historical legacy but a lived reality for many contemporary individuals in the Caribbean diaspora. Its lingering effects may be evident in the higher rates of involuntary detainment in secure psychiatric settings and the greater involvement of the police in this process (see Littlewood, 1986, for a discussion), greater elevated risk (with incidence ratios above 7) of all psychotic disorders when compared to the majority population (Harrison et al., 1997), disproportionate representation among clients diagnosed as schizophrenic (Boast & Chesterman, 1995; Littlewood, 1986, Dunn & Fahy, 1990) and the fact that Caribbeans are 44% more likely to be detained under the Mental Health Act, than their White counterparts, despite this group having similar rates of mental ill health as any other ethnic group (Samuels, 2008). Furthermore this population is far less likely to be offered counseling, rather, they are more often treated with chemotherapy with higher prescribed drug dosage than Whites (Callan & Littlewood, 1998). While these occurrences can be attributed to the stigma associated with mental illness and the beliefs that individuals hold about its causes to some degree, discrimination within mental health services (Samuels, 2008), intergenerational traumatic experiences, a dearth of culturally competent treatment and distrust of conventional establishments (Centre for Addiction and Mental Health, 2008) were also cited as contributing factors to the mental health problems of Caribbean people. Current mental health care practices must reflect a consciousness of these histories and realities in order meet the needs of this population.

Shortcomings of Western Health Care Practices

Critical race and culture scholarship has highlighted the failures and shortcomings of mental health practices in psychiatry (see for example, Fernando, 1988); psychotherapy (see, for example, Moodley & Palmer, 2005); and counseling psychology (see, for example, Helms, 1990; Sue and Sue, 1990; Vontress, 2010). Without exception, all these scholars agree that the current health and mental health care provision for Caribbean, African, and Asian communities falls short of the ethical claims to ensure social justice, equity, and non-oppressive practice. However, some progress is being made by the multicultural and cross-cultural counseling and psychotherapy movement (see, for example, Lago, 2012; Sue and Sue, 1990) to redress these shortcomings.

Historically, mental health counseling has been part of the philosophical traditions of European religion and spirituality. Richards and Bergin (1997) argue that psychology as a whole located itself within a 19th-century naturalistic science that is based on deterministic, reductionist, and positivist assumptions that viewed religious and spiritual beliefs and practices negatively. Hence, spirituality has frequently been overlooked as a representation of diversity in health and mental health care systems. While there has been some significant research attempts to consider a new synthesis between religion, spirituality and traditional healing, and mental health counseling, extending notions of health and well-being to include concern for the spirit (see, for example, Fukuyama & Sevig, 1999; Moodley & West, 2005; Sutherland, 2011; Sutherland & Moodley, 2010; Vontress, 2005), many health and mental health care practitioners persistently choose to maintain their historical ambivalence over cultural competence in this important area of client diversity (Russell & Yarhouse, 2006).

Among minority communities, there is an awareness of the failure of main-stream mental health care systems to treat the whole person. Western models of health care understand illness as located in the body or the mind; consequently, treatment focuses predominantly on the mental and emotional components (see, for example, Duran, 1990; Garrett & Carroll, 2000; Ross, 1992). This compart-mentalization of the individual is a legacy of the dualist Cartesian paradigm which claims that the body and mind are separate entities. This is in sharp contrast to the Caribbean worldview which is based on holism, collectivism, and spirituality. Indeed, clients who hold such worldviews about problems in living often find the process of categorizing personal problems and distress in accordance with a scientifically constructed statistical manual of mental disorders bewildering (see Soulayrol, Guigou, & Avy, 1981, for discussion).

Moreover, in Western approaches to mental health care, there is little attention paid to the larger historical and contemporary contexts that shape and reshape the social lives of these traditional cultural variables, namely, holism, collectivism, and spirituality. There are many historical and ideological forces underlying cultural values, identity, psychological frames of thinking, and approaches to health and well-being in the Caribbean; the colonial past continues to overshadow individuals in respect to self, identity, and social related struggles. Individuals from the Caribbean continue to struggle with issues pertaining to racial identity often referred to as Roast Breadfruit Psychosis (Hickling & Hutchinson, 1999) and Afro-Saxon Psychosis (Best 1999; Maharajh, 2000); in other words, individuals who are Black on the outside but White on the inside. The writings of the psychiatrist and renowned postcolonial theorist Franz Fanon (1965; 1967) were influential in this regard, particularly due to his emphasis on the dehumanizing aspects of colonialism and racism, dissolution of the self and the fragmentation of the psyche.

Similarly, illness representations and conceptualizations of physical and psy-chological distress are predicated on knowledge systems that are often at odds with traditional knowledge systems and wellness ideologies. Intervention models that are based on Eurocentric assumptions and values are often imposed on the Caribbean people; "such imposition is reminiscent of colonialism and can potentially be retraumatizing" (Sutherland & Moodley, 2010, p. 271). Indeed, in seeking to inscribe a liberatory discourse of health, mental health, and well-being, scholars and researchers often run the risk of inadvertently recreating the very trauma that is being critically examined and spotlighted; such endeavors conducted under the guise of an objective and humanistic process to acknowledge and respect the Caribbean and its people end up doing the opposite and prevailing racist notions of the Caribbean people and their cultural and healing traditions are reinforced.

Integrating Caribbean Healing Traditions

As Caribbean populations become more global and their traditional healing practices spread along with them, the need to understand these practices has become an increasingly pressing concern. In many metropolitan cities in Canada, the UK, and the USA it is not difficult to find healers practicing their various Caribbean healing traditions. For example, in the inner city hamlets we find Santeros from the Santeria tradition which is commonly practiced in Cuba; Haitian Hougans and Mambos from the Vodou tradition; Shango and Spiritual Baptist healers from the English speaking Caribbean; Imams and Hindu healers from Guyana, Trinidad, and Surinam; Revival healers from their homeland of Jamaica; Spiritist healers from the Espiritismo tradition practiced predominantly in Puerto Rico; and Rastafari and Christian practitioners who are ubiquitous throughout the Caribbean region, all practicing their type of health and mental health care. Many of these practices represent an amalgamation of religious, spiritual, and social traditions of the Amerindian, African, Indian, and the Europeans and all have incorporated Christian, particularly Catholic rites and rituals, into their practices to varying degrees.

While aspects of ritual, classification of the spirits, the schemas used for identifying ailments, the method of healing, and the use of symbols may differ, Koss-Chioino (2006) contends that these differences are more elaborations of content rather than process; the basic philosophy of the healing process and the role of the healer remain the same. Furthermore, the conceptual distance between body and mind, physical and spiritual healing, or between health beliefs and their treatments is not very vast, in fact, the practices can be considered different hues of each other (du Toit, 2001). In addition, there are several characteristics that are fundamental to these religions. They all represent an amalgamation of monotheism and polytheism with one Supreme Being in addition to a pantheon of gods or deities (Patterson, 1967). Central to these religions and healing traditions is the relationship between human beings and the spirits; spirits of both the ancestors and of other living entities are thought to play a role in the lives of the living (Fernández Olmos, 2003). As well, spirits and power are thought to become centralized into one individual, often the leader or healer, who can then pass knowledge to others, as well as heal various ailments. Inorganic objects can also be permeated with supernatural powers. The connection between the human world and the spirit world is an integral element of Caribbean healing traditions and spirits may be manifested in the bodies of both healers and clients (Fernandez, 2003; Patterson, 1967); all of these traditions draw heavily on rituals, charms, music, dance, and chants as a way to summon the deities from the spirit world.

Moodley, Sutherland, and Oulanova (2008) maintain that when Caribbean clients engage in traditional healing ceremonies and rituals, the fundamental principles of holism and the body–mind–spirit connection upon which their worldviews are predicated are reaffirmed. Hence, this service is not only historically and politically germane but also culturally appropriate. First, the cultural similarity results in a tacit understanding between healer and client and ailments are located within their particular cultural context. This is underscored by NGOMA (2003) who states, "The most effective therapeutic agents are those who embody the culture of their clients. In a sense, the client's culture is the healing instrument" (cited in Vontress, 2005, p. 133). Second, through a collective, undisputed conviction in the powers of the healer, psychological relief from ailments and reduced anxiety are attained (Finkler, 1994). Furthermore, when a patient consults a traditional healer, he or she is expected to have a clear sense of the nature of the presenting ailment and its treatments; in this way, the patient is reassured of the healer's legitimacy in the healing role. Clients also feel confident that the healer knows their anguish because they too have suffered afflictions before becoming healers since it is usually a condition of the initiation process.

This notion of the "wounded healer" (Jung, 1954 [1982]). refers to the process by which a healer connects with his or her own defenselessness to help others suffering from similar experiences (see Koss-Chioino, 2006, for a discussion). This helps to ensure that clients will find a diagnosis that resonates with their understanding of their core issues and they are reassured that the treatment will be acceptable and useful. In addition, clients are expected to be meaningfully engaged with the healing process by being in a state of alacrity as well as to hold a firm belief in the spirits and the techniques of the healer (McCabe, 2007). Other factors include the importance of the quality of the relationship between the healer and the client, as well as the time dedicated to the process (Press, 1978; Ross, 2008). By taking their cues from their clients, traditional healers ensure that the symptoms and illness preferences of their respective clients will be validated.

Traditional healing appears to be an effective, culturally appropriate and widespread form of treatment for physical, mental, and psychological ailments in the Caribbean. This is also true for Caribbean communities in the diaspora. Given its pivotal role in addressing mental health concerns in particular, the underutilization of conventional mental health care services and the prevalence of mental and psychological ailments in this population, it is crucial that these practices are understood in their appropriate historical and cultural context. At the same time, attempting to write about traditional healing in an academic way is in some way counterintuitive to the essence of traditional healing, which is effectively an experiential process. However, if traditional healing is to be integrated into health and mental health care with Caribbean clients, we must find ways of deciphering its non-dual, anti-Cartesian and, at times, contradictory nature into a common clinical lexicon that will enable healers and health and mental health care practitioners to effectively make sense of the system of meanings of the Caribbean client's personal, psychological, and sociocultural experiences. The lack of a common language can often lead to the pathologizing of culturally sanctioned conceptualizations of distress (Sutherland & Moodley, 2011). Hence the collection of chapters in this book is one attempt to promote knowledge and understanding of these healing systems and to articulate the potential of and urgency in integrating Caribbean healing traditions into psychology and the healing professions.

How the Book is Organized

This book is divided into four parts.

Part I: History, Philosophy, and Development of Caribbean Healing Traditions

Part I begins with Chapter 1, The History, Philosophy, and Transformation of Caribbean Healing Traditions by Patsy Sutherland, who explores the specific historical processes of colonialism, slavery, indentureship, and plantation economy, as well as the broad political interests that have shaped and reshaped traditional healing in the Caribbean. Patsy argues that current healing practices are a response to these processes and must be seen as such if they are to have any relevance to the ways in which we deal with the physical, social, and psychological illnesses of the contemporary Caribbean. In Chapter 2, The Evolution of Caribbean Traditional Healing Practices by Wendy Crawford-Daniel and Jicinta M. Alexis, the evolution of traditional healing practices in the Caribbean is explored, as well as the relationship between Caribbean traditional healing practices, the illness beliefs, and health seeking strategies of the people. As many Caribbean societies transitioned from traditional to modern, culturally normative healing practices and beliefs were in conflict with modern Western medicinal practices and beliefs. Chapter 3, Caribbean Traditional Medicine: Legacy from the Past, Hope for the Future by Arvilla Payne-Jackson, discusses how the traditional medical systems evolved in the Caribbean during slavery, with traditional medical and religious beliefs and rituals of Africans forming the primary basis. The chapter also explores the current status of health care provision where the presence of biomedicine and traditional medicine continues to play a significant role in health care throughout the Caribbean. Chapter 4, Herbal Medicine Practices in the Caribbean by Yuri Clement, and details the potpourri of herbal pharmacopeia in the Caribbean which developed primarily from contributions of indigenous Amerindians, enslaved Africans, indentured Asians, and European settlers. Supernatural beliefs and the dichotomous 'hot–cold' concept of health and disease guide the prescriptive use of herbs for simple conditions such as the common cold to complex gynecological conditions.

Part II: Caribbean Traditional Healing and Healers

Part II starts with Chapter 5, Obeah: Afro-Caribbean Religious Medicine Art and Healing, by Nathaniel Samuel Murrell who discusses the art and science of Obeah in traditional religious medicine. He discusses the oppression and persecution of Obeah practices during the colonial governments, driving Obeah underground. He asserts that Obeah practitioners are reluctant to reveal their association with the art, so health care providers may have difficulty merging modern medicine with Obeah healing because of its secrecy. Chapter 6, Vodou Healing and Psychotherapy by Ghislène Méance, is an exploration of Vodou philosophy and its practice of health and mental health. With a particular focus on Haiti the chapter attempts to show that Vodou can be an effective tool in health and mental health care in the West. Ghislène explores how some Haitian immigrants integrate mental health care services and Vodou healing. This chapter will increase readers' awareness of several cultural and religious issues to address when caring for Vodou followers and clients from the Caribbean. In Chapter 7, Sango Healers and Healing in the Caribbean, Stephen Glazier examines Sango rituals and belief systems. He offers a postcolonial critique as a way to situate the resurgence and development of Shango in contemporary Caribbean culture. In Chapter 8, *La Regla De Ocha* (*Santería*): Afro-Cuban Healing Methods in Cuba and the diaspora, Camille Hernandez-Ramdwar explores *La Regla de Ocha* (*Santería*) as an Afro-Cuban religion that has played a central role in the healing of Cuban communities. Camille discusses the common beliefs about illness and well-being from the *Santería* perspective and the resurgence of interest in *La Regla de Ocha* in the Caribbean, particularly in Cuba. In Chapter 9, Puerto Rican Spiritism (*Espiritismo*): Social Context, Healing Process, and Mental Health by Jesus Soto Espinosa and Joan D. Koss-Chioino, the cultural and historical context of Spiritism (*Espiritismo*), as a philosophical, "scientific," and ethical movement, is reviewed. The focus on Spiritism and its underlying principles in Puerto Rico are explored. In Chapter 10, Revival: An Indigenous Religion and Spiritual Healing Practice in Jamaica, William Wedenoja and Claudette Anderson discuss Revival as a religious tradition with an African foundation and Christian influences that is indigenous to the island of Jamaica. Healing is central to the practice of Revival and takes place in sacred places called "balmyards," where it is usually performed by women called Mothers who have received the power of healing as a spiritual gift. Wedenoja and Anderson argue that Revival healing has been marginalized by the medical profession and criminalized by the law. They assert that Revival is an authentic and popular form of folk psychiatry or spiritual counseling that should be legalized. In Chapter 11, Spiritual Baptists in the Caribbean, Wallace Zane brings to our attention the complexities of the Spiritual Baptist religion as an Afro-Caribbean Christian tradition. The religion is revelatory, with differences in practice between the various Caribbean islands and between local traditions within islands.

Part III: Spirituality, Religion, and Cultural Healing

Part III begins with Chapter 12, Christian Spirituality, Religion, and Healing in the Caribbean by E. A. Allen and Abrahim Khan, who explore an integrative model of Christianity as a whole person healing ministry within a traditional and Afrocentric cultural matrix in the Caribbean. In Chapter 13, RastafarI: Cultural Healing in the Caribbean by Kai Morgan, the philosophy of RastafarI is discussed. The origins and development of RastafarI as well as its current challenges, development, and experiences are explored. Chapter 14, Hindu Healing Traditions in the Southern Caribbean: History and Praxis by Keith McNeal, Kumar Mahabir, and Paul Younger, explores Hindu healing traditions in the West Indies by situating practices of religious and popular healing within changing social and historical contexts. It examines the two most prominent forms of contemporary Indo-Caribbean Hindu therapeutic praxis: the psychosomatic healing technique known as *jharay*, as well as trance-based catharsis and exorcism offered by heterodox *Shakti Puja*. The colonial legacy and postcolonial dynamics are discussed with regard to implications for health and mental health. In Chapter 15, Islamic Influence in the Caribbean: Traditional and Cultural Healing Practice by Abrahim Khan, Islamic healing practices are discussed as an adjunctive therapy in the cultural and political economy of the Caribbean. Khan explores the connections between counseling psychology and spirituality, between religion and medicine.

Part IV: Traditional Healing and Conventional Health and Mental Health

Part IV begins with Chapter 16, Community Mental Health in the English Speaking Caribbean by Gerard Hutchinson, who describes the development of community mental health services in the English speaking Caribbean. He argues that the driving force behind this process has been the training of mental health professionals with an initial focus on psychiatry and a more recent emphasis on psychology, thus ignoring Caribbean indigenous or traditional healing methods. In Chapter 17, Psychology, Spirituality, and Well-Being in the Caribbean, Omowale Amuleru-Marshall, Angela Gomez, and Kristyn Neckles discuss the contexts and processes by which traditional healing practices can be a part of Western counseling and psychotherapy. Chapter 18, Practical Magic in the US Urban Milieu: Botánicas and the Informal Networks of Healing, Anahí Viladrich discusses the role of Latino healers as informal counselors among diverse groups of Latino immigrants in New York City (NYC). The chapter explores these issue through empirical research conducted in NYC. The study explored the convergence of spirituality, the social and the physical realms, in conceptualizing their main therapeutic approaches and the resulting treatments. And finally, in Chapter 19, Caribbean Traditional Healing and the Diaspora, Roy Moodley and Michel'e Bertrand explore the evolution and development of Caribbean healing traditions in the West, the complexities, confusions, and contradictions within which Caribbean traditional healing practices survives. The chapter also explores how these healing traditions can be integrated into mainstream mental health care practices.

References

Best, L. (1999). How long it go take? *The Trinidad Express,* p.7

Boast, N., & Chesterman, P. (1995). Black people and secure psychiatric facilities. *British Journal of Criminology, 35*(2), 218–235.

Callan, A., & Littlewood, R. (1998). Patient satisfaction: Ethnic origin or explanatory model? *International Journal of Social Psychiatry, 44*(1), 1–11.

Centre for Addiction and Mental Health, Clarke Institute of Psychiatry (2008). International experts examine the causes of mental illness in African and Caribbean Communities in Canada. Retrieved on April 16, 2008 from http://www.camh.net/News_events/News_releases_and_media_advisories_and_backgrounders

Dunn, J., & Fahy, T. (1990). Police admissions to a psychiatric hospital: Demographic and clinical differences between different ethnic groups. *British Journal of Psychiatry, 156,* 373–378.

Duran, E. (1990). *Transforming the soul wound.* Delhi: Arya Offset Press.

du Toit, B. M. (2001). Ethnomedical (folk) healing in the Caribbean. In Magarite Olmos Fernández (Ed.), *Healing cultures: Art and religion as curative practices in the Caribbean and its diaspora.* London: Palgrave.

Fanon, F. (1965). *The wretched of the earth.* New York: Grove.

Fanon, F. (1967). *Black skin, White masks.* New York: Grove.

Fernando, S. (1988). *Race and culture in psychiatry.* London: Croom Helm.

Fernández Olmos, M. (2003). *Creole religions of the Caribbean: An introduction from Vodou and Santería to Obeah and Espiritismo.* New York: New York University Press.

Finkler, K. (1994). Sacred healing and biomedicine compared. *Medical Anthropology Quarterly, New Series, 8*(2), 178–197.

Fukuyama, M., & Sevig, T. D. (1999). *Integrating spirituality into multicultural counseling.* Thousand Oaks, CA: Sage.

Garrett, M. T., & Carroll, J .J. (2000). Mending the broken circle: Treatment of substance dependence among Native Americans. *Journal of Counseling & Development, 78*(4), 379–388.

Gibson, B. G., Morgado, A. J., Brosyle, A. C., Mesa, E. H., & Sanchez, C. H. (2010). Afro-centric religious consultations as treatment for psychotic disorders among day hospital patients in Santiago de Cuba. *Mental Health, Religion & Culture, 1*(1), 1–11.

Handler, J., & Jacoby, J. (1993). Slave medicine and plant use in Barbados. *Journal of the Barbados Museum and Historical Society, 41,* 74–98.

Helms, J. E. (Ed.) (1990). *Black and White racial identity: Theory, research and practice.* Westport, CT: Greenwood Press.

Hickling, F. W., & Hutchinson, G. (1999) Post-colonialism and mental health: Understanding the roast breadfruit. *Psychiatric Bulletin, 24,* 94–95.

Jung, C. G. (1954 [1982]). *The practice of psychotherapy.* R. F. C. Hull, Trans. Collected works (Vol. 16). Princeton, NJ: Princeton University Press.

Koss-Chioino, J. D. (2006). Spiritual transformation, ritual healing and altruism. *Zygon,* *41*(4), 877–892.

Lago, C. (2012). Approaching therapy across cultures: Clemmont Vontress from a British perspective. In R. Moodley, L. Epp, & H. Yusuf (Eds.), *Counseling across the cultural divide: The Clemmont E. Vontress reader.* Ross-on-Wye, UK: PCCS Books.

Littlewood, R. (1986). Ethnic minorities and the mental health act: Patterns of explanation. *Psychiatric Bulletin, 10,* 306–308.

Maharajh, H. D. (2000). Afro-Saxon psychosis or cultural schizophrenia in African-Caribbeans, *Psychiatric Bulletin, 24,* 96–97.

McCabe, G. H. (2007). The healing path: A culture and community derived indigenous therapy model. *Psychotherapy: Theory, Research, Practice, Training, 44*(2), 148–160.

Moodley, R., & Palmer, S. (Eds.) (2005). *Race, culture and psychotherapy. Critical perspectives in multicultural practice.* London: Routledge.

Moodley, R. Sutherland, P., & Oulanova, O. (2008). Traditional healing, the body and mind in psychotherapy. *Counselling Psychology Quarterly, 21*(2), 153–165.

Moodley, R., & West, W. (Eds.) (2005). *Integrating traditional healing practices into counseling and psychotherapy.* Thousand Oaks, CA: Sage.

Patterson, O. (1967). *The sociology of slavery.* London: Associated University Press.

Poortinga, Y. H. (1999). Do differences in behaviour imply a need for different psychologies? *Applied Psychology: An International Review, 48,* 419–432.

Press, I. (1978). Urban folk medicine: A functional overview. *American Anthropologist, New Series, 80*(1), 71–84.

Rahming. M. B. (2001). Towards a critical theory of spirit: The insistent demands of Erna Brodber's Myal. *Revista/Review Interamericana, 31*(1–4), 1–12.

Richard, P. S., & Bergin, A. E. (1997). *A spiritual strategy for counseling and psychotherapy.* Washington, DC: American Psychological Association.

Ross, E. (2008). Traditional healing in South Africa: Ethical implications for social work. *Social Work in Health Care, 46*(2), 15–33.

Ross, R. (1992). *Dancing with a ghost: Exploring Indian reality.* Markham, ON: Octopus

Russell, S. R., & Yarhouse, M. A. (2006). Training in religion/spirituality within APA-accredited psychology predoctoral internships. *Professional Psychology: Research and Practice, 37*(4), 430–436.

Samuels, Z. (2008). Stigma should not sideline racial decimation in the drive to improve mental health care. *Black Mental Health UK.* Retrieved from http://www.blackmental health.org.uk/index.php

Soulayrol, R., Guigou, G., & Avy, B. (1981). L'adolescent immigré [The adolescent immigrant]. *Psychologie Médicale, 13*(11), 1793–1795.

Sue, D. W., & Sue, D. (1990). *Counseling the culturally different: Theory and practice.* New York: John Wiley.

Sutherland, P. (2011). Traditional healing as a source of resistance, identity and healing among Grenadian women. *Canadian Women's Studies/les cahiers de la femme, 29,* (1, 2), 43–49.

Sutherland, P., & Moodley, R. (2010). Reclaiming the spirit: Clemmont Vontress and the quest for spirituality and traditional healing in counselling. In R. Moodley & R. Walcott (Eds.), *Counselling across and beyond cultures: Exploring the work of Clemmont Vontress in clinical practice.* Toronto: University of Toronto Press.

Sutherland, P., & Moodley, R. (2011). Research in transcultural counselling and psychotherapy. In C. Lago (Ed.), *Handbook of transcultural counselling and psychotherapy.* Berkshire: Open University Press.

Vontress, C. E. (2005). Animism: Foundation of traditional healing in Sub-Saharan Africa. In R. Moodley & W. West (Eds.), *Integrating traditional healing practices into counseling and psychotherapy*. Thousand Oaks, CA: Sage.

Vontress, C. E. (2010). Culture and counseling. In R. Moodley & R. Walcott (Eds.), *Counseling across and beyond cultures: Exploring the work of Clemmont E. Vontress in clinical practice*. Toronto: University of Toronto Press.

PART I

History, Philosophy, and Development of Caribbean Healing Traditions

1

THE HISTORY, PHILOSOPHY, AND TRANSFORMATION OF CARIBBEAN HEALING TRADITIONS

Patsy Sutherland

Introduction

The use of traditional healing practices and rituals can be traced back to the genesis of human history. The Shaman is arguably the first spiritual healer deemed an archetype of the contemporary physician and psychotherapist (Bromberg, 1975). Defined as the practices and knowledge that existed before the beginnings of modern medicine that are used to promote, maintain, and restore health and well-being, traditional healing practices are ubiquitous in diverse societies globally and have, for centuries, met the health care demands of populations (Bannerman, Burton, & Ch'en, 1983). Nevertheless, the particular ways in which these healing traditions have been developed and expressed over time are reflective of varied histories, cultures, environments, resources, and the needs of the populations they serve (Wane & Sutherland, 2010). Caribbean healing traditions are no exception. Any understanding of health, healing, and medical care in the Caribbean inevitably draws our attention to the configuration of history and gives emphasis to the transfer of cultural and healing practices from Africa, India, and Europe.

The different territories that encompass the Caribbean region share a complex and captivating history derived exclusively from the greed and struggle for hegemony by European nations in concert with slavery, indentureship, and plantation agriculture from their inception (De Barros, Palmer, & Wright, 2009; Mintz, 1975). As a general rule, oscillating patterns of sugar production are critical to any discussion of traditional healing in the Caribbean as they account for the importation of slaves as well as their eventual destination in the Caribbean. The shifting configurations of sugar production meant that the greatest volume of slaves was dispersed to locations where production was at its climax, most industrially advanced, and protracted. This resulted in the intense process of cultural exchange from which traditional systems of healing were ultimately derived (Fernández Olmos, 2003; Voeks, 1993). Following the abolition of the slave trade, South Asian indentured workers also brought their religious and cultural healing traditions to the Caribbean thereby, adding to the cultural complexity of these healing systems. Moreover, as tools of colonial power, Christianity, and Western medical science were superimposed on this complex healing system and maintained with remarkable fidelity into the neo-colonial era (De Barros, Palmer, & Wright, 2009). Collectively, these processes have shaped notions of health, healing, and medical care in the Caribbean.

Indeed, the health and medical care of the newly arrived Africans and, later, Indian indentured laborers were gravely threatened by the ghastly life conditions imposed by the European colonizers. Absolute negligence by the colonial masters and the high cost of medical services exposed these individuals to the full violence of diseases and outbreaks, compelling them to tend to their own health care needs (Brizan, 1984; Laguerre, 1987; Voeks, 1993; Weaver, 2002). As a result, they relied on rudimentary knowledge of Amerindian healing systems, their African and Indian traditions, and the utilization of plants that were available to meet their health care needs. According to Laguerre (1987), their survival depended predominantly on their effective use of traditional or folk medicine.

Caribbean healing traditions developed in response to these specific historical forces and represent powerful resources for survival, embody responses to oppression and exploitation, and speak to the determination of the Caribbean people to resist their dehumanizing, life-threatening, and morally offensive conditions (Sutherland, 2011). This chapter begins with an examination of the historical influences that have shaped and reshaped traditional healing in the Caribbean. This is followed by a discussion of the philosophical underpinnings of Caribbean traditional healing systems. Lastly, it explores the broad political interests that have supplanted traditional healing to a reductive place in mainstream society and argue that current healing practices are a response to these processes and have shaped the way in which physical, social, and psychological illnesses are conceptualized, represented, and presented in the contemporary Caribbean.

Historical Background

The study of the Caribbean people has not consistently analyzed the complexity of their historical experiences (Mintz, 1992). The extant historical records represent, in a fragmented and compartmentalized manner, segments of the past that has been expounded from a European perspective. Therefore, any attempt to evaluate the worldviews, spiritual beliefs, and healing practices distinctive to the Caribbean culture, cannot ignore the physical relocation imposed on the people who brought them to the New World (Mintz, 1992). In discussing the Caribbean region, it is important to recognize that while distinct Caribbean societies share many similarities, each is in its own way particular and unique. The historical and cultural development of each country is defined by elements such as the European culture by which it was colonized (English, French, Spanish, or Dutch), the intensity of slavery and the different struggles against it, the degree of economic deprivation, and racial and ethnic heterogeneity and the ensuing identity problems (Mintz, 1989). While these differences may be more evident in the way specific traditions are practiced on the various islands, they must not be overlooked if one is to gain a precise understanding of these societies and their cultural and healing practices.

The Caribbean region, often referred to as part of the New World, is comprised of approximately 50 distinct societies, all of which have endured similar historical experiences (Mintz, 1989). It is the only geographical region in the world where entire societies were brought into existence and sustained by the obliteration of an indigenous population and the massive relocation of an ethnic group from its homeland, Africa, for the purpose of slavery (Patterson, 1967). When Christopher Columbus arrived in the Caribbean in 1492, the region was already inhabited by populations of indigenous people (Brizan, 1984). Geographically disoriented, he erroneously labeled these individuals as "Indians" and characterized them as primitive savages in need of humanizing, thereby justifying European intrusion and subsequent colonization, enslavement, and indoctrination to Christianity (Yelvington, 2000). The indigenous people were unprepared militarily to defend against the invaders. Furthermore, they had no immunity to European diseases and eventually they were eradicated though traces of their ancestry remain in various parts of the Caribbean (Brizan, 1984; Yelvington, 2000). Subsequently, the Europeans imported massive numbers of slaves from Africa and established sugar plantations. It is estimated that approximately 40% of the more than nine million enslaved Africans who survived the Middle Passage to the New World were dispersed throughout the Caribbean[1] (Yelvington, 2000).

Pradel (2000) posits that the African origins of the slaves extended from the coast of Senegal to the south of Angola resulting in a clash of different ethnic groups. She further contends that the magnitude of the slave trade, its intensity, duration, and the lack of any coherent selection process of captives meant that most of the existing rituals from these regions were initiated in the New World. It is not difficult to imagine that many intellectuals and healers ended up the Caribbean as a result of this undifferentiated selection process. According to Voeks (1993) many priests, magicians, and herbalists were included among the newly arrived Africans and they maintained some degree of their previous status, thereby making possible the continued existence of a shaman class in spite of their enslavement. Voeks (1993) added that the practitioners of these African magico-systems were instrumental in reinforcing this collective knowledge in the New World. Enslaved Africans secured a connection with their particular kingdom and home of their gods and it was this continuity that provided the crucial resources for maintaining a sense of identity, culture, and religion (Taylor, 2001).

Both during and after slavery, however, other groups also supplied labor in the Caribbean. For example, more than half a million Indians, of both Muslim and

Hindu faiths, were brought to the region; the majority were sent to Trinidad and British Guyana, with smaller numbers going to Dutch Guyana (Surinam) (Mintz, 1975). Theoretically speaking, indentured laborers were not slaves; however, there are many parallels between the two systems. For example, Samaroo (1987) notes that the recruitment of Indians was conducted by a regularly organized system of kidnapping and/or deceiving unsuspecting individuals into offering themselves for indenture. The absence of a selection process also ensured that the Indians who arrived in the Caribbean originated from various economic castes, religions, village groups, and geographical regions resulting in the creation of a mini India in the Caribbean[2] (Edmonds & Gonzales, 2010) and, thereby deepening the complexity of cultural and healing traditions already present in the region. Similar to enslaved Africans, indentured Indians identified with their ancestral culture and belief systems and looked to India for inspiration in the face of their oppressive conditions; new traditions were created by borrowing from their homeland and incorporating new myths, rituals, and festivals that culminated into vernacular religions that are very distinct from their place of origin (Edmonds & Gonzales, 2010). Many identified with various gods to help cope with the dehumanizing conditions of colonial domination and exploitation. For example, an important aspect of Caribbean Hinduism was the adoption of the Ramayana tradition into everyday life. In the Ramayana tradition, the main protagonist Ram was exiled from his home; Hindu labourers identified with the character Ram and saw themselves as exiled from their motherland, anticipating their eventual return (Mahase, 2008).

The Caribbean, therefore, represents an ethnically, racially, and culturally diverse region influenced by Amerindian, European, African, Asian, and East Indian cultures. These waves of migration of people from virtually everywhere have made this region the site of an unparalleled collision of different ethnic groups. Hobsbawm (1973) described the Caribbean region as a

> curious terrestrial space-station from which fragments of various races, torn from the world of their ancestors and aware both of their origins and of the impossibility of returning to them, can watch the remainder of the globe with unaccustomed detachment.
>
> *(p. 8; as cited in Mintz, 1975)*

At the same time, it is important to note that these horrific events did not result in "social death" even though the Middle Passage, slavery, and indentureship dehumanized all enslaved Africans, indentured Indians, and their offspring in the most injurious way possible (Nishida, 2003). It seems that people of African and Indian descent demonstrated a remarkable degree of resilience and resourcefulness. Indeed, the paradox is that it was the dislocation, transportation, and insertion into the plantation economy by Western colonialism that integrated these populations, despite their differences, in as much as it severed direct retrieval of and connection to their past (Hall, 1994), and gave rise to the profusion of healing traditions and symbols of resistance present in the Caribbean region today. According to Fernandez (2003) it was the fluidity of these religions that enabled individuals to draw on spiritual power from wherever it was generated to acclimatize to their new milieu. Notwithstanding, neither cultural components nor historical factors alone can capture the entire significance of these healing traditions. An exploration of spiritual beliefs, as well as beliefs about the causes of illness and their functional roles, are important for a broad understanding of Caribbean healing traditions.

The Philosophical Basis of Traditional Healing

It seems that over time different cultural groups have developed their own explanations and conceptualizations of illness, mental health, and well-being, and, consequently, identified culturally sanctioned coping strategies (Lee & Armstrong, 1995). At the heart of the collection of hybrid or creolized healing traditions in the Caribbean is the worldview that everything in the universe is of one source and will, and that the world is animated by numerous ancestral spiritual entities, gods, and deities that frequently intervene in the everyday lives of individuals (Vontress, 1991; Wane & Sutherland, 2010). For example, it is believed the body, mind, and spirit are all interconnected and whatever affects one, impacts the other. From this perspective, illnesses and disorders may derive from many sources including natural, social, spiritual, or psychological disturbances that create disequilibrium which can be expressed in the form of physical, social, or mental ill health (Laguerre, 1987; Wane & Sutherland, 2010). Causality for natural illness is typically attributed to elements in the natural environment and can be prevented by maintaining humoral balance within the body or health can be restored with the use of herbs and regulated diets (Miller, 2000). On the other hand, super-naturally engendered illness may originate with the spirits, a rupture in the reciprocal relationship with the ancestors, or be inflicted by a malevolent person; consequently, they are treated by spiritual or traditional healers (Laguerre, 1987). During the colonial epoch, issues around mental health were deemed to have a supernatural basis, making the interventions of traditional healers most critical in the treatment of mental illness (Laguerre, 1987). This trend has persisted into the neocolonial era.

In addition to the philosophy of holism, traditional healing systems are grounded in a philosophy that is intrinsically empowering. The belief that the etiology of adversity is with demons and spirits, regardless of whether the adversity is within the family or the society at large, serves two functions. First, it positions the healer as the one with the power to detect, eradicate, or placate the offending spirit, and second, it creates a sense of order in the context of instability and insecurity (McGuire, 1991). This is an essential element in healing. Clearly, the particular stresses that the Caribbean people experienced reflected the repressive social conditions under which they existed; accordingly, traditional healers understand ailments and, therefore, their cures as encompassing the social realm. By locating causality outside of the individual, these rituals help to contain disorder and trauma by creating a sense of healing and control. This was particularly relevant during the periods of slavery and indentureship as individuals struggled to gain some semblance of agency over their lives (Sutherland, 2011).

Another crucial function of traditional healing that is inextricably linked to its philosophy of connectedness and the essential role of the body is that of assuaging the trauma associated with the process of enforced acculturation (Press, 1978). The physical and psychological dislocations produced by slavery, indentureship, and ensuing chronicles of violence and rupture have resulted in what Sweeney (2007) describes as an "unvoiced" history among Caribbean people that is grounded in a central notion of absence and loss. Any attempt to heal these historical wounds would be remitted without a comprehensive understanding of how these psychological injuries have been consolidated in the collective memories of the Caribbean people and reenacted transgenerationally (Apprey, 1999). The challenge for the Caribbean people is that the nature of their historical injury has produced a predicament in that the collective traumatic experience cannot be translated into narrative. Given that the assimilation of trauma is a central component to healing, without an avenue for expression, it is ultimately manifested as a "latent symptomatic injury" (Sweeney, 2007, p. 51). This specific kind of historical trauma was captured by Knadler (2003) who described it as "a reflexive memory of the body that refuses to 'pass' into any recognizable story" (p. 75).

In Caribbean healing traditions, the body is perceived as a conduit through which individuals can unearth the latent causes of their symptoms. In her analysis of energy healing and psychotherapy Woessner (2007) states,

> The body becomes, in a sense, a record of everything that has ever happened, is happening, will happen . . . You take a journey through the body, because everything will be held in the body . . . and in the journey you find the story that is manifesting in symptoms.
>
> *(p. 62)*

In the Caribbean context it is a particularized story that seems to disallow the discursive negotiations of conventional psychotherapy. Indeed, in her influential work on trauma, Cathy Caruth (1995) explains, "to be traumatized is precisely to be possessed by an image or an event" (p. 5). This notion of "possession" and consequent casting out of "demons" or exorcisms are pivotal to Caribbean healing traditions; anyone who has ever witnessed a Caribbean healing ceremony can attest to central role of the body with its rituals and dances that often culminate in trance-like states where healers and clients engage in a dialogue with the body and spirits to bring about a sense of healing (see Moodley, Sutherland, & Oulanova, 2008, for a discussion). In these healing rituals and ceremonies, according Sartre (1961), they dance . . . the dance secretly mimes, often unbeknownst to them, the No they dare not voice, the murders they dare not commit. In some regions they use the last resort: possession. What was once quite simply a religious act, an exchange between the believer and the sacred, has been turned into a weapon against despair and humiliation.

(p. Iiii)

It seems that this unique healing process is accomplished through what Dow (1986) describes as a complex sequence of exchanges that transpire in a mythic world that is shared by healers and clients. He explains the term "mythic" to denote that that there are cultural experiential certainties delineated in this world that are symbolic of human experiences as well as solutions to these experiences. Healing is accomplished by the reformation of traumatic events replicated in this mythic world through a particular mechanism in which the healer acts as a conciliator between the spirit world and the client; through the chants, dances and trance-states that epitomize Caribbean healing traditions, painful emotions are expressed to bring about a sense of healing and resolution. What is possible in these bodily metaphors and rituals is that a certain kind of history can be "voiced," traumatic experiences and aspirations of liberation can be "acted out," and the imagined community and traditions of the ancestral homeland, whether it is Africa or India, can be symbolically reconstructed to bring about healing and empowerment (Dow, 1986: Hall, 1994; Sutherland, 2011). At the same time, these traditions were not preserved in their pure form; rather, it is their transformation that forces us to interrogate the configuration of power entrenched in the processes of knowledge production, justification, and utilization of these healing traditions.

The Transformation of Caribbean Healing Traditions

Dominant discourses have marginalized Caribbean healing traditions and pushed them to the fringes of society where they have had to transform themselves to adapt to ever-shifting sociocultural and political milieus. The implications of slavery and indentureship were not simply intense labour on the plantations and absolute dehumanization by the slave master, a rich body of literature explores how the colonial subject was created through elaborate systems that measure, compare, and explain human difference (see Bhabha, 1994; Fanon, 1961; 1967; Said 1978). More specifically, Said (1978) argued that Western scholarship's complicity with Western colonial and imperial hegemony, particularly in its representation of non-Western cultures as subjects in need of civilization and acculturation, served the European exercise of power. These processes, predicated on the assumption of the colonizer's obvious superiority in all aspects of culture, history, political and social systems, and religion, justified the extreme imposition on the colonized as people in need of intervention. For example, traditional healers are often referred to as "witchdoctors,' a common nomenclature that was constructed under colonialism (Wane and Sutherland, 2010). This derogatory categorization erroneously defined traditional healing as witchcraft and perpetuated the perception of these poorly understood practices as evil, thereby justifying forced conversion into the sanctity of Christianity.

While Christianity has always been a basic tenet of life in the Caribbean, Fanon's (1961) contention was that the church in the colonies did not call the colonized to the ways of God, but to the ways of the colonial masters. Fanon's analysis of the colonial project was echoed by Grier and Cobbs (1971) who note, "Christianity in the hand of the slave-owner held a potentiality for wickedness that is terrifying, and one that is awed by its perfection for evil purposes"(p. 165). The original purpose of Christianity in the Caribbean drew on its principle of the afterlife to keep slaves enslaved; it provided the motivation for slaves and indentured workers to work themselves to death in the present life (Grier & Cobbs, 1957). Indeed, slaves and indentured labourers were indoctrinated into Christianity and prohibited from practicing their own religions; the tradition of Obeah, for example, was unequivocally proscribed and resulted in either death or transportation (Brizan, 1984). As a result, enslaved Africans engaged in a covert systematic process of preserving African religions in the New World by syncretizing them with elements of Catholicism. The shared philosophy of polytheism made it possible to mask African deities with Catholic saints, and for every African god or deity there is a corresponding Catholic saint (Fernandez, 2003; Voeks, 1993). Similarly, the majority of the indentured labourers did not simply embrace the religion of the colonizers but resisted, however possible, and perpetuated the cultural and traditional healing practices that they brought with them to the New World.[3] The Hosay Riots in Trinidad in 1884 was a clear example of such resistance (see Mahase, 2008 for a discussion). It was this actuality that transformed Caribbean healing traditions into the hybrid, and at times, perplexing collection of religions that exist in the modern day Caribbean.

Another important factor in the transformation and marginalization of traditional healing is its relationship with modern medicine which is grounded in an intercourse of domination with traditional healing representing subjugated or rejected ideology. The power and authority of the natural science paradigm from which biomedicine draws its legitimacy are incontrovertible and the rhetoric of scientific objectivity is alluring (Brodwin, 1998). Consequently, the universality of its model is often speciously accepted in the assumption that it is or ought to be appropriate in the assessment of the effectiveness of traditional healing systems in spite of divergent epistemologies regarding illness and health (Waldram, 2000). Traditional healing or medicine is clearly a cultural phenomenon; therefore, its configuration and purpose are obscured by the application of the allegedly culture-free language of science, as Waldram (2000) notes, "even the basic concepts of *traditional* and *medicine* are fraught with Eurocentrism and English-language biases, and they may be little more than very crude approximations, at best, of complex indigenous thought" (p. 607). What is at issue here is that the hegemonic practices of conventional medicine have distorted conceptualizations of the efficacy of traditional healing rendering it rejected knowledge to be scoffed at by the larger society, condemned on the pulpits of established churches, demoted by the education system, and, at times, prohibited by the authorities (Laguerre, 1987). Traditional healing in the Caribbean represents a structured nosological classification of diseases and ailments with notions of causality and treatment similar to the biomedical model which is clearly one of many healing traditions (Kleinman, 1995; Moodley & Sutherland, 2010). Hence, the marginalization of Caribbean healing traditions appear to be a deliberate strategy in colonizing the elements of human experience over which medical practitioners can allege authority and maintain control by promoting the practices and ideologies of their respective fields (Mishler et al., 1981; Waldram, 2000).

The emergence of mental health research and practice has followed a similar trajectory which parallels the subjugation of the Caribbean people and their healing traditions. The mental health paradigm in the Caribbean also became apparent in the context of plantation economy when slaves who attempted to run away from their dehumanizing conditions were diagnosed with drapetomania[4] or the impulse to run away (Cartwright, 1851). This is a clear example of the influence of political ideology on psychopathology and mental health; from the colonizer's perspective one had to be mentally ill to contemplate escaping the conditions of slavery and indentureship. Conventional psychiatry and psychology advances the idea that psychological, social, and emotional problems are a function of some underlying biological pathology, hence mitigating every feasible kind of psychiatric intervention (Barker, 2003). This is in sharp contrast to the philosophical underpinnings of traditional healing which attributes the etiology of mental illness to the social and spiritual realm. Furthermore, manifestations and presentations of spirit possessions, visions, curses, and spells are consistent with the Diagnostic and Statistical Manual's (DSM) criteria for psychotic disorders upon which Western notions of psychopathology are determined. The result for Caribbean clients who endorse traditional systems of etiology are often inaccurate diagnosis, poor compliance, overrepresentation in involuntary detainment in secure psychiatric settings, and higher prescribed psychotropic drug dosage than their white counterparts (Callan & Littlewood, 1998; Harrison, Barrow, & Creed, 1995).

Indeed, there is an entire movement and a body of literature which challenges dominant psychiatric and psychological thinking and practice on a range of issues, including religion and spirituality, with the goal of enhancing mental health care with diverse populations. This has given rise to an initiative within this field of multicultural counseling and psychotherapy aimed at integrating traditional healing practices into counseling and psychotherapy (Fukuyama & Sevig, 1999; Moodley & Sutherland, 2010; Moodley & West, 2005; Sutherland, 2011); however, this may be a double-edged sword for Caribbean healing traditions. Regardless of their intentions, the ideologies and theoretical approaches of researchers will always determine what gets studied, the findings that are obtained, and, ultimately, how they are implemented (Hutchinson & Sutherland, 2012; Sutherland & Moodley, 2011). What this means is that Caribbean healing traditions may once again have to transform and reconstruct themselves under the guise of culturally appropriate mental health care for Caribbean clients. These and other issues will continue to haunt these traditions and their very existence must be subsumed under the rubric of Western scientific paradigms regarding health and mental health where political power, rather than effectiveness, is pivotal to legitimacy (Laguerre, 1987). It is only when we view these healing practices in their wider historical, sociocultural, and political contexts that we can understand the profound extent to which they represent the unending interplay of interconnected spheres of power, and their remarkable capacity for transformation. Current healing traditions in the Caribbean are a direct consequence of these processes and must be viewed as such if they are to have any relevance to the manner in which we deal with the physical, social, mental, and psychological ailments in the present context (Moodley, Sutherland, & Oulanova, 2008).

Conclusion

What is articulated in the preceding discussion is that Caribbean healing traditions have been a source of resistance, identity, and healing since the beginning of the slave trade. The direct reference to history is at the core of understanding the transformation of these healing traditions in their repeated confrontation with the insidious machinations of colonialism. The Caribbean region has always represented a contested site in which the African and Indian presence have been in a quiet and, at times, not so quiet struggle with the European presence for self-assertion, a struggle spanning the entire period of encounter, slavery, indentureship, colonialism, and neocolonialism. Religion, health, illness, and, consequently, current healing traditions are symbolic of this struggle for agency, control, and survival. Grounded in the principles of holism and a connection with the gods, spirits, deities, and ancestors, traditional healing transcends everyday experiences of diseases and its cures to confront historical wounds of absence and loss. Through its rituals and metaphors, individuals are symbolically reconnected to their places of origins which lie at the center of their experiences of rupture, dislocation, fragmentation, and trauma. By extension, these traditions are resources with which to confront the pathological ways in which these experiences have been reconstructed within the dominant discourses of Western science, medicine, psychiatry, psychology, and Christianity.

Clearly, there is renewed interest in traditional healing practices globally. This renewed interest may be due in part to the failure of conventional health and mental health systems to effectively address the physical and existential ailments of the population. In spite of a growing consciousness of the need to integrate traditional healing into conventional health and mental health care, a lack of knowledge about Caribbean healing traditions has promoted a view of these healing systems as witchcraft, sorcery, primitive, and evil, and its adherents as pathological. These erroneous beliefs have resulted in a particular focus on specific categories of abnormal behavior that are classified as psychoses and disordered personalities among Caribbean populations. While conceptual frameworks regarding health and mental health may vary according to particularized socio-cultural milieus, ironically the overarching agenda must remain constant. Any ethical engagement with traditional healing and the Caribbean people as clients will seek to expand modes of health and healing beyond the discourses of Western health and mental health to account for particular contexts like the Caribbean where conditions of oppression and trauma and, consequently, patterns of resistance and healing are shaped by Western incursion. Such a process would reposition traditional healers from the margins to the centre, and situate traditional healing in its rightful place alongside the other healing traditions such as bio-medicine, psychology, counseling, and psychotherapy.

Notes

1. For a breakdown of the distribution of slaves and patterns of sugar production see Fernandez 2003; Voeks, 1993; Yelvington, 2000.
2. Indians who arrived in Trinidad alone, for example, immigrated from Bihar, Utter Pradesh, Bengal, Punjab, Himachal Pradesh, Kashmir, Tamil Nadu, Kerala, and Andhra Pradesh (Edmonds & Gonzales, 2010).
3. For instance, in Trinidad in 1891 only 12% of the total Indian population were converted to Christianity while 88% continued to practice religions transported from India – Hinduism, Islam, and Buddhism; by 1911, only 3.3% of the total number of Indians who were brought to the Caribbean had converted to the various Christian sects (Mahase, 2008).
4. Drapetomania or the disease causing slaves to run away was coined by an American physician Cartwright, and described as a disease of the mind, as any species of mental alienation only much more curable, that induces the Negro slave to run away from service. Cartwright further identified a preventative measure called "whipping the devil out of them" (p. 708).

References

Apprey, M. (1999). Reinventing the self in the face of received transgenerational hatred in the African American community. *Journal of Applied Psychoanalytic Studies, 1*(2), 131–143.

Bannerman, R. H., Burton, J., & Ch'en, W. C. (Eds.) (1983). *Traditional medicine and health care coverage*. WHO: Geneva.

Barker, P. (2003).The Tidal Model: Psychiatric colonization, recovery and the paradigm shift in mental health care. *International Journal of Mental Health Nursing 12*, 96–102.

Bhabha, H. (1994). *The location of culture*. London: Routledge.

Brizan, G. I. (1984) *Grenada: Island of conflict: From Amerindians to people's revolution 1498–1979*. London: Zed Books.

Brodwin, P. (1998). The cultural politics of biomedicine in the Caribbean. *New West Indian Guide, 72*(1/2), 101–109.

Bromberg, W. (1975). *From Shaman to psychotherapist: A history of the treatment of mental illness.* Chicago, IL: Henry Regnery.

Callan, A., & Littlewood, R. (1998). Patient satisfaction: Ethnic origin or explanatory model? *International Journal of Social Psychiatry, 44*(1), 1–11.

Cartwright, S. A. (1851) Report on the diseases and physical peculiarities of the Negro race, *New Orleans Medical and Surgical Journal, 7*, 691–715.

Caruth, C. (1995). *Trauma: Explorations in memory.* Baltimore, MD and London: Johns Hopkins University Press.

De Barros, J., Palmer, S., & Wright, D. (2009). *Health and medicine in the circum-Caribbean, 1800–1968.* New York, Routeledge

Dow, J. (1986). Universal aspects of symbolic healing: A theoretical synthesis. *American Anthropologist, 88*, 56–69.

Edmonds, E. B., & Gonzalez, M. A. (2010). *Caribbean religious history: An introduction.* New York: New York University Press.

Fanon, F. (1961). *The wretched of the earth.* New York: Grove.

Fanon, F. (1967). *Black skin, white masks.* New York: Grove.

Fernández Olmos, M. (2003). *Creole religions of the Caribbean: An introduction from Vodou and Santería to Obeah and Espiritismo.* New York: New York University Press.

Fukuyama, M., & Sevig, T. D. (1999). *Integrating spirituality into multicultural counseling.* Thousand Oaks, CA: Sage.

Grier, W. H., & Cobbs, P. M. (1971). *The Jesus bag.* New York: McGraw-Hill.

Hall, S. (1994). Cultural identity and diaspora. In P. Williams and L. Chrisman (Eds.), *Colonial discourse and postcolonial theory: A reader.* New York: Columbia University Press.

Harrison, J., Barrow, S., & Creed, F. (1995). Social deprivation and psychiatric admission rates among different diagnostic groups. *British Journal of Psychiatry, 167*(4), 456–462.

Hobsbawm, E. (1973). Review of Irene L. Gendzier (Ed.), *Frantz Fanon: A critical study.* New York Review of Books, p.8

Hutchinson, G., & Sutherland, P. (2013). Counselling and psychotherapy in the (English speaking) Caribbean: fidelity, fit or a cause for concern? In R. Moodley, U. Gielen, & R. Wu (Eds.), *Handbook of counselling and psychotherapy in an international context.* New York: Routledge.

Kleinman, A. (1995). *Writing at the margin.* Berkeley, CA: University of California Press.

Knadler, S. P. (2003).Traumatized racial performativity: Passing in nineteenth-century African-American testimonies. *Cultural Critique, 55*, 63–100

Laguerre, M. S. (1987). *Afro-Caribbean folk medicine.* South Hadley, MA: Bergin & Garvey Publishers.

Lee, C. C., & Armstrong, K. L. (1995). Indigenous models of mental health interventions. In J. C. Ponterroto, J. M. Casas, L. A. Suzuki, & C. M. Alexander (Eds.), *Handbook of multicultural counseling* (pp. 441–456). Thousand Oaks, CA: Sage.

Mahase, R. (2008). "Plenty a dem run away" – resistance by Indian indentured labourers in Trinidad, 1870–1920. *Labor History, 49*(4), 465–480.

McGuire, M. B. (1991). *Ritual healing in suburban America.* New Brunswick, NJ: Rutgers University Press.

Miller, N. L. (2000). Haitian ethnomedical systems and biomedical practitioners: Directions for clinicians. *Journal of Transcultural Nursing, 11*(3), 204–211.

Mintz, S. W. (1975). The Caribbean region. In S. W. Mintz (Ed.), *Slavery, colonialism and racism: Essays.* New York: W.W. Norton & Co Inc.

Mintz, S. W. (1989). *Caribbean transformations.* New York: Columbia University Press.

Mintz, S. W. (1992). *Anthropological approach to Afro-American past: A Caribbean perspective.* Boston, MA: Beacon Press.

Mishler, E. G., Amarasingham, L. R., Osherson, S. D., Hauser, S. T., Waxler, N. E., & Liem, R. (1981). *Social context of health, illness and patient care.* Cambridge: Cambridge University Press.

Moodley, R., & Sutherland, P. (2010). Psychic retreats in other places: Clients who seek healing with traditional healers and psychotherapists. *Counselling Psychology Quarterly, 23*(3), 267–282.

Moodley, R., Sutherland, P., & Oulanova, O. (2008). Traditional healing, the body and mind in psychotherapy. *Counselling Psychology Quarterly, 21*(2), 153–165.

Moodley, R., & West, W. (Eds.) (2005). *Integrating traditional healing practices into counseling and psychotherapy.* Thousand Oaks, CA: Sage.

Nishida, M. (2003). *Slavery and identity: Ethnicity, gender and race in Salvador, Brazil, 1808–1888.* Bloomington, IN: University Press.

Patterson, O. (1967). *The sociology of slavery.* London: Associated University Press.

Pradel, L. (2000). *African beliefs in the New World: Popular literary traditions of the Caribbean.* Asmara, Eritrea: World Press.

Press, I. (1978). Urban folk medicine: A functional overview. *American Anthropologist, New Series, 80*(1), 71–84.

Said, E. W. (1978). *Orientalism.* London: Routledge & Keagan Paul.

Samaroo, B. (1987). Two abolitions: African slavery and East Indian indentureship. In D. Dabydeen, & B. Samaroo (Eds.), *India in the Caribbean.* London: Hansib Publishing.

Sartre, J.-P. (1961) Preface. In F. Fanon (Ed.), *The wretched of the earth.* New York: Grove Press.

Sutherland, P. (2011). Traditional healing as a source of resistance, identity and healing among Grenadian Women. *Canadian Women's Studies/les cahiers de la femme, 29,* (1, 2), 43–49.

Sutherland, P., & Moodley, R. (2010). Reclaiming the spirit: Clemmont Vontress and the quest for spirituality and traditional healing in counselling. In R. Moodley & R. Walcott (Eds.), *Counselling across and beyond cultures: Exploring the work of Clemmont Vontress in Clinical Practice.* Toronto: University of Toronto Press.

Sutherland, P., & Moodley, R. (2011). Research in transcultural counselling and psychotherapy. In C. Lago (Ed.), *Handbook of transcultural counselling and psychotherapy.* Berkshire: Open University Press.

Sweeney, C. (2007). The unmaking of the world: Haiti, history and writing in Edouard Glissant and Edwidge Danticat. *Atlantic Studies, 4*(1), 51–66.

Taylor, P. (2001). *Nation dance: Religion, identity, and cultural difference in the Caribbean.* Bloomington, IN: University Press.

Voeks, R. (1993). African medicines and magic in the Americas. *Geographical Review, 83*(1), 66–78.

Vontress, C. E. (1991). Traditional healing in Africa: Implications for cross-cultural counselling. *Journal of Counseling and Development, 70*(1), 242–249.

Waldram, J. B. (2000). The efficacy of traditional medicine: Current theoretical and methodological issues. *Medical Anthropology Quarterly, 14*(4), 603–625.

Wane, N., & Sutherland, P. (2010). African and Caribbean healing practices in therapy. In Centre for Diversity in Counselling and Psychotherapy (Ed.), *In building bridges for wellness and psychotherapy.* Toronto: CDCP Press.

Weaver, K. K. (2002). The enslaved healers of eighteenth-century Saint Domingue. *Bulletin of History and Medicine, 76,* 429–460.

Woessner, E. M. (2007). *The integration of energy work and psychotherapy* (Psy.D. dissertation). Available from ProQuest Digital Dissertations database. (Publication No. AAT 3265866)

Yelvington, K. A. (2000). Caribbean crucible: History, culture, and globalization. *Social Education, 64*(2), 70–77.

2

THE EVOLUTION OF CARIBBEAN TRADITIONAL HEALING PRACTICES

Wendy Y. Crawford-Daniel and Jicinta M. Alexis

Introduction

The Caribbean has a rich heritage that extends not only to the cultural practices, but also knowledge and experiences of the benefits of the use of traditional medicine. This rich heritage is comprised of diverse cultures that coexisted whether forcibly or voluntarily, and can be traced back to the original inhabitants of the islands. The settlers who hailed from Europe, Africa, Asia, and the Middle and Far East all brought with them traditions that eventually creolized over the years (Brereton, 1989).

The earliest known inhabitants of the Caribbean, the Kalinago and the Tainos, have had their own indigenous systems of caring for the health and well-being of their people which included rituals, festivals, spiritual ceremonies, rites of passage, and dietary habits all contained within their own indigenous political organization (Steele, 2003). They believed that the natural world possessed all that was needed to sustain their existence (Wilson, 1997). It was the common belief that each person had a good or protective spirit looking over them from birth. Most feared were the evil spirits upon who were blamed for all sickness, accidents, and misfortunes of the individual, community, and the tribe (Khan 2003).

The healers were highly respected by all and considerably gifted with the knowledge of medicinal herbs, as well as the power to perform spells to heal the sick and injured (Makinde, 1988). The indigenous people made extensive use of the juices of roots, the use of tobacco for special ceremonies, festivals, and rites, and herbs for healing and spiritual ceremonies. Balms and oils were used, among other practices, in the preparation of the dead. Today many of these herbs, plants, and roots still have widespread use in many islands of the Caribbean.

Immediately following Christopher Columbus' voyage to the Americas in the 15th century, the European powers (Portugal, Spain, England, The Netherlands, and France) came to the Caribbean in search of gold and to set up profitable colonies. Realizing the limited gold deposits and the potential for agriculture, the colonial powers introduced a plantation system, which was initially manned by an indigenous workforce but eventually supplanted by forced African labor. The European colonialists brought a different philosophy and orientation to health care and healing than existed in the indigenous Caribbean. Contrary to the indigenous view the Europeans saw nature as a phenomenon to be scientifically understood, controlled, manipulated, and transformed (Basalla, 1967). In this regard they embarked upon an assault of the cultural traditions and healing practices of the inhabitants including the enslaved Africans they brought to the Caribbean.

The settling of the Caribbean region by the European colonizers and the ensuing lucrative, labor-intensive sugar industry gave rise to the need to import labor from Africa (Brereton, 1989). Thus, in the 17th century, a new workforce, the Africans, who were mainly culled from the west coast of Africa, were introduced to the Caribbean sugar plantations to provide the essential labor required to make the sugar industry sustainable (Brereton, 1989). The African slaves, though removed from their homeland, retained their medicinal knowledge which was inexorably tied to their religious beliefs (Goldberg, 2000). The slaves believed that illness and death had a spiritual causation which occurred as a result of a cosmic imbalance in an individual's aura (Handler, 2000).

The colonial administration and plantation owners were convinced that the cultural heritage which included the religion, music, and traditional healing practices of the enslaved were in fact evil, pagan rituals practiced by the healer and his adherents. In the French Caribbean, the terminology to refer to the African slave beliefs and practices was Quimbois, Voodoo or Vodun, in the Spanish Caribbean and in the Dutch Caribbean, the terminology used was Santería, Regla de Ocha, or Lukumi (Khan, 2003). Whether the term was Obeah, Voodoo, or Santería, there was a negative connotation associated with it.

Following the abolition of slavery, indentured servants from west and south Asia were enticed to the Caribbean to replace the labor force on the plantations, vacated by the recently freed Africans. The indentured workers comprising mainly East Indians were distributed to 14 colonies in the Caribbean and British, Dutch, and French Guiana between 1836 and 1917 (Clarke, 1990). They were primarily of Hindu and Muslim religions, the majority of which settled in Trinidad and Guyana, and who later converted to Christianity, much like their predecessors, the Africans. For the Hindu there was a strong belief that one's life was predetermined by his or her good or bad deeds in a previous life. When ill, a diviner may be consulted to determine which spirit is angry and what ceremony might appease it. Some of the practices that have survived to date include a pageantry of rituals, balancing of body system through diet and emotions, herbs, meditation, self-restrain, acupuncture, and rhythmic music, all of which are integral aspects of traditional healing practices in the Caribbean (Moore, 1995). These practices, however, were not as widespread and pervasive. The practices of the indentured attracted little attention from the colonialists unlike the practices of the former enslaved Africans.

The current health belief system of the people of the Caribbean demonstrates a coexistence of practices of the various civilizations who occupied the islands over the centuries, (Abrahams, 1967). Healing practices of the indigenous people and the many civilizations that occupied the Caribbean have resulted in a multiplicity of health belief systems and healing practices. Some of these practices are mutually exclusive, some coexist in a reciprocal referral system at formal and informal levels, and others have incorporated various aspects of each other in a plethora of approaches to healing (Abrahams, 1967).

This chapter will illustrate how these practices, referred to as traditional, have evolved from a position of primacy prior to modern medicine to being feared, discredited, and outlawed during the colonial and postcolonial era (Paton, 2009). It begins by discussing the influence of West Africa, this is followed by an exploration of traditional healing in the colonial and postcolonial eras, and finally the gradual return to significance in the Caribbean, in light of the shortcomings of modern medicine (Aarons, 1999).

Influence of West African Traditional Healing

West African traditional medicine adopts a tripartite approach to healing which includes herbal medicine, divination, and incantations (Makinde, 1988). In the West African tradition, the healer's knowledge is believed to be derived from Ifa, a Yoruban deity who is responsible for embodying the knowledge of all sciences, including social, natural, and spiritual (Makinde,1988). Akin Makinde noted that "Ifa" was considered an angel of God, who embodied wisdom and knowledge of physics, zoology, botany, herbs, oral incantations, and medicine (Makinde, 1988). Apart from the aforementioned sciences, Ifa's gift of knowledge, including the healing properties of herbal medicine, is imparted to the world through a medium known as an "Orunmila" (otherwise referred to as Osanyin or Onisegun), who is credited with being the father of traditional healers (Makinde, 1988). The typical healing process will include the Ifa priest who would divine the nature of the illness or disease, and the Onisegun who would prepare the herbal remedy in consultation with an Ifa priest, otherwise called a Babalawo. In some instances, the Babalawo may also be an Onisegun, which would result in a complete cure for the patient because herbal medicine, divination, and incantations were employed (Makinde, 1988). The complete cure can be achieved only as a result of Ifa's knowledge of the origins of diseases, the names by which they are called, and the power behind the diseases (Makinde, 1988). Therefore, an understanding of the root cause of disease coupled with prescribing the most effective traditional remedy to treat it, whether herbal, divination, incantation, or any combination of the three, according to the Yoruban standard, was best practice medicinally.

According to the Yoruba, a human being has three main elements: Ara, otherwise called the body; emi, otherwise called the soul; and the ori, otherwise called the inner head. The ori has the distinction of being the bearer of human destiny, and, as such, in some instances, the patient would be expected to sacrifice to the ori as part of the treatment to avert death (Makinde, 1988). There are instances of sacrifices in the African traditional medicine milieu. Due to the belief that one's soul was immortal, and the need to appease the ancestral spirits to intercede on the living's behalf, sacrifices would be offered to the spirits to aid the treatment process (Green, 1980).

Another key aspect of the Yoruban belief system is the belief in evil forces, otherwise known as willful maleficia. This evil force is responsible for illness, disease, and death. Thus, in an effort to appease the evil forces that are at work, sacrifices, otherwise known as ebo/etutu, are offered as a countermeasure. Protective measures to guard against the ill-effects of evil forces include amulets or madarikan, curses or epe, and incantations or ofo/ase/afose (Makinde, 1988).

It was this encapsulation of traditional medicine cultural heritage that migrated into the Caribbean with the arrival of the slaves. The slaves brought both tangible and intangible links to their past, as they began the odyssey of transmigration and slavery. In order to preserve their sense of cultural identity (Goldberg, 2000), the slaves maintained their language, religious, and traditional medicine heritage.

Early Traditional Healing in Colonial Caribbean

After the indigenous workforce was depleted, the European colonizers devised an ingenious scheme for labor replacement. Slaves primarily from West Africa were introduced to the plantation economies of the Caribbean. The slave population was far larger than the plantation owners, and as a result the few European medical practitioners could not provide medical care to the slaves (De Barros, 2007). It was therefore the traditional healers in the Caribbean who were recognized as the prime providers of health care. The healing practices of West Africa, brought to the Caribbean by the enslaved Africans, quickly became the predominant method of healing. Thus, it was necessary for the majority of slaves to rely on their traditional healers to deal with their medical and/or spiritual issues (Handler, 2000). Apart from the limited access to Western medical practitioners, the slaves did not trust their captors to provide medical assistance. The healers had to treat physical illness and spiritual malaise alike (Roach, 1992).

The healers called on their previously acquired knowledge of healing, and though many of the original herbs, plants, and roots were not readily available, they were able to adapt to the new environment and utilize substitutes wherever necessary (Roach, 1992). The healers had to treat physical illness and spiritual malaise alike. They were responsible for providing healing treatments and remedies

in the following areas of medicine: obstetrics, pediatric, gastrointestinal, psychological, and spiritual maladies, to name a few (Roach, 1992).

Over time the healers were also treating the plantation owners and their
overseers. Due to the fact that the African healers were familiar with tropical
climates and diseases, they were able to provide a more effective cure than the
Western trained physicians (Handler, 2000). However, though the healers were
providing an invaluable service by improving and maintaining the physical and
spiritual well-being of the slaves, albeit that they were considered mere commodity, the plantation owners developed an underlying mistrust of the importance
of the role that healers played in the slaves' lives (Goldberg, 2000). Apart from
being the spiritual and healing authority, they were also the cultural repository of
the African heritage. Thus, the healer was perceived as a threat to the conditioning
measures implemented by the plantation owners to make the slaves amenable to
their present condition. The plantation owners grew to fear the healer's ability to
inspire resistance among the adherents, and, more importantly, the healer's ability
to incite the slaves to passively resist the owners control by alluding to a threat far
worse than what the owners intimated (Goldberg, 2000). The psychological hold
of the healer over their adherents, as well as the belief in the power of the healer,
was more potent than any physical threat or torture that the plantation owner
could inflict. Consequently, a concentrated effort to discredit the effectiveness of
traditional medicine and its healers, as well as weaken the hold that the healers had
over their adherents, was implemented by the colonial institutions in the British
Caribbean.

To this end, the Europeans from the British administrated colonies coined the
term Obeah, which referred to the slave acts and practices which were considered
supernatural or evil in nature (Goldberg, 2000). Eventually, the term Obeah was
used as a "catch-all term for a range of supernatural ideas and behaviors" (Handler,
2000, p. 87). This term, however, was a misnomer of a valid religious belief of the
slaves. For the Africans, Obeah practices had a "positive or morally neutral
meaning" which emphasized the spiritual aspect of the healing process (Khan,
2003). In fact, the term Obeah may have been derived from Obi, a Yoruban deity
(Handler, 2000).

Traditional Healing in the Post-Emancipation Era

Two of the foremost, formidable British institutions led the way in the attempt to
officially rein in traditional medicine in the British Caribbean: the judiciary and
the church (Paton, 2009). Both institutions were successful in further advancing a
negative stereotype of the traditional healing/religious beliefs of the slaves and,
circa the post-emancipation era, the recently introduced indentured servants.
There was already a generally held view that Africans were primitive, subhuman
pagans that frequently engaged in evil rituals designed to cause supernatural harm
to adherents and non-adherents (Goldberg, 2000). That perception was further

modified to encompass the point of view that 1) the traditional healers or Obeah men were in fact charlatans trading on the susceptibility of the believers, and 2) once the believers adopted the Christian teachings, they would be less vulnerable (De Barros, 2007). Hence, by prosecuting the healers/ Obeah practitioners, the adherents would recognize that their perception of the healer's omniscience and supernatural power was flawed. The struggle between the Obeah man and the British institutions intensified approximately around the time that calls for emancipation were echoing around the sugar plantations in the Caribbean, as well as the House of Parliament in Britain in the early 19th century (Brereton, 1989).

After repeated allegations of the Obeah man using the supernatural to intimidate adherents and non-adherents, legislations were enacted to criminalize the practice of Obeah in many British Caribbean islands (Brereton, 1989). The statute's wording may have been amended according to each country's specific needs; however, the basis remained the same. The emancipated slaves' and indentured laborers' ability to freely practice their traditional beliefs were now strictly regulated. In light of the fact that the healers (Obeah men) faced the possibility of prosecution for practicing their healing in their customary traditional manner (Roach, 1992), it was necessary for them to covertly perform their healing rituals. Healing rituals in urban communities were incorporated into religious services which insulated the practitioners from being legally charged.

The church also played a key role in the societal regulation of the role of the healer and traditional medicine. The Africans and East Indians were taught the Christian doctrines. However, though these doctrines contradicted the traditional cultural values of the slaves and indentured servants, it was in their best interest to maintain the façade of accepting the plantation owners' religious belief (Brereton, 1989). Eventually, the slaves incorporated some of the Christian doctrines into their traditional belief system (Henry, 2003). As a result, a tenuous duet of a dual worship relationship was danced by the slaves, which involved covertly maintaining their traditional beliefs, while overtly adopting the Christian teachings.

Emancipation saw a resurgence of independent thought among the Africans. The exhilaration of being able to worship freely was celebrated with the opening of Orisha enclaves (Henry, 2003). Orisha was an amalgamation of the traditional Yoruban religion and the newly introduced Christian doctrines. However, Orisha's underlying belief system was predominantly African, and as such retained the traditional healing practices of yesteryear. Unfortunately, the legislative and societal regulatory bodies continued to work to drive the African belief system underground (Roach, 1992), thereby maintaining control of the major ethnic segment of the Caribbean population.

The Obeah Act was passed in the Anglophone Caribbean between the late 1800s and early 1900s (Antigua and Barbuda, Dominica, Grenada, St. Lucia, and St. Vincent 1904; Trinidad, Jamaica, and Barbados 1898). These Acts prohibited the practice of Obeah on the islands. Violation of these Acts was punishable by imprisonment with hard labor and whipping (Handler, 2000). This punishment was meted out to practitioners and users of the service alike, and men and women equally.

Many of the bona fide healers were unable to practice their chosen profession openly in the urban communities, which grew rapidly with the onset of emancipation. They faced one major barrier with many repercussions to the continued practice of their trade: social upward mobility (Brereton, 1989). However, in rural communities, which were mainly agricultural communities, the practice continued relatively unchecked (Wong, 1976).

In the interest of longevity, it was customary to pass on the traditions orally from generation to generation. More importantly, the knowledge of healing was learnt as an apprentice to an experienced healer (Green, 1980). Though in some instances the apprentices may have shown a calling for healing, they were still expected to train for years under skilled, experienced healers. As a result of the criminalization of Obeah and the attendant stigma and discrimination associated with the continued practice and belief, the healers were hard-pressed to find willing applicants to fill the vacant role of apprentice, particularly in the urban communities. Consequently, the extensive knowledge of traditional healing died with the healer practitioners, who embodied the link to the adherents' African heritage as well as being the cultural repositories.

Sociocultural Dilemma in Contemporary Caribbean Healing Practices

A major factor that was a deterrent to the healer practitioner was the drive for respectability among the middle class Africans in urban communities. The rush to transmigrate from the agricultural communities to the urban communities was significant to the Africans, because it meant an escape from the plantations and the horrendous memories of that period of their lives (Allahar, 2005). Rural to urban migration meant the possibility of better jobs and a better way of life in the industrial sector. Education was embraced as one of the means to improve their social standing, thereby moving up the social ladder (Hall, 1994). These educated Africans hoped to achieve middle class respectability; however, for that to materialize it was necessary to disassociate themselves from the cultural beliefs that they had known all their lives.

Thus, in an attempt to acquire respectability, Africans worshipped and engaged in activities within the Catholic and Protestant churches (Allahar, 2005). It was an important criteria for social advancement to be seen worshipping at the right church. Additionally, the traditional healing beliefs and other components of their cultural heritage was laid aside to adopt the Eurocentric culture of the elite, colonial upper class (Allahar, 2005).

Even the age-old utilization of traditional healing was relegated to the uneducated masses with the educated, upwardly mobile segment electing to choose Western medicine (Roach, 1992). In some instances, the ambitious social climbers were the harshest critics of the traditional African culture. They had internalized the negative perception of traditional healing that the British plantation owners and legislators had generated. In this regard, the institutions were indeed able to discredit the traditional practices; however, they overlooked one major aspect of the belief system. Regardless of the advances of society, the population continued to believe in the spiritual causation of illness (Roach, 1992). In this case the adherents, i.e. patients, in some instances would suppress their beliefs in order to conform. Hence, in an attempt to present an acceptable image of self to others, they would visit Western trained physicians, receive treatments, and either self-treat with herbal medicines or use them in conjunction with Western medicines. If healing occurred, subconsciously they would attribute it to the traditional medicines, while simultaneously giving their physicians the impression that it was the Western medicines that worked. On the other hand, the denouncers who had acquired the tool, education, which would eventually facilitate social upward mobility, needed to present a scientific, modern, rational image, which was befitting of the ascribed roles. Hence, the actions of the denouncers reflected their social ambitions. As a result, the healers were still called on, albeit in a covert manner, by persons of varying ethnicities and social standings to treat their ailments (Raphael, 2005).

Implications for Health and Mental Health

The health beliefs which have evolved after centuries of institutionalized conditioning represent the sociocultural and psychological dilemma that exists today in the Caribbean with regards to healing practices. Traditional or cultural knowledge had a conflicting but meaningful relationship between the people's values and social reality. Traditional medicine surpasses the action of self-treatment; it assists the user to maintain ties to social relationships by calling on the wisdom of their ancestors and elders for treatment (Sigerist, 1951). Firstly, the practice of traditional medicine was sustained by the illness belief of the people. The belief that illness had a spiritual connotation which required alternative approaches to treatment was consistent in the Caribbean region. Secondly, the people's trust in traditional medicine was absolute; it was passed down from generation to generation and consequently it had an established historical basis. As a result, the practice of traditional medicine as a social action was occurring because of the attached meaning.

Despite all of the institutional, legal, and psychological strategies embarked upon to promote modern medicine and discredit traditional healing practices, the people of the Caribbean continue to hold to the traditional beliefs system. In a similar vein in which Christianity and traditional religions have found ways to coexist in modern society, so have traditional and modern medicine. The use of divination, herbal medicine, spiritual counseling, and modern medicine or different permutations of these methods is very much alive in the healing practices of the Caribbean.

Modern medicine on its own accord is failing to meet the health needs of the people of the Caribbean, both in scope and quality of care. The cost of modern medicine, particularly specialized care, puts it out of the reach of the average Caribbean citizens (Aarons, 1999). In recent years there has been a significant return in the English-speaking Caribbean to the philosophy and healing practices of traditional medicine to address many of the modern and chronic illnesses both at a preventative and curative level (Aarons, 1999).

Modernity and its emphasis on multiculturalism and cultural relativity have created and encouraged a climate of tolerance and appreciation for differences in culture, in worldview, and in ways of life. This cultural awareness is creating a shift away from the negative attitudes towards traditional medicine. Accomplished Caribbean scholars and researchers, like cultural anthropologists, historians, psychologists and sociologists, are engaging in research and scholarship focusing on traditional medicine in the Caribbean (Payne-Jackson & Alleyne, 2004; Quinlan & Quinlan, 2007). For instance, various universities and institutes throughout the Caribbean are dedicating research grants to furthering research in the field of traditional medicine, as well as incorporating the conducted studies into their formal curriculum.

These developments at the academic level coincide with the development at the general public level where there is a significant resurgence of traditional religions and traditional healers, and a renewed appreciation for the cultural heritage of the region.[1] The antagonistic nature of the previous relationships that existed between formal and informal medicine is gradually diminishing in the Caribbean as modern medicine increasingly embraces the bio-psychosocial model of care—the biological, psychological, and social components that are essential components of traditional medicine, hence long subscribed to by traditional healers.

It is important to factor in the cultural practices of a people in any attempt to develop an efficacious health model. Kleinman, Eisenberg, and Good (2006) posited that illness was culturally shaped; hence perception honed by experiences and social standing would influence an individual's ability to cope with illness (Kleinman et al., 2006).

Consequently, any health model that is not cognizant of the people's beliefs will experience resistance in application. The imposition of the biomedical model as a stand-alone approach did not have any cultural relevance in the psyche of the Caribbean people. This approach resulted in a lack of adherence to Western medical treatment, and widespread prevalence of self-treatment with traditional medicines. The more recent forging of formal and informal medicine into official practices from reciprocal referral systems to treatment regiments are indications of the growing collaboration (Dresang, Brebrick, Murray, Shallue, & Sullivan-Vedder, 2005). Further, due to the fact that traditional medicine promotes health by preventing illness (Lowenberg, 1989), whereas Western medicine focuses on treatment of illness, the logical health model should incorporate traditional and

Western medicines. A concerted thrust towards a complete integrative approach would ensure improved health outcomes.

An integrative health model which would unite the traditional medical approach, which embraces the psychological, physiological, and spiritual well-being of the individual, with the biomedical approach, which focuses on the biological and physiological well-being of the individual, would best serve to incorporate the health beliefs of the Caribbean people. However, this integrative model would require the revoking of existing legislature, thereby allowing traditional healers to legally practice. Further, regulation of the practitioners ensures that the field would be limited to the qualified who have honed their abilities either by apprenticeship or formal training at institutions that offer alternative medicine training.

Conclusion

As Caribbean societies moved towards modernity, traditional medicine experienced consistent and systematic attempts to eradicate the psychological and spiritual stronghold it had on its adherents. Though the educated, legislature, church, modern medicine, and other institutions deployed covert and overt mechanisms to achieve cultural erasure, they all proved unsuccessful. Unfortunately, these institutions/individuals did not acknowledge that traditional medicine is a cultural system which has meaning to the people (Geertz, 1973). In identifying traditional medicine as a cultural system, it would therefore establish a degree of consistency in the practice.

Additionally, traditional medicinal knowledge and practices were internalized and reinforced by repeated reenactment for centuries. Interestingly, some of the individuals that publicly denounced the practice of traditional healing were, in fact, covert believers/users. The growing reciprocity between traditional medicine and modern medicine will have positive outcomes for the health and well-being of the people of the Caribbean.

Note

1. Many of the practitioners are now advertising their services on audio, print, and electronic media. In fact the Jamaican Gleaner newspaper carried an article on a "scientist" (traditional healer) who has opened a supermarket in Kingston selling Obeah and the tools of the trade on the open market. Not to be outdone, many Western trained doctors in the Caribbean are increasingly developing formal and informal referral systems between themselves and traditional healers (Aarons, 1999).

References

Aarons, D. E. (1999). Medicine and its alternative. *The Hastings Report, 2* (4), 23.
Abrahams, R. D. (1967). The shaping of folklore traditions in the British West Indies. *Journal of Inter-American Studies 9*(3), 456–480.

Allahar, A. (2005). Identity and erasure: Finding the elusive Caribbean. *Revista Europea de Estudios Latinamericanos y del Caribe*, 125–134.

Basalla, G. (1967). The spread of Western science. *Science, 156*(3775), 611–622.

Brereton, B. (1989). Society and culture in the Caribbean: The British and French West Indies. In F. W. Knight & C. Palmer (Eds.), *The modern Caribbean* (pp. 85–110). London: Chapel Hill.

Clarke, C. (1990). *South Asian overseas migration and ethnicity*. New York: Cambridge University Press.

De Barros, J. (2007). Dispensers, Obeah and quackery. *Social History of Medicine, 20*(2), 243–261.

Dresang, L. T., Brebrick, L., Murray, D., Shallue, A., & Sullivan-Vedder, L. (2005). Family medicine in Cuba: Community-oriented primary care and complementary and alternative medicine. *Journal American Board of Family Practitioners, 18*(4), 297–303.

Geertz, C. (1973). *The interpretation of culture*. New York: Basic Books.

Goldberg, V. (2000, June 20). *Religion: Spirists, demons and mental illness in Trinidad & Tobago*. Retrieved May 29, 2009, from http://www.trinidad-tobag.net/Article.aspx?PagezId=42

Green, E. C. (1980). Roles for traditional healers in mental health care. *Medical Anthropology 4*, 489–522.

Hall, S. (1994). Cultural identity and diaspora. In S. Hall (Ed.), *Discourse and post-colonial theory: A reader* (pp. 390–401). London: Harvester Wheatsheaf.

Handler, J. (2000). Slave medicine and Obeah in Barbados, circa 1650–1834. *New West Indian Guide/Nieuwe West-Indische Gids. 74*(1/2), 57–90.

Henry, F. (2003). My life with Ebenezer Elliot (Pa Neezer). In F. Henry (Ed.), *Reclaiming African religions in Trinidad: The socio-political legitimation of the Orisha and spiritual faiths* (pp. 202–210). Barbados: University Press of the West Indies.

Khan, A. (2003). Isms and schisms: Interpreting religion in the Americas. *Anthropological Quarterly, 76*(4),761–774.

Kleinman, A., Eisenberg, L., & Good, B. (2006). Culture, illness and care: Clinical lessons from anthropologic and cross-cultural research. *FOCUS The Journal of Lifelong Learning in Psychiatry, 4*(1), 140–149.

Lowenberg, J. S. (1989). *Caring and responsibility: The crossroads between holistic practice and traditional medicine*. Philadelphia, PA: University of Pennysylvania Press.

Makinde, A. M. (1988). African traditional medicine: Principles and practice. In A. M. Makinde (Ed.), *African philosophy, culture and traditional medicine* (pp. 87–91). Athens, OH:. Ohio University Press.

Moore, B. (1995). *Cultural resistance and pluralism, colonial Guyana 1838–1900*. Montreal: McGill University Press.

Paton, D. (2009). Obeah acts: Policing the boundaries of religion in the Caribbean. *Small Axe, 13*(1), 1–18.

Payne-Jackson, A., & Alleyne, M. (2004). *Jamaica folk medicine: A source of healing*. Jamaica: UWI Press.

Quinlan, M. B., & Quinlan, R. J. (2007). Modernization and medicinal plant knowledge in a Caribbean horticultural village. *Medical Anthropology Quarterly, 21*(2), 169–192.

Raphael, C. (2005). *In defence of bush baths*. Port of Spain: Trinidad Publishing Company Limited.

Roach, R. (1992). *Obeah in the treatment of psychiatric disorders in Trinidad: An empirical study of an indigenous healing system*. Montreal, Quebec: McGill University Press.

Sigerist, H. E. (1951). *A history of primitive and archaic medicine*. London: Oxford University Press.

Steele, B. A. (2003). *Grenada: A history of its people*. Oxford: Macmillan Publishers.

Wilson, S. M. (Ed.) (1997). *The indigenous people of the Caribbean*. Gainsville, FL: University Press of Florida.

Wong, W. (1976). Sine folk medicinal plants from Trinidad and Tobago. *Economic Botany,30*(2), 103–142.

3

CARIBBEAN TRADITIONAL MEDICINE

Legacy from the Past, Hope for the Future

Arvilla Payne-Jackson

Introduction

The World Health Organization (WHO) defines traditional medicine as: "the sum total of knowledge, skills and practices based on theories, beliefs, and experiences indigenous to different cultures that are used to maintain health, as well as to prevent, diagnose, improve or treat physical and mental illness" (WHO, 2012, p.1). In this chapter the term traditional medicine is used to refer to healing practices developed prior to the advent of biomedicine, the dominant cultural system of medical care today.

The traditional medical systems that evolved in the Caribbean during the colonial period and that persist today are in large part a continuation of generalized practices of West African traditional religious and medical practices combined with the colonial European humoral medical system and Amerindian medical systems (Bilby,1993; Laguerre,1987; Lowe, Payne-Jackson, & Beckstrom-Sternberg, 2002; Payne-Jackson, & Alleyne, 2004). Factors such as the herbal and medicinal knowledge brought to the New World by Europeans and Africans, the physical environment, and the flora and fauna found in the New World have influenced the development of these medical systems (Laguerre, 1987; Lowe, Payne-Jackson, & Johnson, 2009).

Contemporary traditional medical systems provide a microcosm through which Caribbean culture and healing practices can be understood. The social dynamics of

> the interplay between ethnic community and separateness, on the one hand, and the emergence of some integrated "creole" socio-cultural system, on the other hand, are reflected in the existence and practice of generalized traditional medical belief systems. The role of the supernatural and natural

elements in traditional etiology reflects the general worldview of the populations they serve.

(Payne-Jackson and Alleyne, 2004, p. 6; see also Alleyne, 1988)

In this chapter traditional medicine in the Caribbean is discussed including the social, historical, cultural, and functional context of traditional medicine. This is followed with a discussion on beliefs, perceived etiologies, types of practitioners, and treatments used in treating illness. Finally, the reasons for the tenacity and resurgence of traditional medicine and implications for collaboration and/or integration with mainstream health and mental health are examined.

Social, Historical, Cultural, and Functional Context of Caribbean Traditional Medicine

Traditional medicine has been the primary source of healing for people in the Caribbean since before slavery, throughout slavery, and up until to today. Official medicine while present during slavery was basically inaccessible to enslaved Africans both before and after emancipation and in many instances even today. However, the relationship between traditional medicine and biomedicine is complex and is affected by social, political, historical, and economic factors. For example, the conditions under which enslaved Africans were brought to the New World and the health care available throughout slavery were horrendous. During the Middle Passage slave ships were breeding grounds for a long list of diseases, injuries, and wounds (Sheridan, 1985)

The unavailability of European doctors contributed to the lack of health care. Sheridan (1985) estimates the ratio of doctors to enslaved Africans in British colonies was 1:1600. Other factors were the high cost to plantation owners to use the services of medical doctors, doctors' reluctance to reside outside the main cities, and the lack of their success in treating many of the illnesses and diseases encountered in the New World (Payne-Jackson & Alleyne, 2004; Lowe et al., 2002). Another major factor contributing to the dependence on traditional medicine was the enslaved Africans' mistrust of white doctors. The methods of treatment used by white doctors included blood-letting, purging, sweating, and the use of mercury, opium, and antimony. These methods were often both unsuccessful as well as dangerous (Genovese, 1976; Payne-Jackson & Alleyne, 2004; Sheridan, 1985). White doctors also did not recognize the African-based supernatural etiology of disease and this in turn did not meet the social or spiritual needs of the enslaved Africans (Payne-Jackson & Alleyne, 2004).

Once restrictions were placed on the slave trade, plantation owners established black hospitals (call hothouses). Medical doctors were paid to visit the hospitals once a week. These hothouses were attended by black doctors, nurses, midwives, and attendants, who administered the orders and prescriptions of the white doctors. Unlike the fear and distrust of white doctors, patients and families had close ties and trust with the hothouse practitioners (Eisner, 1961; Gardner, 1873; Lunan, 1814; Sheridan, 1985; Thomson, 1820). Some medical doctors acknowledged the efficacy of slave medicines. Thomson (1820) wrote: "I must candidly acknowledge that the effects of my most laboured prescriptions have not unfrequently been superseded by the persevering administration of their [slaves'] most simple remedies" (p. 10). The presence or absence of owners was another contributing factor to the development of traditional medical systems. For example, Jamaica had a greater incidence of absentee owners and a greater proportion of Africans to Europeans than in Barbados. The result was a stronger presence and influence of the Africans' practices than the Europeans. Also the number of poor whites and indentured servants present in a society was a factor in the social dynamics and social structure of a society. In Jamaica this influence was weak but, on the other hand, for 40 years, Barbados was a société d'habitation (of small holdings) before being replaced by the plantation society (Payne-Jackson & Alleyne, 2004). Furthermore, subsistence farming, where practiced, allowed enslaved Africans to develop a wider range of therapies. A contributing factor to this was the recognition of flora and fauna common to both African and Caribbean countries, which provided a basis of familiar medicinal herbs (Ayensu, 1981; Payne-Jackson & Alleyne, 2004). The constant resupply of Africans to the New World provided a continual flow of African medical rituals, therapies, practitioners, and plants (Ayensu, 1981; Berlin, 1980; Payne-Jackson & Alleyne, 2004).

The health care situation in the 19th century post-emancipation period presented the same basic question that existed during slavery. Were the freed enslaved Africans going to continue to rely on their traditional medical systems as a result of the absence of, difficult accessibility to, and mistrust of the formal government medical systems? Bryan (1991) postulates that both the absence of political will and the declining socioeconomic environment during the 19th century hindered colonial administrations from carrying out improvement to health facilities and health care. This was further hampered by transportation issues and the shortage of medical personnel. These conditions contributed to the preservation of traditional medical practices.

The poor socioeconomic conditions that existed in the post-emancipation period resulted in an ever increasing distance both culturally and ideologically as well as geographically between the freed slaves and the white and brown classes. As freed slaves left the plantations they established villages in remote areas and had little contact with the ruling classes. Missionary activity promoted the continuation and in many instances the deepening of Afro-Jamaican religions (Payne-Jackson & Alleyne, 2004). The neglect and/or failure of colonial administrations to provide basic essential services to the freed enslaved Africans contributed to the preservation and strengthening of traditional practices (Payne-Jackson & Alleyne, 2004).

Many people throughout the Caribbean operate within a continuum between traditional medical systems, at one end of the continuum, and the biomedical medical system at the other end. The continuum reflects the social dynamics and interplay between ethnic continuity and separateness, on the one hand, and the emergence of some integrated "creole" socio-cultural system, on the other hand. Individuals differ in the ways in which aetiology, practitioners and treatments correlate; they differ in the range of illnesses attributed to different causes; they differ in the priority given to different practitioners for the treatment of different illnesses.

(Payne-Jackson & Alleyne, 2004, p. 8; also see Alleyne, 1988),

Independence brought new pride in ethnic identity and traditional culture. The result has been an intertwining of traditional and biomedical ideas. The constantly evolving system is flexible enough to include the occult and spiritual as well as new diseases (Snow, 1993). This flexibility allows the urban, educated, elite and rural, poorly educated, poor to accommodate their needs and beliefs about illness whether predominantly from the biomedical worldview or from the traditional worldview or a combination of both depending on where on the continuum of culture the individual identifies him/herself.

Traditional Medical Beliefs and Practices

Traditional healing systems throughout the Caribbean recognize natural, spiritual, and occult causes of diseases and illnesses. Natural illnesses result from an imbalance in the human body caused by natural elements such as heat, cold, wind, and dew or impurities in the food, water, and air. However, a strong belief exists in the supernatural as a causal factor in illnesses and accidents. Supernatural causes of illness fall into two categories—spiritual and occult. Spiritual causes of illness result from humans who break social and moral taboos of the culture. Illnesses of this nature are seen as punishment sent by God for sins. Yet another source of spiritual illness is malevolent forces of the supernatural world such as Satan, demons, fallen angels, and wandering spirits of the deceased—duppies or Jumby/Jumbe. Spiritual illnesses are also seen as ways to witness for the faith or as calls to service (Payne, 1991; Payne-Jackson & Alleyne, 2004).

Occult causes of illness in the Caribbean are those illnesses that have been intentionally sent by human agents such as an Obeah wo/man. In the Caribbean Obeah is a learned art and is associated with black magic and sorcery and is seen as a form of witchcraft. It was so feared by the Europeans that laws were instituted in the 19th century banning its practice. Occult practitioners, however, can use their powers to bring health and benefits to their clients as well as to cause harm and death (Payne-Jackson & Alleyne, 2004).

Traditional practitioners receive their call to serve through a variety of experiences: dreams, visions, encounters with supernatural beings (e.g., mermaids), or near death experiences. Some are recognized as healers due to special gifts or characteristics at birth, such as being born with the veil/caul (placenta over the face), or being born with teeth. Often times the roles of traditional healers are passed down family lines. No set age is established for when a practitioner can begin his/her work. Training for practitioners may be formal or informal. An apprenticeship is often required. Training entails learning the medicinal value, quality, and use of different herbs and other objects used in treating illness as well as the needed rituals. Practitioners are trained in how to diagnose the cause of an illness or suffering, what treatment is required to treat an illness, and what preventive measures to recommend for the relief of illness or suffering. Practitioners need to be versed in how to diagnose and treat magic, witchcraft, and sorcery. Spiritual and occult healers in particular must also be versed in the nature of and how to handle spirits and the living-dead (Payne-Jackson & Alleyne, 2004).

Traditional practitioners are consulted for treatment of all forms of illness from the common cold to chronic illnesses such as diabetes and hypertension as well as new illnesses such as HIV/AIDS. The perceived cause of an illness determines which practitioner is sought out for healing. An illness thought to be of a natural cause can be self-treated or treated by a herbalist (bush doctor, leaf doctor, etc.). Illness thought to be of a spiritual or occult cause can be treated by a spiritual healer or an Obeah wo/man. Practitioners may be consulted simultaneously. For example, a person with an illness may consult a herbalist for a bush remedy and the Obeah wo/man to determine who sent the illness and what medicine to take to reverse the curse. In many cases a biomedical doctor is consulted concurrently. Failure on the part of the biomedical practitioner to successfully diagnose and/or treat an illness often validates for a patient the need to seek the help of a spiritual and/or occult practitioner (see Patrick & Payne-Jackson, 1996).

The primary form of treatment for physical, mental, and spiritual illnesses in the Caribbean includes a wide array of concoctions made from herbs such as teas, poultices, baths, tablets, ointments, powders, and oils. A primary method of treatment for illnesses of a spiritual or occult nature includes the exorcism of evil spirits in addition to herbal remedies. Exorcism by transference (direct, indirect, or symbolic), incantation and prayers, and intimidation to drive out the evil spirits are three examples of methods used to force evil spirits to leave the body. Deities are also called upon to aid in the exorcisms (Hand, 1980; Lowe et al., 2009).

The Tenacity of Traditional Medicine

Medical systems are closely integrated with the social, cultural, and political institutions of a society. The resurgence and tenacity of traditional medicine can be contributed in part to social, economic, and ecological factors and government policies. Rising costs for health care and health insurance, and the global economic crisis have created a serious decrease in the availability and accessibility of modern health care services and personnel. As a result the use of traditional medicine is increasing as people are relying more on their extensive knowledge of and use of the bush teas for both the more common types of illnesses such as colds as well as chronic illnesses.

The ever increasing decline in economic and moral situations has led people to turn to religion to find fulfillment through spiritual pursuits. The holistic approach of traditional medicine addresses and reinforces the importance of the use of herbs and spiritual and community support in healing the mind/body/spirit as a whole. The perception of disease and illness is perhaps one of the most important contributing factors to the tenacity of traditional healing. As Snow (1993) points out,

> Traditional ways of healing are still to be found because they serve a purpose. They allay the physical ills of the body, of course, but they heal the spirit and mind and heart as well . . . Traditional practices are not simply old ways of treating old problems, for better or worse they are also used to deal with the newer scourges of drugs and AIDS. They may not offer the "cure" sought by biomedicine but they do provide the individual with explanation and accommodation in an increasingly difficult world. They offer empowerment to those who, on the surface, have not much power at all.
>
> *(p. 279)*

Biomedicine is recognized as the modern, scientific approach to treat illness. This cultural approach treats the mind and body as separate entities. The biomedical etiology is based on natural explanations and excludes the supernatural. Patients have minimal input into the diagnosis, treatment, and management of their illness as the power and control over the illness resides in the hands of the biomedical practitioner. However, three questions a biomedical practitioner cannot answer is "why," "how," and "who sent the illness."

The culture of traditional medicine is based on a "holistic approach" (mind/body/spirit) which incorporates the natural and supernatural as explanations for illness. Patients are encouraged to take an active part in the diagnosis (why/how/who) and treatment of their illness and encouraged to use magico/religious items and rituals to aid in regaining balance in their lives. The psychological impact of this approach is that it empowers patients and provides explanations for and gives a sense of control over the illness.

A complex relationship exists between a culture, its cosmology, and its health-related beliefs and actions taken. Religion permeates the lives of people in the Caribbean and is used to explain personal, social, and natural events (Payne-Jackson & Alleyne, 2004). As Pachter (1994) notes,

> Personal experiences, family attitudes, and group beliefs interact to provide an underlying structure for decision making during illness. These factors may also affect communication between the sufferer and others who may be recruited to provide support during illness . . . [E]ffective communication is maximized when the patient and the health care provider share beliefs about the sickness.
>
> *(p. 690).*

The attitudes of biomedical practitioners (including other health care professionals such as nurses and health aides) have, perhaps, the greatest impact on a patient's choice of health care system and his or her compliance with the prescribed treatment. The asymmetries of social status and power such as education, socioeconomic class, and rural/urban provenance are directly related to dialectal differences within the Creole continuum and have been shown to lead to ineffective communication between biomedical practitioners, who use only scientific/medical jargon, and their patients, who use varieties of language along the Creole continuum. This lack of communication in turn affects patients' health behavior and confidence in doctors' abilities (Alleyne, Gregg, Crell, Cruickshank, & Morrison, 1991; Fisher & Todd, 1993; Payne-Jackson, 1999). Moreover, biomedical practitioners tend to hold traditional medical practices and beliefs in spiritual and occult causes of illness in contempt, referring to it as that "mumbo-jumbo." Patients, not wanting to be humiliated by physicians or be treated as foolish or unintelligent, do not tell their doctors of their beliefs or their consultation with traditional healers or using their treatments (Payne-Jackson & Alleyne, 2004). The relationship between traditional practitioners and their patients is of equal importance. As the practitioner and patient are usually of the same social and cultural level and use the same language of communication the results are better communication and understanding.

Implications for Integration

The WHO recognizes four conditions that need to be met for the successful integration of traditional medicine into national health care systems. They suggest that first, traditional medicine should be supported and integrated into national health systems in combination with national policy and regulation for products, practices, and providers to ensure safety and quality; second, the use of safe, effective, and quality products and practices should be ensured; third, traditional medicine should be acknowledged as part of primary health care, to increase access to care and preserve knowledge and resources; and lastly, patient safety should be ensured by upgrading the skills and knowledge of providers of traditional medicine (WHO, 2012).

Mills (1991) suggests a review of the role of traditional health care practices and beliefs is needed.

> [A] positive reason for looking again at health care as our ancestors did . . . [is] we shall see how their perspective was essentially a whole-world view, with each part irreplaceably contributing to a pattern: diseases were seen as imbalances to be corrected rather than as alien invasions to be attacked. Herbal remedies were judged by their ability to adjust patterns of disorder, not by any conventional "antidisease" or allopathic activity. In times when germs and the other usual "bad guys" of disease are proving harder and

harder to attack, we may be ready to look again at medicines that treat illness differently.

(p. 7)

Discrepancies in beliefs and behaviors are often greatest when the physicians and patients have different cultural orientations and explanations of the etiology and treatment of illness. Reconciling and/or adopting the cultural differences in traditional and biomedical approaches will be a major part of the process if integration is to be achieved. It can be expected that appropriate use of health services, compliance with therapeutic interventions, and improved health outcomes have a higher likelihood of being realized when the health care provider and the patient acknowledge and respect each other's beliefs about illness, even though these beliefs may not be wholly concordant (Payne-Jackson & Alleyne, 2004).

Lowe et al. (2002) note that health educators face two major problems in attempting to integrate traditional medicine and biomedicine. First, they must educate people about both the positive and harmful aspects of traditional medical practices and how the community can benefit from modifying some practices. Second, they need to educate biomedical health practitioners (doctors, nurses, midwives, etc.) and social workers as to the advantages, disadvantages and public health implications of traditional practices. Lowe et al., note:

> Within this framework will be the need (for the benefit of patients) to investigate, identify and offer information concerning: (1) the types of illnesses for which patients consult a doctor or ethnopractitioners; (2) the illnesses which patients prefer to treat at home; (3) the attitudes of patients towards health facilities and health professionals in general; and (4) the reasons for the attitudes.
>
> *(p. 35)*

At the same time, biomedical personnel will need to be trained in the premises of traditional medicine and how to integrate this knowledge with biomedicine so that they can communicate effectively with patients without denigrating their beliefs and practices. The impact of science and technology, the increase in the use of herbs in medicine, and the incorporation of herbal medicine into the legislative laws of many countries has resulted in a change of traditional medicine as oral traditions to a commercial enterprise (Lowe et al., 2009, p. 61).

A major issue for the integration of herbal medicine is the problem of standardization. The scientific process focuses primarily on determining the phytochemicals in different herbs and the potency of the chemical effects. This ignores and loses vital information about mixtures of herbs and the cultural and social relations linked to rituals, faith, and the patient's experience in the treatment of illnesses by traditional healers (Pool & Geisler, 2007).

The international recognition of the healing qualities of many herbs has resulted in patients having more confidence in traditional remedies. A review of the literature has shown that many herbs are safe to use and have significant clinical implications; however, other herbs are considered unsafe or unfit for human consumption. If the establishment of standards related to indigenous drugs in pharmaceutical preparations is to be effective, then proper quality control must be established and maintained (Lowe et al., 2002). Lowe et al. (2002) propose a model for the development of an indigenous drug industry and the incorporation of herbal medicines into current biomedical training and practices. This would involve developing an infrastructure for research and development to determine the chemistry and pharmacology of herbal materials including screening programs and intensive research into those areas that show greatest promise and relevance to the health requirements of the people.

The pragmatic merit of integration of biomedicine and traditional medicine is that "it already exists in part even though unplanned and unprogrammed" (Payne-Jackson & Alleyne, 2004, p. 168). The challenge is to facilitate modernization but not at the expense of the traditional cultural base which can be seen as "the spiritual and moral force which drives the development process and can become the springboard for scientific technological development" (Payne-Jackson & Alleyne, 2004).

Conclusion

The traditional medical systems found in the Caribbean that evolved as a result of contact among Amerindians, Africans, and Europeans are a rich source of healing knowledge and are a common bond across the cultures in the Caribbean. The value of and use of herbs by traditional practitioners bridges cultural, religious, and ethnic differences.

Traditional practitioners today, as in colonial times, receive their calling through recognized special features (e.g., being born with the veil), dreams, visions, and/or near death experiences. Training is primarily informal, passing down family lines, or more formally through apprenticeship. The worldview of traditional practitioners includes a tripartite etiology of illness—natural, occult, and spiritual. As in colonial times, practitioners today are consulted for all forms of illness from the chronic disease, to the common cold, to the new scourge.

The persistence of traditional medicine across cultures and across time can be understood by looking to the past. Local conditions during slavery were significant in accounting for the development and prevalence of traditional medicine among the enslaved Africans. The lack of medical services for the enslaved Africans led to reliance on traditional practices, including magico-religious practices and rituals to treat illness. Emancipation saw no improvement in accessibility to health care.

Health care for many today, especially those of lower socioeconomic classes of urban and rural provenance, continues to be traditional medicine. Contributing factors to this tenacity include the lack of medical facilities, inaccessibility either logistically or financially, the high cost of transportation and medication, socio-cultural and linguistic barriers, mistrust of doctors, miscommunication between patients/practitioners, perceived cause of illnesses, and incompatibility of world-views and religious beliefs. The holistic approach of traditional practitioners allows them to empower patients to have more input in the diagnosis and treatment of their illness.

An important contributing factor to the resurgence of reliance on traditional medicine today is that many consumers do not trust modern biomedicine to have all the answers and they believe that natural products are "naturally" safe as they have been used for centuries. This contrasts with biomedical medicines that come with myriad warnings about side effects, some of which can be fatal. These warnings often come several years after a product has been on the market. However, the dosage and toxicity of traditional remedies, either self-subscribed or subscribed by traditional practitioners, is a major concern for biomedical practi-tioners as is the fact that some bush teas can be harmful while others can mask symptoms of serious illnesses such as diabetes. Development of an indigenous medical system that can provide standardization of herbal remedies would promote integration of the two systems together with a side benefit of an economic boost to local economies.

The WHO has called for integration of traditional medical systems and practitioners into health care. To accomplish this, education of both biomedical and traditional healers is needed to address differences in worldviews, beliefs, and treatment practices. This includes re-evaluation of the cultural differences that underlie the two traditions including the dual (mind/body) approach of bio-medicine and the holistic approach (mind/body/spirit) of traditional medicine to health and wellness. As religious belief and ritual are an important part of traditional healing, it is for biomedical practitioners to understand the importance of recognizing both natural and supernatural etiologies, the natural and supernatural properties of herbs used to treat illnesses, and incorporate methods of treatment and rituals that address both perceived etiologies. Using herbal remedies, under-standing and appreciating differing worldviews and explanatory models of illness, and formally integrating traditional healers into the health care systems are important steps to bringing health care to all peoples throughout the Caribbean.

References

Alleyne, M. (1988). *Roots of Jamaican culture*. London: Pluto.
Alleyne, S., Gregg, R., Grell, K., Cruickshank, J. K., & Morrison, E. Y. (1991). Jamaican patients' understanding of diabetes mellitus. *West Indies Medical Journal, 40*(60), 60–64.
Ayensu, E. (1981). *Medicinal plants of the West Indies*. Algonac, MI: Reference Publications.
Berlin, I. (1980). Time, space, and the evolution of Afro-American society on British mainland North America. *American Historical Review, 85*(1): 44–78.

Bilby, K. (1993). The strange career of "Obeah": Defining magical power in the West Indies. Paper presented at Johns Hopkins University, Institute for Global Studies in Culture, Power, and History.

Bryan, P. (1991). *The Jamaican people, 1880–1902.* Warwick University Caribbean Studies, London: Macmillan.

Eisner, G. (1961). *Jamaica 1830–1930: A study in economic growth.* Manchester: Manchester University Press.

Fisher, S., & Todd, A. (1993). *The social organization of doctor-patient communication.* (2nd ed.) Norwood, NJ: Ablex Publishing Corporation.

Gardner, W. (1873). *A history of Jamaica from its discovery by Christopher Columbus to the present time.* London: E. Stock.

Genovese, E. (1976). *Roll, Jordan, roll: The world the slaves made.* New York: Vintage Books.

Hand, W. (1980). *Magical medicine. The folkloric component of medicine in the folk belief, custom, and ritual of the peoples of Europe and America.* Berkeley, CA: University of California Press.

Laguerre, M. (1987). *Afro-Caribbean folk medicine.* South Hadley, MA: Bergin & Garvey.

Lowe, H., Payne-Jackson, A., & Beckstrom-Sternberg, S. (2002) *Jamaican ethnomedicine: Its potential in the health care system* (2nd ed.). Kingston: Pelican Press.

Lowe, H., Payne-Jackson, A., & Johnson, C. (2009). *The legacy of African, African-American & Caribbean traditional medicines: Mind, body and spirit.* Kingston: Pelican Press.

Lunan, J. (1814). *Hortu Jamaicensis or a botanical description and an account of the virtues, & c. of its indigenous plants hitherto known as also of the most useful exotics* (2 vols.). Jamaica: St. Jago de la Vega Gazette.

Mills, S. (1991). *The essential book of herbal medicine.* Arkana: Penguin Books.

Pachter, L. (1994). Culture and clinical care. *Journal of the American Medical Association, 271,* 690–694.

Patrick, P., & Payne-Jackson, A. (1996). Functions of Rasta talk in a Jamaican Creole healing narrative: "A bigfoot dem gi' me". *Journal of Linguistic Anthropology, 6*(1), 1–38.

Payne, A. (1991). The traditional concepts of Jamaican folk medicine. *Latin American Essays, 3,* 147–160.

Payne-Jackson, A. (1999). Biomedical and folk medical concepts of adult onset diabetes in Jamaica: Implications for treatment. *Health, 3*(1), 1–46.

Payne-Jackson, A., & Alleyne, M. (2004). *Jamaican folk medicine: A source of healing.* Kingston: The University of West Indies Press.

Pool, R., & Geissler, W. (2007) *Medical anthropology.* New York: Open University Press.

Sheridan, R. (1985). *Doctors and slaves: A medical and demographic history of slavery in the British West Indies, 1680–1834.* Cambridge: Cambridge University Press.

Snow, L. (1993). *Walkin' over medicine: Traditional health practices in African American life.* Boulder, CO: Westview Press.

Thomson, J. (1820). *A treatise on the diseases of Negroes as they occur in the island of Jamaica.* Kingston: A. Aikman.

World Health Organization. (2012). *Traditional medicine.* Retrieved from http://www/who.int/mediacentre/factsheets/fs134/en/

4

HERBAL MEDICINE PRACTICES IN THE CARIBBEAN

Yuri Clement

Introduction

There is a long heritage of medicinal plant use in the Caribbean. Before the 15th century arrival of Europeans into the region, native Amerindians practiced indigenous health care rituals which included the use of endemic plants for medicinal purposes. Over the last five centuries these peoples have been largely displaced by Europeans, enslaved Africans, indentured Indian labourers, and other minority ethnic groups. These migrant peoples brought with them indigenous health care practices which incorporated the local flora and over time a potpourri herbal pharmacopoeia emerged (Mischel, 1959; Simpson, 1962; Wong, 1967).

Although over 20,000 vascular plants exist in the Caribbean, with about 7,000 endemic species (Davis, Hywood, Herrera-MacBryde, Villa-Lobbs, & Hamilton, 1997), only a small number are used in traditional medicine. For instance, 170 species (including just 8 endemic species) were used in herbal remedies (Cano & Volpato, 2004) in Eastern Cuba, where over 3,000 species of vascular plants have been identified. Similarly, surveys in Jamaica (Meeks Gardner, Grant, Hutchinson, & Wilks, 2000) and Trinidad (Clement et al., 2007) identified only a small fraction of the plants being used in herbal preparations.

In this chapter I will review the traditional concepts of health and disease in the Caribbean and the use of herbs for the treatment of disease and health maintenance in this context. I will also discuss the spectrum of herbal remedies ranging from the treatment of minor self-limiting conditions such as the common cold to the treatment of non-communicable chronic diseases, such as hypertension and diabetes mellitus.

Traditional Concepts of Health and Disease in the Caribbean

The various peoples who came to the region practiced health care based on their cultural concepts of health and disease, with varying degrees of incorporation of some aspects of resident Amerindian concepts on the different islands. Two dominant concepts included the belief that there was an involvement of the supernatural and the balance between "hot" and "cold" humors in physical well-being.

In traditional Afro-Caribbean healing practices there was always the link between natural and supernatural with respect to disease and health, with little distinction between body, mind, and spirit (McCarthy Brown, 2003). In this context, herbal use facilitated the relief of symptoms while spiritual rituals addressed underlying supernatural causes. Many enslaved Africans had confidence in their "self-help" spiritual healers and "herbalists/doctors" (Handler, 2000) where "bush bathes" or "bush teas" were accompanied by songs, chants, drumming, dancing, and prayers to deities in communal ceremonies. Although many of these rituals originated in African cultures, such as Yoruba from Nigeria, most of the herbs used were from the region (Handler, 2000).

Enslaved Africans in the Caribbean existed under brutal conditions where sickness and premature death were constant companions, especially during the early periods of chattel slavery where slaves were an expendable commodity. Consequently, Africans with residual "hands-on" experience and those "apprenticed" locally provided health care for their counterparts in the face of scarcity of medical attention from plantation overseers (De Barros, 2004).

With forced European indoctrination of Western religious practices, a fusion between West/West Central African religions and Christianity/Roman Catholicism emerged. The European "hot–cold" humoral concept of medicine became incorporated into the Afro-Caribbean medicinal systems. For instance, the Afro-Cuban *Santería* rituals (an amalgamation between the Nigerian Orisha religion and Roman Catholicism) incorporated a wide range of herbs to treat spiritual and health conditions (Brandon, 1991; Wedel, 2009). In Trinidad and Grenada the "bush doctor" of the Shango cult, an amalgamation of Yoruba beliefs and Roman Catholicism, integrated ceremonial rituals with the use of herbs in healing practices (Mischel, 1959: Simpson, 1962).

In many Caribbean islands the term "Obeah" was originally associated with varied African ritualistic practices, but over time it was largely relegated to the use of the supernatural for evil magic especially by the colonial European plantation overseers (Ordenson, 1842). In many of these territories the colonial authorities moved swiftly to outlaw such practices and practitioners were punished, some being killed to deter others. This environment has had a lasting impression over time. In the contemporary Caribbean the use of "bush" medicine is sometimes associated with these negative 'Obeah' connotations.

During the period of slavery, the "hot–cold" dichotomy of health and disease was widely accepted and practiced in Western medicine (Foster, 1979; 1988). An imbalance in "hot" or "cold" humors resulted in excessively "hot" or excessively "cold" diseases (Jackson, 2001). Restoration of good health was achieved when "hot" diseases were treated with "cold" remedies and "cold" diseases treated with "hot" remedies.

"Hot" conditions included fever, infections, diarrhea, constipation, kidney problems, rash and skin ailments, sore throat, liver problems, ulcers, and menstruation and were treated with "cold" plants. Herbs were categorized according to taste and colour of flowers, with bitter or bad tasting plants being "cold" and used as "cooling" to treat "hot" conditions (Anderson, 1984; Schoental, 1957). A survey by Wong (1967) in a remote village in Trinidad identified 214 plants as being either "hot" or "cold," with 31 "cooling" recipes being used as "blood cleansers" and "purifiers." Most "cooling" plants were termed "cold" and were used to treat or prevent disorders such as rashes, measles, yaws, and sexually transmitted infections.

With the abolition of chattel slavery in 1845 indentured labourers from the Indian subcontinent entered the Caribbean sociocultural landscape. These transplanted people brought with them many aspects of the centuries-old traditional medicinal systems, such as Ayurveda and Unani, which resembled the European "hot–cold" humoral concept. Several plants used in Hindu rituals and for the treatment of conditions such as fever, skin infection, women's health problems, and diabetes mellitus now constitute a significant portion of the region's herbal pharmacopoeia. These include *Tamarindus indica, Momordica charantia, Mangifera indica, Curcuma domestica, Cannabis sativa, Cymbopogon citrates,* and *Ocimum gratissimum* (Payne-Jackson & Alleyne, 2004).

The first Chinese emigrants arrived in Trinidad in 1806 and they brought many aspects of established traditional Chinese medicine, as well as herbs. A recent survey in Trinidad showed that several medicinal plants currently used for skin and stomach problems have their origins in Chinese traditional medicine including *Abelmoschus moschatus, Achyranthes aspera, Eupatorium macrophyllum, Phyllanthus urinaria,* and *Portulaca oleraceae* (Lans, 2007a).

Herbs used for the Common Cold, Fever, and Flu

Traditional "bush tea" remedies for the common cold, fever, and flu symptoms abound in the Caribbean. In a survey in Trinidad, 42 plant species were cited for the treatment of the common cold and cough and included *Leonotis nepetifolia, Zingiber officinale, Chromolaena odorata, Cymbopogon citrates,* and *Neurolaena lobata* (Clement et al., 2007). In Wong's (1967) survey, plants such as *Lantana camara, Pimenta racemosa, Myristica fragrans,* and *Bambusa vulgaris* were used to treat cold fever, and it is interesting to note that most of these plants were classified as either "hot" or "very hot" according to classical humoral definition.

A survey in six geographically diverse Jamaican communities showed that 33 plant species were used to treat fever and 22 for the common cold, with overlap use of *Annona reticulata*, *Argemone mexicana*, *Cymbopogon citratus*, *Ocimum basilicum*, and *Momordica charantia* (Payne-Jackson & Beckstrom-Sternberg, 2006). Among Haitian communities *Momordica charantia*, *Bidens pilosa*, *Costus speciosus*, and *Phyllantus procerus* were popular for fever (Volpato, Godínez, Beyra, & Barreto, 2009).

Herbs as "Blood Purifers" and Anthelmintics

The blood plays a central role in the maintenance of health and the medico-cultural concept of "bad blood" is firmly rooted in many Caribbean traditional beliefs. "Bad blood" leads to diseases such as skin disorders and sexually transmitted infections. According to Haitian folk medicine, abnormalities of the eyes, fingernails, and skin would necessitate the administration of a herbal "blood purifier" to "cleanse" the liver, kidneys, spleen, and bowels. Among immigrant Haitians in Cuba *Erythoxylum havanense*, *Roystonea regia*, *Momordica charantia*, and *Senna occidentalis* were frequently used as "blood purifiers" (Cano & Volpata, 2004; Volpata et al., 2009). In another survey in Trinidad, *Aloe vera* was the most commonly used herbal "blood cleanser" (Clement et al., 2007).

There is the medico-cultural construct of intestinal worms thought to be located within a "worm bag." It is also believed that these intestinal worms either confer health benefits, such as aiding in digestion, or harm and cause "gripe," flatulence, or even seizures when there is an overabundance. Yet other communities believe that excessive worms are associated with the supernatural. Herbal preparations are given over a few days to either kill or cause worms to "sleep" so that they could be expelled in the feces.

A survey in Dominica identified *Chenopodium ambrosioides*, *Aristolochia trilobata*, *Ambrosia hispida*, and *Portulaca oleracea* as herbs commonly used to treat intestinal worms (Quinlan, Quinlan, & Nolan, 2002). Another survey in Haitian immigrants and descendents in Cuba corroborated the use of these plants and also cited *Cocus nucifera*, *Crescentia cujete*, and *Momordica charantia* L. as being commonly used for intestinal worms (Volpato et al., 2009). In Trinidad and Tobago, Lans (2007a) identified the use of *Citharexylum spinosum*, *Cucurbita maxima*, *Tagetes patula*, and *Eupatorium triplinerve* for the treatment of intestinal worms.

Herbs used for Sexual, Women's Reproductive, and Child Health

Herbs play a major role in the traditional management of the reproductive health of women in the region, ranging from alleviation of menstrual pain to "womb cleansing." A literature review and fieldwork in the Dominican Republic revealed that herbs were used to treat many women's health conditions including uterine fibroids, excessive uterine bleeding, endometriosis, and hot flushes in menopause. In this study, 87 plant species were cited including *Agave* sp., *Beta vulgaris*, *Saccharum officinarum*, and *Kalanchoe gastonis-bonnieri* (Osaski et al., 2002).

In the Caribbean, sexual potency and vitality are highly valued. In the recent past a man's ability to father many children and a woman's ability to bear children were highly esteemed in society; and infertility is still considered taboo. In Trinidad, a survey by Lans (2007b) identified *Chamaesyce hirta* and *Cola nitida* as useful plants commonly used to treat female infertility. In the Dominican Republic, *Allium cepa*, *Petroselium crispum* and *Serenoa serrulata* were cited as being useful to treat infertility (Osaski et al., 2002).

Throughout the Caribbean the prized *bois bandé* (loosely interpreted from the French to mean "potency wood") has been used traditionally to aid sexual performance with assumed potent aphrodisiac qualities. In Trinidad, *bois bandé* in fact represents two distinct plant species: *Parinari campestris* and *Richeria grandis* (Lans, 2007b). In eastern Cuba several plants have been identified as being used to treat impotence and enhance sexual performance, the most common being *Stachytarpheta jamaicensis*, *Chiococca alba*, and *Roystonea regia* (Cano & Volpato, 2004). In this survey *Scoparia dulcis*, *Ageratum conyzoides*, *Gomphrena globosa*, and *Cucurbita maxima* were also cited as plants useful in the treatment of prostate problems.

Among the Surinamese Maroons the popular practice of "dry sex" is facilitated by female genital herbal steam baths which dry and tighten the vagina to the increase sexual pleasure for the male partner. A survey in Suriname identified over 177 herbs used in genital herbal baths, including *Vismia macrophylla*, *Piper marginatum*, and *Xylopia frutescens* (van Andel et al., 2008).

The traditional use of herbs to treat sexually transmitted infections is a common practice throughout the region and is believed to be caused by "bad blood." A recent survey in eastern Cuba identified several herbs as being used to treat sexually transmitted infections including *Erythoxylum havanense*, *Chiococca alba*, *Roystonea reglia*, *Senna occidentalis*, *Solanum Torvum*, *Cassia fistula*, and *Swietenia mahogoni* (Cano & Volpata, 2004).

In this survey several plant species were also identified that treat menstrual irregularities including *Cissus sicyoides*, *Senna occidentalis*, and *Cassia fistula* (Cano & Volpata, 2004). In the tradition of Surinamese Maroons, vaginal baths commonly use the leaves of *Mangifera indica* to "cleanse" the uterus and vagina after childbirth (Ruysschaert, van Andel, van de Putte, & van Damme, 2009; van Andel, de Korte, Koopsman, Behari-Ramdas, & Ruysschaert, 2008). In Trinidad and Tobago, *Abelmoschus moschatus*, *Aristolochia rugosa*, and *Aristolochia trilobata* are given as "bush teas" to expel the "afterbirth" or placenta and cleanse the uterus after delivery (Lans, 2007b).

The control of fertility to regulate their reproductive capacity, especially during the period of chattel slavery, was an area of grave concern for enslaved African women. Many herbs were employed to "regulate" menstrual flow and may also have been used as abortifacients by enslaved African women ". . . to abort their children, so that they will not become slave like themselves . . ." (Schiebinger, 2008, p. 718). Many herbs in the Caribbean have been identified which induce abortion or "increase uterine flow." In eastern Cuba *Cocus nucifera*, *Roystonea regia*, and *Cinnamomum verum* were the most commonly cited abortifacients, whereas in Trinidad *Ambrosia cumanensis*, *Aristolochia rugosa*, and *Aristolochia trilobata* were cited (Cano & Volpata, 2004; Lans, 2007b). About 20 herbs have been identified in Haiti with traditional use as abortifacients or emmenagogues which included *Casearia ilicifolia*, *Eleutherine bulbosa*, *Rhoeo spathacea*, and *Stemodia durantifolia*; and extracts of these plants have demonstrated significant activity against in vitro mouse uterine smooth muscle (Weniger, Haag-Berrurier, & Anton, 1982).

Herbal remedies, especially those for oral consumption, are used cautiously in children, with "stronger" herbs being reserved for adults. These "bush teas" were used as tonics and to self-treat commonly occurring ailments such as cough, fever, and intestinal worms. In a survey in Dominica, *Chenopodium ambrosioides* (which was considered safe) was the preferred antihelminthic medicinal remedy for intestinal parasites in children, with limited use of *Aristolochia trilobata*, which has known toxicities (Quinlan et al., 2002). A survey in a pediatric clinic in Jamaica showed that 71% of mothers gave their children "bush teas" (Michie, 1992). Medicinal plants commonly used included *Mintha viridis*, *Momordica charantia*, *Annona muricata*, and *Cymbopogon citratus*.

Surinamese Maroon communities have a rich herbal pharmacopoeia where herbal baths are commonly used in newborns and infants to strengthen, promote health, and protect against malevolent supernatural forces. A recent survey showed the use of over 400 preparations using 178 plant species by Maroon mothers in childcare in Suriname (Ruysschaert et al., 2009). The most commonly used medicinal plants included *Anacardium occidentalis*, *Gossypium barbadense*, *Rolandra fruticosa*, *Eleusine indica*, *Paspalum conjugatum*, *Stachytarpheta cayennensis*, and *Stachytarpheta jamaicensis* for herbal baths for infants. Herbal baths are also used in these communities to "cleanse the belly" as an effective purgative, where babies are given small amounts of the bath water to drink.

Herbs used for Diabetes Mellitus and Hypertension

There has been an increasing prevalence of chronic lifestyle diseases in the Caribbean, such as hypertension and diabetes mellitus, and over recent decades herbal remedies have been applied to alleviate associated symptoms. In Morton's (1981) guidebook of medicinal plants several species useful in the management of diabetes mellitus were identified and include *Ageratum conyzoides*, *Aristolochia trilobata*, *Bixa orellana*, *Borreria verticillata*, *Caesalpinia bondou*, *Cassia fruticosa*, *Chromolaena odorata*, *Eryngium foetidum*, *Gomphrena globosa*, and *Scoparia dulcis*. A survey of public primary health care facilities in Trinidad and Tobago revealed that 24% of patients used herbs for diabetes-associated symptoms, particularly for the burning sensation or numbness in the feet (Mahabir & Gulliford, 1997). Another survey several years later in a larger sample at similar public health care facilities in Trinidad showed that just 9.3% of diabetic patients reported the use of herbs

(Clement, 2009). Plants most commonly used in these patients included *Momordica charantia*, *Aloe vera*, *Catharanthus roseus*, *Allium sativum*, and *Panax ginseng*. It is noteworthy that all herbs mentioned by Trinidadian patients in this survey originated in Asia and Europe. In Dominica, "bush teas" for diabetes were made using *Pluchea symphytifolia*, *Stachytarpheta jamaicensis*, and *Chaptalia nutans* (ACCT, 1985). Additionally, *Anacardium occidentale* and *Artocapus altilis* were cited as useful anti-diabetic herbs in Jamaica (Payne-Jackson & Beckstrom-Sternberg, 2006).

Allium sativum (garlic) was the most popular herb used by hypertensive patients attending public primary health care facilities in Trinidad (Clement, 2009). In another survey in eastern Cuba a small number of respondents identified *Annona muricata*, *Annona reticulata*, *Citrus aurantifolia*, and *Bidens pilosa* as ingredients of traditional herbal mixtures used in hypertension (Cano & Volpato, 2004). Among Haitians in Cuba *Citrus sinensis*, *Tamarindus indica*, and *Thevetia peruviana* were most commonly used for hypertension (Volpato et al., 2009). In Jamaica, other herbs used for hypertension were *Artocarpus altilis*, *Catharanthus roseus*, *Persea americana*, and *Sechium edula* (Payne-Jackson & Beckstrom-Sternberg, 2006).

Documenting and Preserving the Caribbean's Herbal Legacy

A vast amount of traditional knowledge of herbal remedies has been lost due to a combination of lack of intergeneration transfer and disinterest by the current generation. Although many ethnobotanical surveys have been conducted in several islands, TRAMIL (Traditional Medicine in the Islands) is by far the most coordinated and comprehensive effort to document and preserve the Caribbean herbal legacy. It is a region-wide research network which attempts to document commonly used herbs and objectively assess safety and efficacy using pre-clinical methods (Robineau & Soejarto, 1996).

The TRAMIL program was started in 1982 in the Dominican Republic and has since conducted over 50 ethnopharmacological surveys in over 27 territories. The ethnopharmacological survey is designed to identify medicinal plants used for common self-limiting conditions and to date monographs have been prepared for 99 plants. Although many plants are identified in these surveys only those with over 20% citations or "significant use" for a specific condition are included in the TRAMIL Caribbean herbal pharmacopoeia. It is interesting to note that over 40 of these 99 documented plants were introduced into the region from Asia, Europe, and Africa, with only two species (*Bignonia longissima* and *Pimenta racemosa*) being endemic to the Caribbean islands. It has been shown that some of the "significant use" plants have actually been shown to be toxic by scientific methodology and TRAMIL provides warning against their use. Some of these plants include *Argemone mexicana*, *Datura stramonium*, *Lantana camara*, *Piper auritum*, *Pouteria sapota* and *Thevetia peruviana*.

In some territories such as Cuba, Dominican Republic, Honduras, Nicaragua, and Panama some commonly used plants (with satisfactory safety and efficacy testing) have been integrated into primary health care programs.

The Future of Traditional Herbal Medicine in the Caribbean

In addition to the lack of knowledge transfer, traditional herbal knowledge has also been lost due to the combined effect of the institutionalized post-emancipation suppression of African cultural practices (which utilized various herbal remedies) and the emergence of and reliance on the dominant evidence-based Western medicine culture in the last century. As there is little intergenerational oral transfer of traditional knowledge, and it has rapidly disappeared without adequate documentation, TRAMIL should be applauded and supported for its efforts. Most territories in the Caribbean Basin have attained certain levels of economic development where individuals have easy access to Westernized public health facilities, and health care workers actively discourage the use of traditional herbal remedies. Many persons using herbal remedies as their primary source of health care have limited access to these public health facilities, or do so without informing their attending clinicians and use concomitantly with conventional synthetic medicines (Clement et al., 2007; Delgoda et al., 2004).

There are many obstacles to the integration of herbs into conventional medicines, ranging from standardization to the lack of sufficient clinical evidence to support their use (Clement, 2008). Unlike developed countries where attempts are made to validate herbal medicines by rigorous scientific inquiry, the use of this modality in the Caribbean remains largely in the domain of the folklore. However, TRAMIL with its ethnobotanical approach to identifying "significant use" herbs and its associated pre-clinical studies should be a used as a springboard to advance to the next level of scientific validation. With the emphasis on evidence-based medicine the inevitable path forward would be to conduct human clinical trials to provide the support for the use of Caribbean herbs for an integrated health care approach in the region.

Conclusion

There is a wealth of traditional knowledge regarding medicinal plant use in the Caribbean which exists as an amalgam of medico-cultural concepts from indigenous Amerindian and European settlers, enslaved Africans, indentured Asian Indians, and other minority groups that have arrived over the last five centuries. There is significant loss of this traditional knowledge across generations as the oral tradition has been severely eroded and pervasive evidence-based Western medicine has taken root in Caribbean societies over the previous century. There is an urgent need for the preservation of this folkloric knowledge and TRAMIL has begun the work to document and validate "significant use" plants using pre-clinical models. This validation needs to be carried further using clinical trials to facilitate integration into the highly Westernized health care systems that currently exist in the Caribbean.

References

ACCT (1985). *Medecine traditionnelle et pharmacopee. Contribution aux etudes ethnobotaniques et floristiques a la Dominique (The Commonwealth of Dominica).* Paris: Agence de Cooperation Culturelle et Technique (ACCT).

Anderson, E. N. (1984). "Heating and cooling" foods re-examined. *Social Science Information, 23*(4/5), 755–773.

Brandon. G. (1991). The uses of plants in healing in an Afro-Cuban religion, Santeria. *Journal of Black Studies, 22*(1), 55–76.

Cano, J., & Volpato, G. (2004). Herbal mixtures in the traditional medicine of Eastern Cuba. *Journal of Ethnopharmacology, 90*, 293–316.

Clement, Y. N. (2008). Challenges facing the integration of herbal remedies into mainstream conventional medicine. In P. I. Eddington & U. V. Mastolli (Eds.), *Health knowledge, attitudes and practices.* (pp. 247–263). New York: Nova Publishers.

Clement, Y. N. (2009). Herbal self-medication at primary health care facilities in Trinidad. *Journal of Alternative and Complementary Medicine, 15*(1), 6–7.

Clement, Y. N., Morton-Gittens, J., Basdeo, L., Blades, A., Francis, M., Gomes, N., Janjua, M., & Singh, A, (2007). Perceived efficacy of herbal remedies by users accessing primary healthcare in Trinidad. *BMC Complementary and Alternative Medicine, 7*, 4.

Davis, S. D., Hywood, V. H., Herrera-MacBryde, O., Villa-Lobbs, J., & Hamilton, A. C. (1997). *Centres of plant diversity.* Volume 3. The Americas. Cambridge: WWF/IUCN.

De Barros, J. (2004). "Setting things right": Medicine and magic in British Guiana, 1803–1838. *Slavery & Abolition, 25*(1), 28–50.

Delgoda, E., Ellington, C., Barrett, S., Gordon, N., Clarke, N., & Younger, N. (2004). The practice of polypharmacy involving herbal and prescription medicines in the treatment of diabetes mellitus, hypertension and gastrointestinal disorders in Jamaica. *West Indian Medical Journal, 53*(6), 400–405.

Foster, G. M. (1979). Humoral traces in United States folk medicine. *Medical Anthropology Newsletter, 10*(2), 17–20.

Foster, G. M. (1988). The validating role of humoral theory in traditional Spanish-American therapeutics. *American Ethnologist, 15*(1), 120–135.

Handler, J. S. (2000). Slave medicine and Obeah in Barbados, circa 1650–1834. *New West Indian Guide, 74*(1&2), 57–90.

Jackson, W. A. (2001). A short guide to humoral medicine. *Trends in Pharmacological Sciences, 22*(9), 487–489.

Lans, C. (2007a). Comparison of plants used for skin and stomach problems in Trinidad and Tobago with Asian ethnomedicine. *Journal of Ethnobiology and Ethnomedicine, 3*, 3–14.

Lans, C. (2007b). Ethnomedicines used in Trinidad and Tobago for reproductive problems. *Journal of Ethnobiology and Ethnomedicine, 3*, 13–24.

Mahabir, D., & Gulliford, M. C. (1997). Use of medicinal plants for diabetes in Trinidad and Tobago. *Pan American Journal of Public Health, 1*(3), 174–179.

McCarthy Brown, K. (2003). Healing relationships in the African Caribbean. In H. Selin (Ed.), *Medicine across cultures: History and practices of medicine in non-Western cultures* (pp. 285–303). London: Klumer Academic Publishers.

Meeks Gardner, J., Grant, D., Hutchinson, S., & Wilks, R. (2000). The use of herbal teas and remedies in Jamaica. *West Indian Medical Journal, 49*(4), 331–336.

Michie, C. A. (1992). The use of herbal remedies in Jamaica. *Annals of Tropical Paediatrics, 12*, 32–36.

Mischel, F. (1959). Faith healing and medical practice in the Southern Caribbean. *Southwestern Journal of Anthropology, 15*, 407–417.

Morton, J. F. (1981). *Atlas of medicinal plants of middle America: Bahamas to Yucatan.* Springfield, IL: Charles C. Thomas.

Ordenson, J. W. (1842). *Creoleana: Or, social and domestic scenes and incidents in Barbados in days of yore.* London: Saunders & Otley.

Osaski, A. L., Lohr, P., Reiff, M., Balick, M. J., Kronenberg, F., Fugh-Berman, A. & O'Connor, B. (2002). Ethnobotanical literature survey of medicinal plants in the Dominican Republic used for women's health conditions. *Journal of Ethnopharmacology, 79*, 285–298.

Payne-Jackson, A., & Alleyne, M. C. (2004). *Jamaican folk medicine: A source of healing.* Kingston: UWI Press.

Payne-Jackson, A., & Beckstrom-Sternberg, S. (2006). Traditional remedies: Legacy from the past – implications for the future. In Y. N. Clement, & C. E. Seaforth (Eds.), *Advancing Caribbean herbs in the 21st century. Proceedings of the 7th international workshop on herbal medicine in the Caribbean.* (pp. 50–77). Trinidad & Tobago: MPC Printers.

Quinlan, M. B., Quinlan, R. J., & Nolan, J. M. (2002). Ethnophysiology and herbal treatments of intestinal worms in Dominica, West Indies. *Journal of Ethnopharmacology, 80*, 75–83.

Robineau, L., & Soejarto, D. D. (1996). TRAMIL: A research project on the medicinal resources of the Caribbean. In M. J. Balick, E. Elizabetski, & S. A. Laird (Eds.), *Medicinal resources of the tropical forest (biodiversity and its importance to human health)* (pp. 317–325). New York: Columbia University Press.

Ruysschaert, S., van Andel, T., van de Putte, K., & van Damme, P. (2009). Bathe the baby to make it strong and healthy: Plant use and child care among Saramacan Maroons in Suriname. *Journal of Ethnopharmacology, 121*, 148–170.

Schiebinger, L. (2008). Exotic abortifacients and lost knowledge. *The Lancet, 371*(9614), 718–719.

Schoental, R. (1957). Herbal medicines and disease. *The Journal of Tropical Pediatrics, 2*(4), 208.

Simpson, G. E. (1962). Folk medicine in Trinidad. *Journal of American Folklore, 75*, 326–340.

van Andel, T., de Korte, S., Koopmans, D., Behari-Ramdas, J., & Ruysschaert, S. (2008). Dry sex in Suriname. *Journal of Ethnopharmacology, 116*, 84–88.

Volpata, G., Godínez, D., Beyra, A., & Barreto, A. (2009). Uses of medicinal plants by Haitian immigrants and their descendents in the Province of Camagüey, Cuba. *Journal of Ethnobiology and Ethnomedicine, 5*, 16.

Wedel, J. (2009). Healing and spirit possession in the Caribbean. *Stockholm Review of Latin American Studies, 4*, 49–60.

Weniger, B., Haag-Berrurier, M., & Anton, R. (1982). Plants of Haiti used as antifertility agents. *Journal of Ethnopharmacology, 6*(1), 67–84.

Wong, W. Y. (1967). *The folk medicine of Blanchisseuse, Trinidad. Anthropology 300a.* Waltham, MA: Brandeis University.

PART II

Caribbean Traditional Healing and Healers

5

OBEAH

Afro-Caribbean Religious Medicine Art and Healing

Nathaniel Samuel Murrell

Introduction

Obeah is a secretive medicine art that involves a range of religious practices, activities, and beliefs designed to help persons in distress deal with crisis response to tragedy, battle psychological and physical illness, withstand or protect themselves against human abuse, and fight for survival. In this Afro-Caribbean religious tradition, believers use herbal remedies and mystical or unnatural means to address their physical, social, and emotional needs. Practitioners blend their practical knowledge of pharmacopeia with beliefs in divine powers and psychological conditioning as a means of securing physical well-being and social justice. Through this religious art, uprooted Africans, in the past, tapped into traditional medicines to deal with misfortunes, trauma, and historical contradictions of their lives under colonialism and slavery.

The meaning and existence of Obeah, quite naturally, have been contested in Caribbean history; though its influence may still be felt psychologically in areas of law, politics, religion, culture, and even health care economics (Murray, 2007). Since historically Obeah has been a secretive and "transgressive" medicine art (it worked outside of the endorsement and control of society against colonialism), its existence continues to generate debate as to whether it is: a figment of some Caribbean people's imagination, the destructive use of ritual objects and practices on the simpleminded, a naive appeal to spiritual powers in a community for good or ill fortune, or (for British colonials), "almost the entirety of African Caribbean religions" (Paton, 2009, p. 4).

This chapter examines the practice of Obeah in the Caribbean. It begins with a discussion of Obeah as a Creole healing phenomenon in Caribbean religious consciousness, its evolution, legal proscription, and practice as a medicine of defense under British colonialism. The chapter discusses also the transgressive nature of Obeah, its healers, their training in preparation to deploy Obeah medicine, and the role of pharmacopeia in this healing tradition. The chapter concludes by noting the challenges posed for a collaborative relationship between modern medicine and Obeah healing; and the difficulties Obeah poses for students in mental health.

The Obeah Phenomenon

Obeah, as an atypical phenomenon, does not have its own identifiable religious system or organization. It is an oral culture that thrives on different religious traditions and among varying ethnic groups (Case, 2001). The results of that versatility are Creole practices that practitioners draw on through a rich variety of religious traditions. Obeah is practiced in traditional religions and cultures, in remote and impoverished communities where alternative medicine is a last lifeline, as well as in upscale or middle-class society. During slavery, Obeah was practiced among the Maroons, slaves, free Africans, and poor whites. Later, it knew no boundaries; it found reception among peoples of different faiths, ethnicity, and social standing. Its practitioners were Jamaican Myalists, Pocominists, and Kuminists; it is among the Trinidad and Tobago Spiritual Baptists and Orisha (or Kabbalists) avatars; it is found in Guyanese Hindu Kali Mai Pujah, as well as Muslim and Christian sects. Obeah appeals to descendants of indentured immigrants, people of African and European descent, and other Creole peoples; so Obeah is not a religion of illiterate maladjusted Africans. Caribbean people of all hue and faith may visit Obeah men—to receive pharmacopeia or to be corralled by their blessings and receive their amulets of fixed trinkets, beads, necklaces, and other good luck charms. A politician may discreetly visit the Obeah practitioner during a political campaign; business people occasionally seek spiritual baths for protection from the "evil eye," or to come into good fortune.

Obeah operates outside of constricted boxes of traditional ways of being and conceiving the religious and human health care. This script-evading religious tradition is not publicly embraced. Because of the long history of suppression, proscription, and punishment (not to mention the stigma associated with the art), people do not openly admit their association with Obeah or identify themselves as an Obeah woman or Obeah man to an informant. Few people will admit to practicing Obeah and, as Katrin Norris (1962) said, "For the same reason that an obeah-man is rarely convicted in a court, it is difficult for sociologists to learn a great deal about the obeah-man's influence" (p. 16). Unlike the avatars of Vodou, Candomble, Santería, or Orisha, whom a researcher may interview in person, Obeah practitioners are difficult to identify with certainty. Rather than carry the title Obeah woman, or Obeah man, one may take the title "health provider," "facilitator of good health," or "servant of God." One may also claim another Afro-Caribbean religion as his/her religious affiliation and base. As traditional medicine in a broad sense, Obeah is not restricted to one modus operandi; it uses medicines for causative, therapeutic, protective, and punitive effects—its medicines aim at treating psychological (spiritual, mental, social) and physical health while offering protection against detractors and punishment for offenders—it works like medical provision, psychiatric help, and law enforcement combined.

Evolution of Obeah in Colonialism

Obeah originated in West Africa as one of the continent's least significant religious traditions but was an obscure practice in the Caribbean until its obliteration from society became a phobic preoccupation of colonial governments. The African practices "were transformed in the crucible" of colonialism and slavery "into spiritual support for the Afro-Caribbean community" (Savory, 1999, p. 218); it provided the oppressed alternative avenues through which they could procure medical treatment and access their African powers for psychological reinforcement to survive the wretchedness of plantation life. During slavery, Africans also used Obeah to intimidate others who habitually plundered their meager huts, hog sties, and garden plots; to them, Obeah was an indispensable defensive medicine weapon. After emancipation, the poor property-less, and unemployed, ex-slaves— wards of the British Crown—were *personae non grata*, estranged in colonial society, and had to rely on African traditional religions and medicines to fight poor health, injustice, new forms of oppression, and other colonial miseries.

The British helped to perpetuate Obeah's existence by adopting the name as a label for a number of religious traditions of African origin in the Caribbean. Before Vodou, Santería, Myal, or Shango entered common vocabulary, Obeah meant any African religion or "superstition" and was assigned many sinister designations (Murrell, 2010). This is partly because Obeah was African, disquietingly secretive and stealthy, vaguely understood, and historically transgressive in nature— officially, it constituted outlawed alleged iniquitous superstitious African beliefs and practices that did not follow the European-Christian ilk; it made colonists nervous of Africans given to slave uprising (see, for example, Richardson, 1999; Patterson, 1967); and it was seen as working against the harmony and welfare of colonial society. So since the 1700s, Obeah was criminalized throughout the Anglophone Caribbean and remained that way until recent times in many island states (Murrell, 2010; Paton, 2009). Of course, the laws did not stop uprooted Africans from contemplating and embracing "transgression" for their own survival and freedom in the strange colonial world of the Americas.

British Robinson and Walhouse (1893) referred to Obeah as a "science" possessed only by "natives of Africa" who brought it with them to the colony, "where it is so universally practiced, there are few of the large estates, possessing native Africans, which have not one or more" Obeah men (p. 207). To these colonials, Obeah "science" constituted neither a subject worthy of study nor *religion*, terms reserved for "civilized" society. As Murray (2007) observes, "it is very unlikely that any African-derived traditions, such as British West Indian *obeah* . . . would have qualified as appropriate for research as a science" (p. 813) or a religion. Many colonials saw Africans as uncivilized, backward, primitive, and void of "religion" and "culture;" so African Obeah was not to be given such privileged designations reserved for established institutions and systems of beliefs and practices of "civilized and enlightened" peoples of European origin. Even some modern scholars are not ready to accord Obeah the title religion. British colonial society feared, despised, and relentlessly pursued Obeah and its practitioners for over 200 years. Whites feared Obeah because of its clandestine activities, dreaded poisons, its alleged relation to secret deaths and slave revolts, and the fact that it was irrational to the scientific worldview of Enlightenment Europe. This fear often worked to the advantage of slaves, largely on small plantations, who were able to garner better treatment from their masters overcome by fear of Obeah.

The British brought Obeah to prominence in the English-speaking Caribbean through the concern over its subversive nature as a transgressive force against the "drum and beat" of the colonial plantation. Among the many non-conventional weapons available to slaves in the fight against slavery were: secret revolts, arson, poisoning, suicide, and spiritual science (Obeah) which slaves had known in Africa or creolized in the Caribbean to meet their needs. As a facilitator of resistance and revolt, Obeah "provoked an "ideological rallying point" in sanctioning rebellion, afforded meeting places and leaders, and formed a repository for the collective memory of the slaves by preserving African traditions which could be opposed to the dominant colonial culture" (Richardson, 1999). Its peculiar acts of resistance occasionally necessitated violence: aiding slave revolts, poisoning a master or a slave snatcher, or "fixing" an overseer with a fatal illness or paralysis. This subversive character of Obeah was evident in the slave revolts of the 1700s. In a Caribbean arena that constantly brewed "new and unpredictable challenges," virtually every group had to be creative to survive (Murray, 2007, p. 818), even subversively transgressive.

Myths of evil Obeah and claims of its use as a dreaded science in black resistance to slavery were enough to keep legislative prohibitions in place and feed satire and racial and religious stereotypes even to modern times. As Murray (2007) noted, "The English were constantly creating new institutions to control the enslaved Africans, protect their plantations and . . . themselves. The slave court and its laws was one . . . such British innovations" (p. 818). Regarding Obeah works as detrimental to colonial Caribbean society, the authorities made the practice a primary target for legal proscription and control. Between 1760 and 1792, Obeah became a criminal act in Jamaica through a series of laws prohibiting Obeah practices on penalty of death upon conviction (Bisnauth, 1989; Newall, 1978). In the early 1800s, the official view of Obeah shifted from being exclusively related to witchcraft, as a "primitive" religious activity, to charges of fraud, deception, and pretention (Paton, 2009) and carried serious punishment under draconian laws. In a British courtroom, Obeah was "non-falsifiable"; one could not rationally believe in the factuality of Obeah, and thus officials regarded the art as primitive African superstitious pretensions (Murray, 2007). As a result, the legal prohibition against Obeah sought to punish practitioners' "pretentions"; an odd crime in the field of jurisprudence but, as Paton (2009) says, "In this law and others passed during slavery, the primary definition of obeah was 'pretending to have communication with the devil' or 'assuming the art of witchcraft'" (p. 4).

Scholars noted that from 1838 governments maintained Obeah laws in force in British Caribbean colonies by also linking the practice to "vagrancy" laws, specific Obeah acts, deception by "rogues and vagabonds," so-called "persons pretending or professing to tell fortunes, or using any subtle craft, means, or device, by palmistry or otherwise, to deceive and impose" and attempt to secure "financial gain" (Paton, 2009, p. 6). The legal prohibitions extended throughout the Anglophone Caribbean, where other colonies followed Jamaica's lead in legislating against Obeah: Barbados adopted Vagrancy Acts 1840 (CO 111/30/2) and 1897 (CO 30/35). "An Act for the Punishment of Idle and Disorderly Persons, and Rogues and Vagabonds in British Honduras" was passed 1863 (26 Vict. C. 5), Grenada enacted "Summary Conviction Ordinance 1897 (CO 103/22, no 2), and Trinidad and Tobago adopted several anti-Obeah laws between 1838 and 1888. From 1872 to 1905 St. Lucia, Dominica, and the Leeward Islands passed nine ordinances all targeting Obeah (Paton, 2009, p. 17); and Obeah conviction carried the death penalty in St. Vincent (Newall, 1978, p. 29). Despite legislative instruments for punishment of Obeah works, British law and its penal threats failed to eradicate the secret but highly influential art; in spite of the severe penalties, post-slavery Obeah continued to play a significant role in colonial culture (Bridger, 1973, p. 51; Norris, 1962, p.15), a role though exaggerated and made prominent by a colonial Obeah obsession through legislation.

Resurgence of Obeah

The many controversies surrounding Obeah, the question of its existence or lack thereof, its widely "differentiated meanings" (Paton, 2009, p.1) in Africa and the African diaspora, and its seemingly ephemeral legacy in Caribbean people's consciousness, account for the significant resurgence of interest in the subject in popular culture and the academy, especially in the United States since the mid-20th century. In the last few decades, health-care providers also have taken a new interest in the study of Obeah relative to mental health and healing; and economic circumstances have driven many Caribbean people to explore alternative means of health care (Aarons, 1999; McClure, 1982; Wing, 1998). Colonial governments' attempt to obliterate Obeah from its proto-Christian society drove the art underground where it became most potent and given to stealth. Obeah comes to public attention and scrutiny only in times of economic hardship, stress, sickness, and critical need.

In the postcolonial cultural zeitgeist of Caribbean nationalism, many colonial religious regulations, including those on Obeah, were repealed. In 1951 Trinidad and Tobago repealed its Obeah ordnances and St. Vincent followed suit in 1965. In 1973, Forbes Burnham's socialist government abrogated Obeah laws in Guyana, with a proviso that it was not to be used for "capitalist gains" (Paton, 2009). Leonard Barrett (1988) still made the claim that Obeah "is the most dreadful form of Caribbean witchcraft plaguing both blacks and whites in the days of slavery and continuing to haunt Jamaicans today" (p. 28). This is partly because a culture of Obeah paranoia or obsession still prevails—largely among African peoples on both sides of the Atlantic—and is encouraged in horror movie-stories, myths, and stories of missing persons, suspicious afflictions, mysterious deaths, and in legends of Obeah-fixed persons, objects, and places. Occasionally, packages allegedly containing magic potions, accessories suspected of Obeah "works" are intercepted in the mail by authorities. The anxiety and curiosity that surround these suspected "bundles" preserve the aura of the Obeah practitioners' personae as "terrifying figures" (Newall, 1978) with respect in their communities. Another stimulus that keeps the aura of Obeah alive comes from the academy. There is a well-spring in the study of Obeah, as evident in the substantial scholarly production on this transgressive medicine art, seen partially in the sources that significantly informed this chapter. So the religious medicine art is alive and well in 21st century Caribbean people's consciousness, in popular literature, and in Hollywood. Karla Frye (1999) says, "the pull of Obeah remained strong enough to foster doubt in the minds of even the staunchest disbeliever and naysayer" (p. 199) and its tools—spirits, natural objects, pharmacopeia, magic, fear, fantasia, and faith—continue to maintain their efficacy in peoples' cultural subconscious.

In modern times, peoples with Caribbean ancestry (some of whom live in Britain, the United States, and Canada) who believe in Obeah's efficacy, use the religious medicine art to seek personal desires, treat poor health, secure good fortune, win a tough litigation battle, discourage conjugal infidelity or unfaithfulness, protect their property from larceny, and settle scores in domestic feuds. Someone may "turn the affections of the objects of his love or lust towards himself, evince revenge upon his enemies, and generally manipulate the spiritual forces of the cosmos in order to obtain his will" (Morrish, 1982, p. 41). Economic distress that depresses medical provisions among Caribbean peoples creates a market for Obeah to marshal natural and spiritual forces to battle poor health and other crises. Aarons (1999) has noted the growing decline in governments' ability to maintain good medical health-care standards in Caribbean states—which "are low-income developing countries with open free market economies" (p. 23) but serving large unemployed and underemployed populations—where "governments try to balance their budgets among competing social goods, such as crime prevention, education, housing, transportation, health, and employment for the less privileged in their societies" (p. 23). At the same time, the cost of Western medical care continues to spiral, requiring "the complex interplay of people's beliefs, practices, and the accessibility" (p. 23) of alternative forms of health care (see also McClure, 1982; Wing, 1998). Afro-Caribbean religions' folk medicine become some peoples' last lifeline; they resort to Obeah, Vodou, Santería, Candomble, and other African-derived medicine traditions "because of poverty, personal beliefs, spiritual awakening, or the inaccessibility" of medical providers (Aarons, 1999, p. 25). Respect for this service, claims of its efficacy, and Obeah's economic returns in hard times perpetuate its success and vitality in Caribbean cultural consciousness.

Obeah Healers and Their Training

By dint of circumstance, Obeah practitioners work undercover and keep secret their "transgressive medicine" out of fear of prosecution. The Obeah man and woman belong to the tradition of healer, medicine man, *conjurer doctor*, root-worker, diviner procurer of cures, and agent or finder. These varied possessors of magical arts are said to be "double-sighted"; they have the ability to see the spiritual world operating in the physical (Baer, 2001, p. 149). Afro-Caribbean religions often combine the roles of healer, priest, medium, herbalist, and medicine woman (man) who work with herbal and other recipes. Healer, Obeah woman, and Obeah man are often one and the same; some Obeah men are more adept at healing medicine than others who might be better at protective and punitive medicine. Clients seek the same practitioners for consultation to securing cures to ailments, solutions to social problems, justice for wrongs, or obtain charms and amulets so to ward off spells cast by an "evil eye." An Obeah initiate undergoes an informal apprenticeship period to develop knowledge of the craft and learn its secrets. However, this training is informal and acquired by observation, "inheritance," or special "endowment." As Baer (2001) observes, one may become an Obeah specialist "in one of three ways: inheritance of the position, apprenticeship under the tutelage of an established practitioner, or a 'calling' from god" (p. 149). Most Obeah healers' knowledge is filial in origin—learnt from a mother, grandmother, grandfather, uncle, and other family members. Some claim a special gift (endowment) from God and might begin healing as a minor (a prodigy may start as early as six to seven years old). Others receive the gift of healing in a vision, dream, epiphany, or in a situation of crisis (e.g., terminal illness or death of a loved one).

Women have always featured prominently in Obeah magic and herbal medicine and they used the system to their own economic and social advantage. Because of their skill in religious magic, knowledge of plant pharmacopeia and other medicines, and partly through their strong leadership roles in African religions, women are highly respected and feared in Afro-Caribbean religions. Historically, Caribbean women were more likely than men to turn to Obeah for social and economic support in the face of inequities, unemployment, underemployment, and the domestic abuse they experienced.

The title Obeah woman represents something far more loathing than Obeah man. To British colonials, Obeah women epitomized the wicked African witch who works dangerous magic with poisons, the fierce Nanny Maroon leader or the Wicked Witch of Rose Hall (Jamaica), and the evil Queen Jezebel in ancient Hebrew tradition; these women used stealth, deception, and aggression to accomplish their ends and so corral a mystic around them that is foreboding. Often the more physically robust, curvaceous, and oversize the woman, the more dread her appearance, and the more effective her remedies, the more respect she commands, and the higher her "donations" (consultation fees). Healing is performed for consultation fees, in cash or kind. For an Obeah practitioner, this "medicine" activity derives a small supplemental income but Obeah can be profitable if done professionally. As Newall (1978) says "The obeah practitioner, who is professional, and performs sorcery [services] at the request of his clients . . . on payment of a fee, is frequently enjoying a higher living standard than the other members of his [or her] community" (p. 35).

Whether male or female, Obeah practitioners are the sole arbiter of their magical craft; they are answerable to no one, fear none, but respect one another. They work in realms of the mysterious and their magic, though apparently miraculous or supernatural, are learned crafts and principles employed to a desired end. To perform the unconventional and "transgressive" services, an Obeah avatar must study and dispense medicine believed endowed with sacred powers for healthy and protective or punitive purposes. An Obeah woman or man must be able to operate with coded magic and co-opt esoteric artilleries of sorcery, prescience, and witchcraft to deploy psychological medicine. This requires special knowledge gained from a natural human talent or through training. The Obeah healer must be "four-eyed," "having developed the gift to see both the visible and the invisible world" (Murphy, 1994, p. 121); she must see in front and behind, in the future and in the past. Divine problems, illnesses, conditions, and situations affecting her clients and prescribe treatment based on a range of acquired knowledge. She depends on "psychological analysis" and the power of suggestion for her success and ability to mesmerize believers with her mystical spells medicines. As specialist in herbal pharmacopeia, the Obeah man must also know and master the use of herbal medicines and their healing potential; Obeah medicine is largely plant based. Pharmacopeia and balmyard works from Caribbean flora are vast and one can take significant time attempting to master the art of producing and applying the right herbal medicines to psychological and biomedical or physical ailments. Skill in Obeah medicine comes from practice and practical knowledge.

Deploying Obeah

Obeah "services" often fall into two general categories: psychological or non-biomedical medicine, which affects mainly the mind and spirit of the client (inquirer), and physical or biological medicine intended to heal or protect the body. Most problems for which people seek Obeah healing might be classified as sociological and psycho-physiological or psychosomatic. Sociological problems include: forcing a harmful person out of a neighborhood or property, stopping a stalker in a fatal attraction, settling a score in a love triangle, salvaging a broken relationship, punishing a malicious enemy, getting even with a landlord or employer, fighting a lawsuit, or increasing one's business chances, etc. The mystique that an Obeah man carries in his community often serves as a deterrent to the acts of nefarious persons who otherwise would have committed offenses/ violence against people who were not "Obeah protected." In this way, Obeah works as a code of conduct in communal morality; it is used to catch thieves and criminals and punish dishonesty or cheating; some women, for example, use Obeah medicine to inhibit the sexual deviance of their partners, others employ it to seal a desired or unrequited relationship. So in a believing community, the belief and practice of Obeah can serve positive functions—and more so among economically stressed peoples who cannot better protect themselves.

Obeah as non-biomedical medicine is outside of traditional scientific verification and may be the most problematic for mental health practitioners. It focuses on restoring relations, a sense of harmony, or accord in the person's conflicted life because of a perceived breach in "yin–yang" type balance in their world; this may be between an individual and the natural world, between lovers, families, enemies, or competitors. Some physical conditions may amend after disharmony is restored. A range of healing paraphernalia is employed in this psychological traditional medicine endeavor. Among those spiritual services are: therapy, prayers, spells, psychological conditioning, oath taking, balms, herbal baths, striking on a sick part of the body "in the spirit," exhorting or counseling, and performing other actions with special words. As the need arises, these are accompanied by spirit-infused objects or things: spiritual entities, amulets, magic potions, charms, trinkets, personal effects, clothing, unusual objects (e.g., birds' feathers, grave dirt, animal parts or offal), powders, love and healing oils, to name a few. Traditional healing also uses herbs to alter a client's behavior, mental imbalance, and demeanor or state. A change in dietary habits, vices, and profession (e.g., a stressful job) may be recommended as effective medicine. A healer may council divorce, remarriage, or change of environment to reduce stress or restore peace and harmony in a client's life. These non-biomedical medicines often are applied with prayers and "rituals of power" involving dancing, singing, magic spells, sorcery, and witchcraft. There may even be meditation, incantations, exorcisms, and curses under spirit possession (Murrell, 2010).

Obeah works involve séance (an ability to communicate with ancestral spirits), intuit cause and effect reality, divine future events, and use magic spells or substances to deal with what Murphy calls "the disintegrative forces of a society under stress" (1994, p. 120). In Caribbean mythology, Obeah practitioners have effected retributive justice and caused disease or other misfortune through sympathetic magic. This involves infusing "fixed energy" into an object or effigy that represents a person and, through a mysterious transference of the energy, the affliction reaches the individual targeted without the "sponsor" making any direct contact with the afflicted. Obeah healers also are consulted for what is called "reading," or "telling," an ancient art of seeing what the stars predict for a business or personal venture; it is magically foretelling one's future or fate. A practitioner might also require a client to perfume herself with the "oil of love," a pharmaceutical that carries a very pleasant fragrance. This perfume is supposed to attract the spirits who then loiter around, like the proverbial fly on the wall that aids the couple in their romance. A client seeking advice on increasing her chances for success in business might receive a solution based on common sense; like putting a mirror or some important object in her shop to attract more customers' attention (Murrell, 2010).

Notwithstanding its use of magic and witchcraft as important psychological healing tools, Obeah medicine is partly biomedical or health related; its healing is largely natural pharmacopeia accessories that have a large plant base (Murrell, 2010). Many Obeah paraphernalia come from plants and animals. The healer uses an array of herbs, some very common and well known but most are unusual and unfamiliar (Aarons, 1999). Some floras are used in mixtures with other herbs while others are applied by themselves to cure a variety of ailments, skin irritations, or diseases. Believers allege that Obeah can treat malfunctions in women's reproductive system as well as a range of other maladies (Seaga, 1963). The marijuana plant (ganja, Indian hemp, or cannabis) has been a major healing pharmacopeia since early colonialism. The practice of smoking ganja in nightly dances and healing rituals, for the curing of a variety of ailments, was very common in West and Central Africa, parts of India and the Caribbean. Herbalist, Obeah men/women, and medicine men use the herb for asthma, respiratory problems, stomach disorders, rheumatism, hot flashes, cramps, overheating, depression, hypertension, and other conditions.

A diversity of citruses is among the common healing folia. The Palma Christi, used internationally to treat colds, is applied as a poultice for cuts, bruises, and some skin infections. It also works as a laxative or purge for constipation and lower bowel irregularities (McClure, 1982, pp. 296–297). Just like the Jamaican Akee when picked before it is ripe, the Palma Christi also can produce a deadly toxin for Obeah defense. Obeah poisoning is medicine for both protection of someone and revenge against another and is deployed with magical powers. According to McClure (1982),

> Poisoning for revenge is a customary ritual among followers of Obeah. In 1809, on the isle of Antigua, poisoning was so frequent that the law intervened to subdue it. The old people were acquainted with both the medicinal and the poisonous plants of the island"

and sold potions at a price (McClure, 1982, p. 298). Although Obeah is thought of more for its "negative" medicine, its poisons are applied only in rare cases and under adverse circumstances. The healing and other services Obeah men offer are usually sought as a last resort; few Caribbean people who are ill turn first to a healer or Obeah man. A patient first applies "bush remedies" (homemade balms), then modern medicine, and only when these fail or are unavailable does she search for a spiritual cause and cure (Seaga, 1963, p. 12) in Obeah or another Afro-Caribbean healing tradition.

Obeah and Conventional Medicine

Perhaps the biggest problem mental health professionals may face in dealing with Obeah healing is the one that researchers encounter, the secrecy–invisibility phenomenon. Obeah is an indistinct religion; its practitioners are difficult to identify with certainty and their operation is often covert—information about their practice is almost always indirect anecdotes from and about clients. The loathing stigma attached to Obeah in the Anglophone Caribbean, alleged association with evil, devil worship, curses, suspicious disappearances and poisonings, and legal proscription keep believers in Obeah under a code of secrecy. Documenting who Obeah clients and practitioners are and precisely what they do and how they perform their healing can be a daunting task; also, although Obeah may address psychological and even psychiatric conditions, they are often not a mental health treatment provider and neither practitioners nor clients may suffer from mental imbalance, cerebral instability, or serious mental illnesses. Normal people's interest in Obeah can be spun by a number of concerns or causes: medical, religious, psychological, social, or economic.

Medical practitioners and mental health students know that much of modern medicine comes from plants and animals and that often some home remedies that evolved from years of experiments with plants and animals in ancestral traditions have proven very effective in treating some illnesses. Such health provision should not be disregarded at face value as mere folklore. Obeah is also an oral tradition that is yet to document its practices as a healing tradition. So students in mental health may be concerned about the absence of documentation and guide for dealing with various herbal remedies and treating health conditions with folk medicine. No official record is available on how many clients receive healing and if any were harmed with permanent damage from Obeah application of herbs with toxic properties. This is another cataract on the path to the merging of modern medicine with traditional healing such as Obeah. Unless practitioners break their code of secrecy and allow for their public identification with Obeah, the art will remain mysterious, indistinct, and off-limits to collaboration between modern medicine and folk healing.

Conclusion

Obeah had a noted existence in Caribbean history and survived every colonial attempt to obliterate it from people's consciousness and society. As an oral tradition that thrived on human imagination especially in times of hardship, trauma, and distress, this art evolved as a medicine of defense against oppression and abuse as well as good health. Though often confined to Caribbean folklore and past primitive African superstition, Obeah still exists in Caribbean people's consciousness as a protective medicine that can be used for a variety of human needs. The art has the potential for significant value derived from herbal medicine, psychological conditioning, and as a medicine that discourages harm and abuse of the vulnerable. The secretive, oral, and mystical nature of Obeah practice poses serious—though not insurmountable—challenges for academic study and use in modern medicine.

References

Aarons, D. E. (1999). Medicine and its alternatives. Health care priorities in the Caribbean. *The Hasting Center Report, 29*(4), 23–27.

Baer, H. A. (2001). *Biomedicine and alternative healing systems in America: Issues of class, race, ethnicity, and gender.* Madison, WI: University of Wisconsin Press.

Barrett, Sr., L. E. (1988). *The Rastafarians,* Boston, MA: Beacon Press

Bisnauth, D. (1989). *A history of religions in the Caribbean.* Kingston, Jamaica: Kingston Publishers.

Bridger, P. (1973). *A West Indian family in Britain.* Kingston, Jamaica: Kingston Publishers.

Case, F. (2001). The intersemiotics of Obeah and Kali Mai in Guyana. In P. Taylor (Ed.), *Nation, dance, religion, identity, and cultural difference in the Caribbean.* Bloomington, IN: Indiana Press.

Frye, K. Y. (1999). Obeah and hybrid identities in Elizabeth Nunez-Harrell. In M. Olmos & L. Gebert (Eds.), *When rock dance, sacred possessions, Vodou, Santeria, Obeah and the Caribbean* (pp. 195–215). New Brunswick, NJ: Rutgers University Press.

McClure, S. A. (1982). Parallel usage of medical plants by Africans and their Caribbean descendants. *Economic Botany, 36*(3), 291–301.

Morrish, I. (1982). *Obeah, Christ and Rastaman: Jamaica and its religions.* Cambridge: James Clark.

Murphy, J. M. (1994). *Working the spirit, ceremonies of the African diaspora.* Boston, MA: Beacon Press.

Murray, D. (2007). Three worships, and old warlock and many lawless forces: The court trial of an African doctor who practiced "Obeah to cure" in early nineteenth century Jamaica. *Journal of Southern African Studies, 33*(4), 811–828.

Murrell, S. N. (2010). *Afro-Caribbean religions an introduction to their historical, cultural and sacred traditions.* Philadelphia, PA: Temple University Press.

Newall, V. (1978). Some examples of the practice of Obeah by West Indian immigrants in London. *Folklore, 89*(1), 29–51.

Norris, K. (1962). *Jamaica: The search for an identity.* London: Oxford University Press.

Paton, D. (2009). Obeah acts: Producing and policing the boundaries of religion in the Caribbean. *Small Axe: A Caribbean journal of criticism, 28,* 1–18.

Patterson, O. (1967). *The sociology of slavery: An analysis of the origins, development and structure of Negro slave society in Jamaica.* London: MacGibon & Kee.

Richardson, F. (1999). Romantic Vodou: Obeah and British culture, 1797–1807. In M. Olmos & L. Paravisini-Gerbert (Eds.), (pp. 216–230).

Robinson, M., and Walhouse, M. J. (1893) Obeah Worship in East and West Indies. *Folklore, 4*(2), 207–218. Republished by Taylor & Francis, Ltd, on behalf of Folklore Enterprises, Ltd. JSTOR 2011.

Savory, E. (1999). Another poor devil of a human being: Jean Rhys and the novel as Obeah. In M. Olmos & L. Paravisini-Gerbert (Eds.), *Sacred possessions, Vodou, anteria, Obeah, and the Caribbean* (pp. 216–230). New Brunswick, NJ: Rutgers University Press.

Seaga, E. (1963). Revival cults in Jamaica, notes toward sociology of religion. *Jamaica Journal, 3*(2), 3–14.

Wing, D. M. (1998). A comparison of traditional folk healing concepts with contemporary healing concepts, *Journal of community health nursing, 15*(3), 143–154.

6

VODOU HEALING AND PSYCHOTHERAPY

Ghislène Méance

Introduction

Vodou is defined as a system of magic that may include sacrifice, divination, and conjuring (Metraux, 1972); however, Vodou rituals may also involve root doctors and herbalists. Practiced predominantly in Haiti, Vodou is an official and organized religion combining elements of African Vodun and Roman Catholicism—revering the spirit world of ancestors and designed to both heal the sick and injured body and soul, promote success and wealth as well as to guide the spirit to God. Haitian families believe in certain forces or principles that comprise an order by which they can live and to which they are subject. It is estimated that about 80% of the Haitian population practice some aspects of Vodou regardless of their religion and socioeconomic status. Vodou healers are consulted when clients are looking for answers for problems that neither medicine, nor other religions are able to answer. In addition to being a religion Vodou is also an art of living, focused on daily life's problems. Haitians usually turn to Vodou for counseling, protection, help, wealth, health, and justice. Aspects of the religion or ways of living are also observed within the Haitian diaspora, particularly in the United States where examples of Vodou practices have been observed.

Haitian Vodou has an affinity with many other religions and mythologies; it is known in Cuba and throughout South America under names such as *Hoodoo, Santería, Chango, Ñañiguismo, Candomble*, and *Macumba*. A Vodou priest cited by Bodin (1990) explains that, "Vodou is an organized religion combining elements of African Vodun and Roman Catholicism—revering the spirit world of ancestors and designed to both heal the sick and injured body as well as to guide the spirit to God" (p. 1). According to local beliefs, families inherit ancestral spirits from Dahomey, West Africa. These spirits are worshiped through elaborate rituals, which include drumming, sacrifice, singing, and praise.

After centuries of persecution and de-valorization by other religions and by some political regimes, Vodou was decreed an official religion by the Haitian government in 2003. Historically, Vodou existed as a subversive political force that fueled the Haitian Revolution from French control in 1804, which may partly explain its marginalization and devaluation by Western society. For several decades, Vodou has attracted attention from social scientists, in part because it has acted as a positive force in promoting Haitian liberation from colonial domination (Bartkowski, 1998). In fact, in 1804 Haiti became the first Black Republic in the world after the Haitian revolution led by Vodou practitioners and followers.

Simpson (1978) found that Vodou followers rely on that religion for solidarity and a sense of belonging. During initiation, followers gain confidence that the spirits will protect them and cast away any harm. Vodou followers also understand that it is considered a blasphemy against God to disclose secrets of Vodou. Bibb and Casimir (1996) explained that Vodou encompasses both the religious and the medical worlds. Haitians, they say, see causes of mental illness as derived from the supernatural external world and Vodou as providing solutions to problems emanating from this world.

This chapter will focus on Vodou as practiced in Haiti where it is also designated as *Vaudou*, *Vodou*, and *Vodu*.[1] It begins with a discussion of the religion and its divinities. This is followed by an exploration of the healers and their healing practices and how illness and wellness are conceptualized in this system. Lastly, the chapter highlights the need for collaboration between Vodou and conventional mental health care systems.

Vodou Religion and Divinities

The Yoruba religion is the most widely spread manifestation of African religions in the New World. Yoruba followers, who live mostly in West African countries such as Togo, Benin, the Ivory Coast, and Ghana, believe in a supreme being, primordial divinities, and spirits that have been deified (Horton, 1989). Bibb and Casimir (1996) note that these forces are not visible and are referred to as *les invisibles* or the "unseen," and they are perceived only when showing concrete signs of their presence through experiences of "possession" during religious ceremonies, and therefore take a numinous or mysterious quality. According to Deren (1970), their personification became known as divinities or *lwas*. A *lwa* which, in the Yoruba language, means *mystery* is a specific spirit such as Legba, the spirit of the gate, Erzuli, the spirit of love, or Gede, the spirit of the dead. In the Vodou religion, worshipping the *lwa*, according to Deren, is to celebrate what he calls "the principle not the matter" in which it may be momentarily or permanently manifest.

De Vos (1988) reported that there are 401 *lwa*. Furthermore, there are different categories of *lwa*. Some of them exist in natural phenomena, such as plants and trees, and animals, such as snakes. A different class or category of *lwa* is thought to reside in situations or special individuals who serve them. These *lwa* need these phenomena or special individuals in order to exist. De Vos reports that, according to the Vodou worldview, as the *lwa* and person live in mutual interaction, mutations in their form and qualities may occur with the passage of time and within the changing environment. Relationships and interactions between *lwa* and people are very important and when there are conflicts between a *lwa* and a person, for example, it can be manifested through symptoms of depression and anxiety.

Michel (1996) understands Vodou teaching and learning as referring to balancing commonalities or universal knowledge with differences to create global harmony and peace among people and between people and Nature as well as the spirits. Indeed, teachers and learners play equally active roles in guiding and facilitating, making the most use of tangible and intangible resources. This "democratic foundation" makes Vodou quite a progressive system compared to other more doctrinaire, authoritarian religions. Unlike other major religions of the world, the Vodou priest or priestess does not necessarily wear a recognizable garb or uniform that conveys their social status. Nevertheless, they are perceived as respectable and important members of society in Haiti.

Vodou Healers and Healing Practices

In Haiti there is one Vodou healer for every 100 Haitians versus one medical doctor for every 100,000 (Cohen, 1997), therefore, Vodou healers and their healing practices are critical. Worship and healing are sustained by adherents led by a Vodou priest called *hungan* or priestess called *manbo*. The main function of the *hungan* or the *manbo* is to heal. It takes about five years to become a Vodou healer followed by years of training before initiation. In order to qualify for this vocation, the person is required to have specific talents and attend various trainings. Above all it is considered an inherited gift from the family's ancestors and spirits.

Haiti attracts a lot of international Vodou apprentices and is considered the best place for formal and informal training in Vodou healing. Vodou practitioners who are non-Haitians and students interested in the religion tend to make the trip to Haiti to be initiated "into the rites of Vodou" and are able to practice various levels of Vodou ritual based on their advanced training. A Yoruban Vodou priestess currently practicing in Louisiana, interviewed by Bodin (1990), confessed that her training in Haiti was a process of getting herself "spiritually straight." This Vodou priestess considers the Haitian Vodou and the Yoruba Vodou as sister religions because both religions treat their ancestors with great respect. Touloute (1998) notes that respect for ethics is highly valued by the Vodou community. Vodou priests and priestesses receive counsel and treatment from one another because "Vodou does not discriminate on the basis of gender, race, age, sexual orientation, national origin requirements or pre-existing religion affiliation" (Touloute, 1998, p. 5). Vodou priests who violate Vodou ethics are called *boko* or evil charlatans. They are said to serve certain *lwa* called *dyab* or wild spirits. These *dyab* and *bòkò* are said to be invoked on behalf of clients for magical compensation, and they may affect a person's demise. The *dyab* is also supposed to protect practitioners from possible acts of random aggression according to Touloute (1998).

It is estimated that the training period may last as long as five years, where the master *ougan* or *manbo* passes along formal knowledge to an apprentice. Then for several more years, the master supervises the work of the apprentice before initiation. The training is considered as a beginning of a long journey because in the Vodou world the growth in knowledge is attained over time and with experience. Moll and Greenberg (1990) note that the Haitian culture believes in the social distribution of knowledge; accordingly, knowledge is not something to be possessed personally because it is available and accessible through different social networks including spiritual inheritance. Following from this logic, there are no written directions or sacred books that contain dogma, formula, and rules.

Healers work at the *hunfo* or Vodou temple, located near churches or markets, to heal, worship, and communicate with the spirits. These *hunfo* can be identified by a flag displayed on the roof of the building, and the style and decoration of the flag indicates which *lwa* the priest or priestess serve. Also in the Vodou world, cemeteries, crossroads, oceans, rivers, chutes, fields, households, and other sites are prominent and meaningful places of worship and treatment according to Michel (1996). According to Touloute (1998), "the Vodou priesthood performs such functions as healing, pacifying the spirits, initiation, foretelling, dream reading, spell casting and creating potions for various purposes like protection love and death" (p. 5).

Illness Representations and Wellness Practices

In Haiti mental illness is considered supernatural and mainly treated with techniques of Vodou healing. According to Charles (1986), in Haiti the majority of people live without any knowledge of psychiatric care. He notes, "Religion, society, family and supernatural belief systems provide resources for dealing with stressors that impinge mental health" (p. 186). In addition, Morrison and Thornton (1999) found that some Haitians simultaneously practice both Christianity and Vodou. However, they might not admit being Catholic/Protestant and *Vodouizan* (Voodooist) at the same time. According Morrison and Thornton (1999), this attitude is related to the fact that white European and American slave masters have painted Vodou with a negative image for centuries. In order to reconcile these exteriorly imposed negative beliefs, Vodou rituals integrate elements of Christian theology in an unusual religious syncretism.

Bibb and Casimir (1996) revealed that it is common for many Haitian Catholics and Protestants to practice and believe in Vodou in varying degrees. Bibb and Casimir (1996) explained that Vodou practice is most commonly associated with the lower socioeconomic classes, which comprises the vast majority of Haitians. Their members practice Vodou more openly than the middle and upper class. This may be because the lower class Haitians are more connected to the African traditions brought over by the slaves, while the upper class identifies more with European cultures. When Haitians suffer from psychiatric and psychological symptoms the healing process starts at the Vodou temples, continues at the Church, and ends at the psychiatric hospital or other mental health facilities (Charles, 1986; Philippe, 1974). Hence, Western forms of healing are used only when traditional medicine and familial resources have been exhausted and unsuccessful. The process is not necessarily linear but this pattern is the one most likely to be observed in rural areas.

Clients visit the Vodou priest or priestess in an attempt to find out the cause of their illness. Charles (1986) defined *foure pye-w nan dlo*, an expression literally meaning "put your feet into the water," as the initial attempt made by the client to find out the cause of the problem. Generally, if the person is too sick to do so by himself or is a minor, a member of the family is supposed to help them seek treatment. They usually make an overnight trip with the mentally ill to the *ounfo* or Vodou temple where the Vodou priest's job is to provide a diagnosis or *pase leson* to find out basically what kind of problem it is, who did it, why the problem exists, and how it can be treated.

During the first visit to the Vodou temple the *pase leson* or diagnostic interview is focused on social relationships and religious beliefs, current or past mistakes. In the Vodou religion, it is believed that nothing happens by chance or accident. A Vodou priest may ask: Do you have any enemies? Have you lost a piece of cloth recently? How well do you do in your job, school? Are you having an affair with somebody's wife/husband? Do you have spirits in your family? Do you respect the traditions?

The healer then suggests some kind of hypothesis on the cause of the client's disease after consulting his or her own spirits or colleagues. Observations reported by Charles (1986) of the interaction between mental patients and Vodou priests indicate that "there are 3 categories of diagnosis: a) *giyon* or bad luck b) *lwa kenbe* or retaliation from the spirits and c) *anvoutman* or possession by a malevolent spirit" (p.188). Brown (2001) identified a subcategory of *giyon* called *dyok*, described as a condition in which a patient suffers from getting too much attention from the public.

Giyon is the Vodou term used to describe what the Western psychologist would call depression. Clients present with a high level of anxiety and also report sensations of weakness and vulnerability. Charles (1986) indicated that the Vodou priest attempts to remove the *giyon* or bad luck by restoring the client's self-confidence. He or she does so by trying to reinforce the coping strength of the client while helping him build a greater sense of personal protection. This process helps convince the client that there are no more obstacles to recovery. Charles found that the following techniques are used in the recovery process:

a) cleansing the person, with ointments, oils, magical potions, bath with plants, wines and perfumes, b) cleansing the client's environment—typically the house—with incense, candles and magical waters, and c) construction of an *amulet* or special necklace that the client will have to wear for personal protection.

(p. 188)

All of these techniques may involve a magical potion that the client is supposed to drink in order to gain greater strength.

Lwa kenbe or retaliation from the spirits is the term used for clients presenting with symptoms similar to those of phobias, hysteria, and overtly paranoid delusions of persecution. Charles (1986) notes that when dealing with *lwa kenbe* the Vodou priest explains to the person that the sickness is related to a failure to keep a specific commitment with a *lwa* or spirit and has discontinued worship. It is believed that certain spirits are protector *lwa* and, in some cases, dead ancestors or guardians who have been neglected. Such offenses are said to occur through violations of taboos or special traditions and according to Charles (1986), "the treatment is then focused on supernatural strengthening, which includes renewing alliances with the *lwa*. This technique also focuses on appeasement of the angry or offended spirits" (p. 188). Treatment includes ceremonies with rituals using foods, animal sacrifices, and cleansing baths. They end with a ritual called the "paying back" in which the client had to throw seven pennies into the left over bathwater, and destroy accessories that were used for the treatment while repeating the formula: "Now I am paying for all my past debts. Now I do not owe anybody anything. I want to be free again, to continue a decent life as a normal human being" (Charles, 1986, p. 189). The Vodou priest then takes all the waste and discards it, typically in the forest or a cemetery. The supposed meaning of this action is an engagement taken by the client to start his life over and focus on the future while acknowledging his past mistakes.

Anvoutman or possession by a malevolent spirit, as described by Charles (1986) includes symptoms of hallucinations, hostile delusional systems, paranoid ideation, pronounced thought disorders, and other symptoms associated with schizophrenia. *Anvoutman* is the loss of control over one's own ego and the loss of protection of the self, and it may be manifested by expression of suicidal and homicidal ideation. According to Charles (1986), in the Vodou worldview "every human being is assumed to have a supernatural shield, which is believed to maintain a balance between positive and negative influences and to constitute a magnetic envelope that protects one from harm" (p. 189). He explains that inherited familial protective spirits supposedly set up this human shield. A client suffering from *anvoutman* would have his supernatural shield penetrated by bad spirits.

At times, the initial intervention of the Vodou priest will focus on making a deal with benevolent spirits that can offer protection to the client and therefore work to restore his supernatural shield. Exorcism is another technique used to fight *anvoutman*. After the initial episode of the illness, if the client experiences the symptoms again, the client is given magical formulas to repeat whenever he/she experiences a feeling of relapse. At other times there are special mandates to be followed as burning a prescribed number of candles, paying a visit to the Church or cemetery or making a charitable gift.

(Charles, 1986, p. 190)

In addition to *anvoutman*, *dyòk* or Bad Eyes is described by Brown (2001) as a particular condition where the client is suffering from the fact that too many people are thinking and talking about him/her. Some of the presenting symptoms are: distractions and lack of awareness preceding potential professional errors because the patient is absorbed with the glory provided by the public attention. In the Vodou philosophy, all this unusual attention can push the person off balance. This diagnosis, however, does not indicate a conscious intent from the public to harm the client.

There is no time limit set by the Vodou healer or the client for treatment; it all depends on how well everybody plays their part in the therapy process, including the spirits (Philippe, 1974). First the client must be kept inside a *peristil* (clinic) that is located in the countryside. Later, the client is sent home where his/her family takes care of him/her and follows the *hungan* or Vodou priest's instructions until complete recovery. In case of failure, the client consults another Vodou healer, but this time one who is considered to be more competent.

In general, Vodou is mostly respected and practiced for its reactive/protective aspects. Techniques such as spiritual reshaping, supernatural strengthening, and exorcism are used to help the client get rid of supernatural symptoms or "reactive rituals" of Vodou. They involve an attempt to eliminate or repair harms made to the individual. But the religion also has some proactive or preventive elements, which help to maintain mental health. Garey (1991) defines possession, or *lwa monte*, as a behavioral manifestation of communication with the spirit where the individual loses complete control over their self and appears to be excited physically and emotionally. In a particular context of ritual involving incantation of drums, singing, and powerful environmental suggestibility, the client is more likely to achieve a trance-like state. Members of the assembly believe that the client is possessed by a specific *lwa* or spirit and may say and do things of which he or she may not be able to later recall. Usually their speech contains a message from the spirit, which can be a warning, a prediction, or advice and as Garey (1991) notes, "through possession of a member of the congregation, spirits can also enter into the midst of the congregants to punish, admonish, reward and encourage them as well as treat and cure their ills and worries" (p. 65). By entering in a trance the body expels stress through shaking and convulsion (Charles, 1986; Garey, 1991). This is in sharp contrast to conventional mental health care.

Vodou and Conventional Mental Health Care

Bibb and Casimir (1996) noted that some Haitians might appear to be unresponsive to Western therapy because they tend to minimize, intellectualize, or relegate their problems to God or spirits. Within the mental health care system, the traditional formulation of some psychotherapy approaches (e.g., psychoanalysis) have operated to maintain inequalities among people even while claiming to address universal human problems. Psychotherapy is less likely to predominate as a healing technology in a collectivistic culture because there are larger organizations such as the church, government, and extended families that will care for individuals in distress. Psychotherapy as a helping mechanism expresses the values of independence and individual responsibility found in the Western culture. Therefore, it may be of limited value when applied to clients from other cultures where these values are a lesser part of the web of significance. Haiti is known to be a country where collectivism as opposed to individualism has helped in shaping its identity as the first Black Republic, and as a resilient nation in the face of poverty and natural catastrophes.

According to Van den Berg (1961), psychotherapy is an attempt to unify two bodies: the community and the individual that were once one. But how can the Western psychology unify the Haitian client, already essentially collectivist, to an essentially individualistic worldview that was never theirs in the first place? To answer this question the reader is referred to Cushman (1995), who describes *philosophical hermeneutics* as an approach to understanding human experience as interpreted in one's historical and cultural contexts. For Cushman, people and things exist only within a certain political and cultural context, and they are not understandable when abstracted out of these contexts. Cushman argued against what he called "psychological imperialism" over a local community or "the act of equating the self-package of one culture with that of another, or to analyze the self-package or frame of reference of one culture solely through the distinctions and understandings of another" (1995, p. 25).

When professionals fail to understand Haitian clients' perspectives of their problem, many times those clients are disappointed, and some give up on treatment. Often, these individuals choose to seek help in the Vodou religion. Therefore, with a better understanding of their worldview, professionals may be able to show more competence in providing psychological treatment to Haitian clients. It is also important that clinicians be culturally sensitive enough to differentiate how their Haitian clients perceive normal and abnormal symptoms; what is considered a psychiatric disorder in Western society might not be considered abnormal in Caribbean communities.

Mental health care professionals should be aware that some alerting symptoms for Western clients, such as symptoms of depression, delusions, and so on may not be interpreted as symptoms by Haitians. So the reasons motivating the first group to seek psychological help will not necessarily motivate the second group.

Therefore, clients' interpretations of their feelings are an important factor toward implementing treatment for the client.

Vodou priests interviewed by Meance (2005) showed genuine willingness to share their knowledge and make themselves accessible to a stranger with "an agenda." In Haiti, they rarely reject invitations to collaborate with psychologists if it is necessary to help a *pitit fèy* or client. Anthropologists and sociologists have painted such a disparaging picture of Vodou that the chance of a frank and genuine collaboration between the Vodou priest and the psychologist at this historical juncture is minimal. Despite the fact that both the psychologist and the Vodou priest are healing the soul and relationships, they frame healing situations or symptoms quite differently. One critical difference between a Vodou healer and a psychotherapist is that the first believes in the existence of spirits and the latter does not need to have such a belief to provide treatment. If Haitian patients consider their *lwa* as real spiritual beings, the explanation and interpretation Western therapists offer does not address their *emic* system (cultural context of their problems), and therefore is not helpful. It is important to ask patients how they perceive their problems in order to understand what psychological function they play in their lives.

One aspect of Haitian Vodou healing that clearly describes the difference in the concept of relationship healing between Vodou healing and psychotherapy is possession. Because the phenomenon often surprises devotees, it is perceived as a sign of approbation by God and that he listens when a group of people gathers to ask for a sign of his existence by sending his spirits. Bourgignon (1976) considers people's wish to be possessed to be positive if the individual embraces the experience and believes that they benefit from it. Brown (2001) argues that this acceptance of being possessed involves a "surrender of self," a passive/receptive relationship not seen in this degree in most Western psychotherapies. This ego-exchange with the spirit seems necessary because it benefits the people around the mountee, and the process of mounting specifically refers to when a spirit mounts a participant. It is called mounting because the spirit takes control of the participant much as a rider takes control of a horse. It is a sacred moment for the assembly to receive messages from their ancestral spirits. It is also an occasion for spirits to communicate to their devotee about what the spirits expect from them. This mutual exchange proves that the spirit needs the Vodou follower as much as they need the spirits. It is a mutual relationship that holds significant meanings to the devotees, and surrender of self to the spirits also contains an active element, a "leap of faith," in contrast to the Western therapy concept of "resistance." When people are possessed, it also implies that their *gros bon anj* or *mèt tèt* (guardian angel) is in good terms with them and will protect them. In that sense, possession can be considered as a renewal of faith, protection, and good physical and mental health.

Conclusion

Vodou is not just a religion but a way of life in some countries of the Caribbean, particularly in Haiti. People refer to Vodou to maintain good health and wealth as well as to heal and soothe when in pain. Vodou followers also refer to Vodou instead of psychotherapy when all else fails to effectively address psychological distress, emotional dysregulation, and existential dilemmas.

Psychotherapists and Vodou healers have a lot in common in their attempt to help clients heal. They both listen carefully to the client's story and their perception of the cause of their suffering, attempt to validate the client in distress and offer supportive comfort, and offer unconditional and genuine empathy while attempting to come up with a collaborative treatment plan. In addition, they both place great emphasis on self-care and protective measures to avoid decompensation and to maintain homeostasis and, above all, they both place great emphasis on relational issues that affect the human psyche and behavior. Without the spiritual aspect in the equation, Vodou healing and psychotherapy seem to be have similar objectives; hence, the reasons why Vodou healing seems to be a substitute for mental health in the Caribbean and in Haiti in particular. Therefore, collaboration between the Vodou healer and the psychotherapist is critical for the benefit of the clients they serve.

Note

1. Different spellings of the word are due to Creole's development from many languages and dialects (Dayan, 1991). For the sake of uniformity and to make the phonetics more accessible to English speaking readers, Vodou will be used throughout this chapter because it is phonetically the closest to the Haitian Creole, an official language in Haiti.

References

Bartkowski, J. P. (1998). Claims-making and typifications of voodoo as a deviant religion: Hex, lies, and videotape. *Journal for the Scientific Study of Religion, 37*(4), 559–579.

Bibb, A., & Casimir, G. (1996). Haitian families. In M. McGoldric (Ed.), *Ethnicity and family therapy*. New York: Guilford.

Bodin, R. (1990). *Vodou: Past and present*. Lafayette, LA: University of Southwestern Louisiana, Center for Louisiana's studies.

Bourgignon, E. (1976). *Possession*. San Francisco, CA: Shandler and Sharp.

Brown, K. M. (2001). *Mama Lola, A Vodou priest in Brooklyn*. Los Angeles, CA: University of California Press.

Charles, C. (1986). Treating the Haitian client. In H. P. Lefley & P. B. Pedersen (Eds.), *Cross-cultural training for mental health professionals* (pp. 183–198). Springfield, IL: Thomas

Cohen, R. (1997). *Global diasporas: An introduction*. Washington, DC: University of Washington Press.

Cushman, P. (1995). *Constructing the self, constructing America: A cultural history of psychotherapy*. New York: Addison-Wesley.

Dayan, J. (1991). Vodoun, or the voice of the gods. *Raritan: A Quarterley Review, 10*(3), 32–57.

De Vos, E. L. (1988) Vodou: Our link with the occult. In Sternback (Ed.), *The Analytic Life*. Boston, MA: Sigo Press.

Deren, M. (1970). *Divine horsemen*. New York: Chelsea House.

Garey, J. (1991). Templo spiritual Luz Divina. *New York Newsday*, 64–67.

Horton, H. (1989). *Yoruba religion and myth*. African Post Colonial Literature in English in the Post Colonial Web. Retrieved January 5, 2005, from http://www.postcolonial web.org/nigeria/yorubarel.html

Meance, G. (2005). A cultural and conceptual comparison of psychotherapy and Vodou healing: Alternative modalities of mental health care. Chicago, IL: CSOPP.

Metraux, A. (1972). *Vodou in Haiti*: New York: Schocken Books.

Michel, C. (1996). Of worlds seen and unseen: The educational character of Haitian Vodou. *Comparative Education Review, 40*(3), 280–294.

Moll, L., & Greenberg, J. (1990). Creating zones of possibilities: Combining social contexts for instruction. In L. C Moll (Ed.), *Vygotsky and education* (pp. 319–348). Cambridge, MA: Cambridge University Press.

Morrison, E. F., & Thornton, K. A. (1999). Influence of southern spiritual beliefs on perception of mental illness. *Issues in Mental Health Nursing, 20*(5), 443–458.

Philippe, J. (1974). *Classes sociales et maladies mentales en Haiti*. Port-au-Prince: Ateliers Fardin.

Simpson, G. E. (1978). *Black religions in the new world*. New York: Columbia University Press.

Touloute, P. (1998). *A glimpse into Vodou*. Retrieved January 5, 2005, from http://www.world-religions.org/voodoo.pdf

Van den Berg, J. H. (1961). *The changing nature of man: Introduction to a historical psychology*. New York: W.W. Orton.

7

SANGO HEALERS AND HEALING IN THE CARIBBEAN

Stephen D. Glazier

Introduction

There is a long-standing interest in religious healing in the Caribbean. During the 1980s, psychiatrist Michael Beaubrun (1924–2002) underscored the therapeutic potential of African-derived religions like Sango (Ward & Beaubrun, 1979).[1]

Sango is the Yoruba god of thunder (Bascom, 1972; Houk, 1995) with devotees throughout the Caribbean and Latin America. As the Yoruba god of thunder, Sango can kill as easily as he can heal.[2] He is sometimes depicted as a mulatto—making him attractive in multiracial societies like Puerto Rico and Brazil. In Haiti (Desmangles, 1992), Cuba (Brandon, 1990), Brazil (Hale, 2009; Matory, 2005), Puerto Rico (Romberg, 2007; 2009), and the Dominican Republic (Deive, 1975), Sango occupied a prominent place from the 17th century onward. In the English-speaking Caribbean, however, Sango was not a major presence until the mid-19th century (Henry 1999; Trotman, 2007). The popularity of Sango has ebbed and waned over time. Sometimes, Sango was practiced openly; at other times, it was practiced in secret. While it is clear that the Sango religion was perceived as a form of "protest" by colonial authorities, it is also clear that many of Sango's earliest followers probably saw themselves as maintaining ties with the collapsed Oyo Empire. In other words, Sango 19th century devotees saw themselves as reaffirming an established, African state religion (Trotman, 2007).

Trotman (2007) has suggested that the designation of all Orisa religion as "Shango" may have come about because in Africa the rulers of the Kingdom of Oyo used the Orisa Sango to consolidate imperial power. Trotman (2007) contends that in Trinidad and Grenada various sub-ethnic Yoruba groups sought to "transcend intra-religious animosities by emphasizing the common symbol of Sango" (p. 219). This may be one reason the Orisa religion was designated as

"Shango" in Trinidad and Grenada, but does not explain why the Orisa religion is not designated "Shango" elsewhere in the New World (Bascom, 1972).

Sango healers travel extensively. Prominent Sango healers consult with clients (and maintain religious centers) on multiple Caribbean islands, in the United States, Canada, and Europe. In Trinidad, nearly half of Sango healers were born and/or raised in Latin America and the Caribbean (Venezuela, Guyana, Grenada, Barbados, St. Vincent, Puerto Rico, and Aruba) (Glazier, 2008).

Prior to the 1980s, many traditional healers in Trinidad, St. Vincent, and Grenada were known locally as "Sango Baptists." The Baptists (also known as Spiritual Baptists) are an international religious movement with congregations in St Vincent, Grenada, Guyana, Venezuela, London, Toronto, Los Angeles, and New York City. Ninety percent of Sango devotees also participate in Baptist rituals, and 40% of Baptists also participate in Sango (Desmangles, Glazier, & Murphy, 2009; Rocklin, 2012). Sango is but one member of a larger pantheon of Afro-Caribbean deities; for example, when researcher Frances Henry (2008) first met Pa Neezer (one of Trinidad's most renowned Sango healers), Henry told Pa she wanted to learn about "Shango." He corrected her responding: "It's not Shango. It's Orisha . . . It's the 'African' work" (Henry, 2008, p. xi). Pa Neezer emphasized that the religion should not be known as "Shango" since other Orisas are always involved in Sango's ceremonies.

This chapter examines Sango beliefs and illness representations with a primary focus on Sango healing practices. In addition, it explores divination and spirit possession within the Sango tradition and examines relationships between Sango healers and biomedical practitioners. Lastly, this chapter documents the resurgence of Sango in contemporary Caribbean societies and implications of this resurgence for biomedicine and mental health care in the region.

Sango Beliefs and Illness Representations

A central idea is that illness and misfortune result from a lack of attention to the Orisas and a belief that the Orisas, when properly attended, care about their devotees and are both willing and able to help them in their daily lives. The Sango universe does not allow for random events, every event is determined at a higher level and is subject to retroactive change (Olupona, 2004).

Orisas' powers, including Sango's, are limited, and many events are outside of their control. But because the Orisas lack bodies and therefore are not bound by time and space, they can journey from the past, to the present and the future, and thereby offer predictions and practical advice to their devotees. While devotees attempt to establish binding contracts with the Orisas, Orisas are not bound to agreements with humans. Relations with Orisas are fluid, and there is a high degree of uncertainty; at times, the Orisas keep their promises and at other times they do not (Glazier, 2003).

For healers and their clients, all illness is interpreted as a "call" to participate in Sango and/or Spiritual Baptist ceremonies. But relatively few clients follow this path because sponsorship of ceremonies demands both time and money. It entails "too much" personal sacrifice (Glazier, 2009). For Sango healers with strong Baptist connections, the most likely suggested "cure" is participation in Spiritual Baptist mourning ceremonies. Psychiatrist Ezra E. H. Griffith (1983; 2010) has suggested that sponsorship of Spiritual Baptist ceremonies may be therapeutic as clients gather necessary ritual items and, in the process, experience positive, mutually reinforcing contact with believers and non-believers alike.

The most popular way to treat afflictions is through private consultations. Consultations allow for direct interactions between the Orisas, healers, and clients. Interactions include ceremonial spirit possession; offerings and sacrifices to gain favor and avoid punishments from the Orisas; divinatory procedures including casting *obi* and *Ifa;* the use of herbal medicines; ritual baths; and employing charms, amulets, and *gris gris* bags.[3]

Sango healing is never free. A client's willingness to sacrifice (whether by a monetary contribution, sponsorship of a Sango feast, or providing a live animal) is seen as integral to the healing process. Sacrifice is a sign of commitment to the Orisas and is considered a first step toward a "cure." Within the Yoruba tradition, all illness is seen as a call to sacrifice. Sacrifices vary (a coin, an ear of corn, a chicken, or a goat), but are the only way to gain the attention of the Orisas. Sometimes, depending on the reputation of the healer and the desperation of the client, payments to Sango healers may be considerable (in the hundreds of dollars over several years) and, in some instances, more costly than biomedical treatment (Paton, 2009).

Since Orisas are gods, they are not obliged to answer all questions posed nor are they obliged to answer questions unambiguously. In my experience, Orisas seldom allow for follow-up questions (Glazier, 2008). An Orisa decides when a session is over; sometimes stating bluntly, "Bring the next child." Orisas' comments can be cryptic, metaphorical, and contain arcane phrases that require further explication. The Orisas reveal only what they wish to reveal, no more or less. At times, they are silent and, at other times, they may answer in an "African" tongue or in "Creole" (Caribbean *patois*). Such answers may be further interpreted for the client (usually for an additional fee). Older Sango healers might know 5–15 "Yoruba" phrases, but many of these phrases are "African" sounding nonsense words which they believe to be of "Yoruba" origin (Simpson, 1965). These words may or may not be understood by Yoruba speakers or understood by other Sango healers (Warner-Lewis, 1989).

Sango Healers and Healing Practices

Some healers prefer Sango over Ogun (who some consider an even stronger healer) because Sango is less demanding of his devotees (Glazier, 2003). Sango healing is fluid, dynamic, transactional, and contractual.

George Eaton Simpson (1965) suggested that "all" leaders in the Sango tradition also acted as healers. If this was an accurate assessment in the 1960s, it was not true by the 1970s. There is little formal training, and most Sango healers claim to have been selected by the Orisas. This contrasts with Ifa diviners (Bascom, 1980; Hucks, 1998; Olupona, 2004) all of whom have undergone extensive training in Trinidad, Cuba, and/or in Africa. A small number of Sango healers have trained under established practitioners, but a majority emphasize that they have been inspired ("called to heal") directly by an Orisas.

Sango healers have participated in a variety of religious traditions during their lifetimes and often borrow healing techniques from each other. Each healer's practices (and/or "operations") reflect his or her personal religious history and travels as well as prior religious affiliations (which might include Roman Catholicism, mainstream European denominations, Pentecostalism, and indigenous traditions like the Spiritual Baptists). What ultimately differentiates Sango healers from all other healers is that they say their healing powers come directly from Sango. Whatever techniques may have been borrowed from other religious traditions, they believe it is Sango who makes these techniques efficacious (Glazier, 2009).

While clients of Sango healers represent all age groups, Sango healers are predominantly "old heads." A few are in their mid-30s, most are in their 50s and 60s with few in their 80s. It takes many years to develop a following as a Sango healer, and clients are reluctant to try anyone new. Healing powers are based on personal reputation, and reputation is largely based on "word of mouth." Healers are not expected to promote themselves and the most powerful healers are those who have been practicing the longest. This is consistent with Max Weber's (1960) prediction that traditional authority usually outweighs personal charisma.

In Trinidad, St. Vincent, and Grenada, Sango healers are male and female; older, and educated, in fact, all are literate and a number have advanced university degrees. Some Sango healers have also received medical training as nurses, chiropractors, and pharmacists. Over time, this has had an impact on Sango healing practices. But there is a high degree of "compartmentalization" and Sango devotees with biomedical training separate their Sango beliefs from their professional duties in biomedical settings. For example, one Sango healer with pharmaceutical training dispenses biomedicines five days a week in a suburban drug store and dispenses traditional 'bush medicines' exclusively at Sango ceremonies.

Sango healers often choose to live considerably beneath their means to avoid being accused of Obeah and/or witchcraft (Paton, 2009). In spite of their prominence, a number of prominent Sango healers choose to live in small wood-frame houses without electricity or running water claiming that this is what the Orisas demand.

Healing practices vary considerably from religious center to religious center, and (sometimes) even from week to week within the same center depending on individual practitioners and the particular needs of clients. Clients make gifts to the healer. Healers, in turn, make gifts to the client. Sango healers always offer clients something to take home: an amulet, a cloth sachet, a candle, a cloth or pebble with the blood of sacrifice, a satchel of herbal tea, a lithography of a saint, pages from a sacred book, a twig, a bag of herbs and spices, bath oils, and so on. Ultimately, healing rituals mobilize specific actions by both healers and their clients including absolutions, observance and/or breaking of taboos, incantations, formal offerings, sponsorship of ceremonies, and animal sacrifice (Houk, 1995; Mischel, 1959).

Within Sango Baptist tradition, "healing" is broadly conceived and, as noted, includes problems that would not ordinarily be treated by biomedical practitioners. Despite myriad differences among practitioners, Sango healing is united by a common focus on the Orisas.

Sango healers meet with some clients once or twice a week. Other clients only consult a Sango healer once or twice during a lifetime. Most Sango healers set aside two or three mornings each week for healing although some very prominent healers receive clients four days a week and consult with as many as 20 clients each day. This is atypical. About 30% of consultations are carried out in Spiritual Baptist churches. Most consultations, however, are carried out at the healer's home. Sango healers who can afford it dedicate separate areas of their homes to the Orisa. Those with smaller residences use their kitchens or *parlours* for consultations (Houk, 1995; Glazier, 2009).

Consultations are by far the most common Sango healing technique. Most Sango consultations are fairly straightforward. Healers are possessed by Sango and carry on conversations with the afflicted; Orisas speak through the healer. The client's job is to listen and follow the Orisas' advice. In many cases, Sango speaks clearly in English. But Orisas' pronouncements are not always clear and forthcoming, and, sometimes, there is considerable ambiguity surrounding the cause or causes of an illness. Consultations are ostensibly private, but often a thin curtain is all that separates other clients (and the visiting anthropologist) from the Orisas' comments. Some consultations are highly informal and brief (less than five minutes). The Orisas express their opinions addressing supplicants on a first name basis. Other consultations with Orisas are more formal. In general, Orisas refuse to deal with clients who they consider disrespectful or who have not followed their advice in the past.

Sango healers also consult with and make referrals to other traditional healers, as previously noted. Sango healers sponsor joint healing ceremonies with devotees of Osun or Oyo (and/or other of Sango's multiple wives). Healers recognize limitations to their techniques and often encourage clients to explore alternative remedies. Sango healers also encourage their clients to consult with Western-trained doctors. For instance, there is little Sango healers can do for clients diagnosed with advanced forms of cancer except to prepare them for the next life. They attempt to make clients comfortable and prescribe soothing herbs, fasting, Spiritual Baptist mourning ceremonies, animal sacrifice, sponsorship of Sango feasts, and performing acts of charity. Nevertheless, collaboration between Sango practitioners and biomedical practitioners is often one way. Sango healers refer their clients to biomedicine, but biomedical practitioners rarely refer their patients to Sango healers.

Access to traditional healers is a persistent problem. In many rural areas, there are more traditional healers than trained health care professionals, but traditional healers do not work "full-time" as healers. Most Sango healers have secular jobs and additional religious obligations that take up much of their time. Sometimes, it is easier to consult an urban biomedical specialist than consult with a well-known Sango healer. Cost is also a factor. Biomedical treatment in the Caribbean is often available at little or no cost. Traditional healers such as Pentecostals, Charismatics, and others provide healing at very low cost (a small contribution is expected, but is not mandatory); however, Sango healing is never free. As noted, a client's willingness to make a monetary contribution, help sponsor a Sango feast, or provide an animal for sacrifice is seen as an integral part of the healing process. It is a sign of commitment to the Orisa and is the first step toward a "cure" (Olupona, 2004).

Divination and Spirit Messengers

Much of Sango healing is centered on diagnosis. The first step is to determine the exact cause of illness. Causes are sought in past behaviors, relations with others, relations with the spirit world, and treatment of ancestors (Elder, 1970). Private consultations are direct and personal while divination is indirect, less personal, and more focused on technique. In those instances where consultations are inconclusive, divination is the first step in the healing process. As in other areas of religious life, Sango devotees are pluralists and experiment with multiple forms of divination; in some cases, the results of divination are unclear forcing them to explore multiple options. There is a sense in which all illnesses are characterized by uncertainty and, as Winkelman and Peek (2004) astutely noted, divination becomes "a broader inquiry into life circumstances and meaning, of which diagnosis of the immediate causes of a malady is a part" (p. 166). Again, healing is defined very broadly; to heal is to address everything that troubles a client: physical illness, anxiety, social disruption, and/or help in making difficult decisions. The assumption is that divinatory procedures reveal information that is accessible to the gods but would otherwise be inaccessible to humans.

For the client, divination is an enormously practical enterprise. But, as noted previously, divination does not automatically resolve uncertainty; at times it raises as many questions as it answers; it is "edification by puzzlement" (Fernandez, 1986). The popularity of a particular divinatory technique is largely determined by its perceived cost, efficacy, and the level of personal commitment engendered.

Healers and clients within the Orisa movement have recourse to a variety of divinatory techniques including Ifa (Hucks, 1998) and "Sixteen Cowries"

(Bascom, 1980). Other options include: Kabala, astrology, a seance, private consultations with Orisa, reading tea leaves, reading animal entrails, breaking chicken bones, dreams, Spiritual Baptist mourning ceremonies, Oiji boards, throwing bones, tossing coins, throwing dice, and consulting Obeah men and/or Obeah women. Many Sango healers utilize a combination of the above techniques although consulting an Obeah man or Obeah woman is usually a last resort because practitioners of Obeah are greatly feared since Obeah is seen as witchcraft (Williams, 1932).

Most divination entails dealings with spirit messengers (intermediaries) in various guises, and some messengers are more reliable than others. Messengers like the Orisa Exu are tricksters and often distrusted. But as Hale (2009) observed, "Without the trickster spirit Exu, one can do nothing" (p. 27). Exu is a key member of the Yoruba pantheon, and is a go-between. Like the Greek god Hermes (Crapanzano, 1992), Exu is impossible to coerce, predict, and/or control. He/she has mixed loyalties and is not bound by human conventions. Therefore, dealing with Exu requires years of training and even more years of experience. It takes a lifetime to establish rapport with Exu and to master the techniques of Ifa. Sango, too, can be something of a trickster. As noted, Sango healers sometimes prefer to deal with other more predictable members of the Yoruba pantheon such as Oyo, Oshun, Sakpana, and Ogun (Glazier, 2003).

Jules-Rossette (1978) deftly outlined what she saw as continuities between discovery processes in divination and discovery processes within Western science. She emphasized that in Africa, divination is the major vehicle for uncovering and relieving social conflict. Jules-Rossette also noted that African diviners offer interpretations that are central to the social distribution of information. At the same time, she acknowledged that some information should never be accessible and/or made public. Healing rites, for example, are not always public events, and most divination is conducted for individuals and is carried out in private settings.

Divination's main goal is to reduce randomness and establish hitherto unrecognized patterns. Clients may have experienced a set of events that they already see as interconnected. Diviners are charged with the task of discerning linkages and commonalities. As Evans-Pritchard (1937) suggested in his study of the Azande poison oracle, divination can be a closed system entailing "circular reasoning" but its results are difficult if not impossible to refute. Similarly, Winkelman and Peek (2004) emphasized that divination constitutes a potent "way of knowing"; it enables its practitioners (diviners and their clients) to see and participate in an alternate, more predictable, coherent world.

Divinatory procedures are accessible while at the same time being deliberately misleading and mysterious. They are simultaneously public and private, clear and opaque, and attempt to bridge the gap between the mechanical and the magical. Furthermore, all forms of divination collapse time and space. In divination, the present partakes of the future as well as the past; everything is contingent on everything else and, most importantly, through divination the future can be changed by blood sacrifice which makes Ifa among the most potent divinatory options. Some Sango devotees, however, are ambivalent about animal sacrifice, as one devotee stated, "the gods call for it, but it vexes me" (Glazier, 2009).

Divination may be impromptu or highly organized. The two major contexts of divination are: preparation of sites for religious ceremonies, and healing. Almost every aspect of preparation for Spiritual Baptist and Orisa ceremonies must be confirmed and reconfirmed by the Orisa before being implemented (see, for example, Houk's (1995) description of Leader Scott's frequent use of *obi*. As Sango healer Scott began preparations for ceremonies, he repeatedly tossed *obi* seeds asking a series of "yes or no" questions to discern the Orisas' preferences. According to Houk (1995), Scott mainly cast *obi* seeds while preparing for Sango ritual; he did not cast *obi* on a daily basis. Other Sango leaders cast *obi* throughout the day.)

Within the Sango tradition, divination also occurs with Bush healers or private consultations and healing constitutes the major occasion for divination. Bush healers mostly read "signs" like tea leaves and bath rings. In his study of Jamaican Bush healers Wedenoja (1989) noted that healers seldom ask patients to describe their symptoms, rather they divine the cause of affliction by "concentration." A competent healer is already expected to intuitively know the cause of a client's problem. They may stare into space, a cup of water in which a coin has been placed or at the direction of a flame; they may pass their hands over the afflicted or just look into a client's eyes to immediately understand what is wrong. Dolls also play a part in Caribbean healing ceremonies (Fernandez-Olmos & Paravasini-Gebert, 2001). Even commercially-produced dolls like Mattel's "Barbie," can be brought into the service of diviners.

Healers are expected to "know" clients' problems in advance. They seldom question their clients since this would constitute an insult to the Orisas and the client, and an open admission of lack of ability as a healer. Some healers have developed a wide network of trusted healers who "help each other out" with diagnoses; however, less senior healers seldom refer clients to other healers, adding formal divinatory procedures (casting *obi*; tea leaves) to their healing rites instead.

Herbal medicines feature prominently in Sango healing and are widely utilized throughout the Caribbean. Each healer has his/her own pharmacopoeia and most herbal medicines are taken as teas or baths (see Barrett, 1976; Stewart, 2005; and Price, 2007 for a description of ritual baths). Sango herbalists are "called" by plants who revealed their healing powers in visions and dreams. Plants "speak" to them, shouting "Pick Me! Pick Me!" as healers pray about a particular client's needs. Gathering plants is an integral part of the healing process and healers typically offer a libation of white rum before each plant is picked followed by salutations. Some Bush medicines may or may not possess biomedical efficacy (Lans, 2007; Mischel, 1959), nevertheless, metaphorical and symbolic connections often override pharmacological properties. For example, one Sango healer rubs ginger root on the hands of her arthritic clients because the root resembles a gnarled hand.

Recently, Trinidad herbal medical practitioners, like aromatherapists, have been organizing to gain greater official recognition (and possible insurance co-payments) for their services; however, so far, Sango healers have not joined in these efforts.

In addition, time is integral to the Sango healing process. Illnesses that stem from bad relations with the Orisa develop over many years. It takes months, and sometimes years, to overcome problems because 1) it takes considerable time to organize Orisa feasts, make preparations for sacrifice, and so on, and 2) outcomes are not immediately apparent. In the Sango tradition, every positive event (good travel connections, successful shopping trips, positive family interactions) indicates an improving relationship with the Orisa. On the other hand, bad travel connections and negative family interactions can indicate worsening relationships with the Orisa. Because it takes years to determine when and if one is sick, it also takes years to determine when and if one has been "cured."

Sango and Biomedical Practitioners

There are perhaps as many as 80,000 Sango healers in the Caribbean indicating that contemporary Sango is on a rebound (Glazier, 2008). This may be due to a number of factors. Much of the time, biomedical professionals (clinical psychologists, counselors, and/or biomedical practitioners) are of a different social class than their clients and do not share a common worldview with those they serve. In this respect, Sango healers may possess an advantage. They are usually of the same social class and possess the same educational backgrounds as their clients. Most important, they share a common worldview. Sango healing is predicated on a holistic view of health and illness (Allen, 2001; Moodley & West, 2005) that includes physical (biological) maladies as well as what biomedicine would classify as "bad luck." For Sango healers, illness is a "call" to serve the spirits; a call to sacrifice, a call to divine, and a call to sponsor a feast honoring the Orisas. Divination (Ifa, Kabala, casting *obi*) encourages clients to take a more active role in their cures. Such a holistic approach is not generally available within Caribbean National Health Systems. Therefore, in order to be most effective, biomedical practitioners need to acknowledge their clients' belief in the Orisas (Glazier, 2009).

Conclusion

Sango has been reported in the Caribbean since the mid-18th century. In the popular mind, Sango healers were lumped with other Caribbean healers like Obeah, and colonial authorities attempted to curtail the spread of Obeah, Sango, and the Spiritual Baptist faiths claiming that these religions were disruptive, uncontrollable, and (potentially) subversive. By the latter half of the 20th century, ordinances against Sango had been abolished and Sango healing was no longer perceived as a threat to the established political order, but instead was perceived as a direct challenge to European medicine.

Currently, Sango is on a rebound. Its persistence and resurgence may be accounted for both in terms of media support and a more prominent place in popular culture. Sango receives favorable coverage in the media and has been the subject of numerous television documentaries and editorials as well as articles and editorials in the *Jamaica Gleaner* and the *Trinidad Guardian*. Clearly, Sango healing provides a mechanism for Caribbean people to validate their past and recover their African "roots." Furthermore, its contribution to health and mental health both historically and in the present context cannot be overlooked. Indeed, a number of Sango healers (some of whom have earned advanced academic degrees) have sought formal affiliations with regional mental health centers and foreign-sponsored faith based organizations and have made contributions to the treatment of some symptoms of mental disorders in an attempt to address the health and mental health care needs of their followers.

Notes

1. Beaubrun was born in Grenada. He received medical training at the University of Edinburgh, and served as a professor of medicine at the University of the West Indies from 1976 to 1988. Simultaneously, he served as director of the psychiatric unit at St. Ann's. Beaubrun served as a Trinidad and Tobago Senator from 1976 to 1981. As a Senator, he actively incorporated indigenous religions into mental health treatment. Another prominent psychiatrist, Trinidad-born Ezra E. H. Griffith of Yale University, has conducted extensive research on the mental health benefits of Sango and Baptist ceremonies (Griffith, 1983; 2010).
2. Once an African king, Sango is sympathetic to human frailties. His magic failed him; he was betrayed by his wives; and, eventually, he lost his kingdom. But Sango is also feared because of his violent temper. Sango seldom holds a grudge. His punishment is swift and severe, but even if offended on one day, he can be asked for assistance on the next. As noted, Sango is sometimes portrayed as a mulatto, but members of the Trinidad Orisa movement perceive him as black (Houk, 1995; Hucks, 1998).
3. *Gris gris* bags are cloth sacks filled with assorted objects such as finger nail clippings, torn pages from books of ancient wisdom, twigs, dirt from cemeteries, human hair, and animal bones.

References

Allen, E. A. (2001). Whole person healing, spiritual realism, and social disruption. *International Review of Missions, 90*, 118–132.
Barrett, L. (1976). *The sun and the drum*. Kingston: Sangster's
Bascom, W. (1972). *Shango in the New World*. Austin, TX: University of Texas.
Bascom, W. (1980). *Sixteen Cowries*. Bloomington, IN: Indiana University Press.
Brandon, G. (1990). African religious influences in Cuba, Puerto Rico and Hispaniola. *Journal of Caribbean Studies, 7*, 201–231.
Crapanzano, V. (1992). *Hermes the thief and other essays*. Berkeley, CA: University of California Press.
Deive, C. E. (1975). *Vodu y Magie en Santo Domingo*. Santo Domingo: Museo del Hombre Dominicano.

Desmangles, L. G. (1992). *The faces of the gods: Vodou and Roman Catholicism in Haiti.* Chapel Hill, NC: University of North Carolina Press.

Desmangles, L. G., Glazier, S. D., & Murphy, J. M. (2009). Religion in the Caribbean. In R. S. Hillman & T. J. D'Agostino (Eds.), *Understanding the contemporary Caribbean* (pp. 289–338) Boulder, CO: Lynne Reinner.

Elder, J. D. (1970). The Yoruba ancestor cult in Gasparillo. *Caribbean Quarterly, 16,* 5–20.

Evans-Pritchard, E. E. (1937). *Witchcraft, oracles and magic among the Azande.* Oxford: Clarendon.

Fernandez, J. W. (1986). Edification by puzzlement. In I. Karp & C. S. Bird (Eds.), *Explorations in African systems of thought.* Bloomington, IN: Indiana University Press.

Fernandez-Olmos, M., & Paravisini-Gebert, L. (2001). *Creole religions of the Caribbean* New York: NYU Press.

Glazier, S. D. (2003). Limin' wid jah: Spiritual Baptists who became Rastafarians and then became Spiritual Baptists again. In A. S. Buckser & S. D. Glazier (Eds.), *The anthropology of religious conversion.* Lanham, MD: Rowman & Littlefield.

Glazier, S. D. (2008). Wither sqango?: An inquiry into Sango's authenticity and prominence in the Caribbean. In J. Tishken, T. Falola, & A. Akinyemi (Eds.), *Sango in Africa and the African diaspora.* (pp. 233–247). Bloomington, IN: Indiana University Press.

Glazier, S. D. (2009). Demanding spirits and reluctant devotees: Belief and unbelief in the Trinidadian Orisa movement. *Social Analysis, 52*(1), 19–38.

Griffith, E. (1983). The impact of sociocultural factors on a church-based healing mode. *American Journal of Orthopsychiatry, 53,* 291–302.

Griffith, E. (2010). *Ye shall dream: Patriarch Granville Williams and the Barbados Spiritual Baptists.* Mona: University of the West Indies Press.

Hale, L. (2009). *Hearing the mermaid's song: The Umbanda religion in Rio de Janeiro.* Albuquerque, NM: University of New Mexico Press.

Henry, F. S. (1999). *Reclaiming the African past.* Mona: University of the West Indies Press.

Henry, F. S. (2008). *He had the power: Pa Neezer the Orisa King of Trinidad.* San Juan, Trinidad: Lexicon Press

Houk, J. T. (1995). *Spirits, blood and drums.* Philadelphia, PA: Temple University Press.

Hucks, T. E. (1998). *Approaching the African god: An examination of African American Yoruba history from 1959 to the Present* (Ph.D. dissertation), Harvard University.

Jules-Rossette, B. (1978). The veil of objectivity. *American Anthropologist, 80,* 549–570.

Lans, C. (2007) *Creole remedies of Trinidad and Tobago.* Lulu.com

Matory, J. L. (2005). *Black Atlantic religion: Tradition, transnationalism and matriarchy in Afro-Brazilian Candomble.* Princeton, NJ: Princeton University Press.

Mischel, F. S. (1959). Faith healing and medical practices in the southern Caribbean. *Southwestern Journal of Anthropology, 15,* 407–417.

Moodley, R., & West, W. (2005). *Integrating traditional healing practices into counseling and psychotherapy.* Thousand Oaks, CA: Sage

Olupona, J. K. (2004). Owner of the day and regulator of the universe. In M. J. Winkelman & P. M. Peek (Eds.), *Divination and healing: Potent vision.* (pp. 103–117). Tucson, AR: University of Arizona Press.

Paton, D. (2009). Obeah acts: Producing and policing the boundaries of religion in the Caribbean. *Small Axe, 13,* 1–18.

Price, R. (2007). *Travels with Tooy.* Chicago, IL: University of Chicago Press.

Rocklin, A. (2012). Imagining religions in a Trinidad Village: The Africanity of the Spiritual Baptist movement and the politics of comparing religions. *New West Indian Guide, 86,* 55–79.

Romberg, R. (2007). Today Chango is Chango. *Western Folklore, 66*, 75–106.

Romberg, R. (2009). *Healing dramas: Divination and magic in modern Puerto Rico.* Austin, TX: University of Texas Press.

Simpson, G. E. (1965). *The Shango cult in Trinidad.* Rio Piedras: Institute of Caribbean Studies.

Stewart. D. M. (2005) *Three eyes for the journey: African dimensions of the Jamaican religious experience.* New York: Oxford University Press

Trotman, D. (2007). Reflections on the children of Shango: An essay on a history of Orisa worship in Trinidad. *Slavery and Abolition, 28*, 211–234.

Ward, C., & Beaubrun, M. (1979). Trance induction and hallucination in Spiritual Baptist mourning. *Journal of Psychological Anthropology, 2*, 479–488.

Warner-Lewis, M. (1989). *Trinidad Yoruba: From mother tongue to memory.* Tuscaloosa, AL: University of Alabama Press.

Weber, M. (1960). *The sociology of religion.* Glencoe: Free Press.

Wedenoja, W. (1989). Mothering and the practice of 'balm' in Jamaica. In C. S. McCain (Ed.), *Women as healers: Cross-cultural perspectives.* New Brunswick, NJ: Rutgers University Press.

Williams, J. J. (1932). *Voodoos and Obeahs: Phases in West Indian witchcraft.* New York: Dial.

Winkelman, M. J., & Peek, P. M. (2004). *Divination and healing: Potent vision.* Tucson, AR: University of Arizona Press.

8

LA REGLA DE OCHA (SANTERÍA)

Afro-Cuban Healing in Cuba and the Diaspora

Camille Hernandez-Ramdwar

Introduction

La Regla de Ocha[1] (otherwise known as *Santería* or *Lucumí*) is a syncretic Afro-Cuban religion derived from the traditions of enslaved Yorubans who were brought to Cuba beginning in the 18th century. The religion played an important healing role for Afro-Cuban communities in the dearth of available health care prior to the 1959 revolution. Post-revolution, practitioners were eventually forbidden from practicing and had to go underground. In contemporary Cuba the religion has undergone a revitalization and resurgence, partly due to the government's support and realization that the religion attracts foreign tourists and is therefore a lucrative state venture. Although *La Regla de Ocha* is the most widely known of the Afro-Cuban religions, one also finds *Regla de Ifá* (also of Yoruban origin, and often practiced in tandem with *La Regla de Ocha*), *Palo Monte*, *Abakuá*, and *Vodou* in various parts of the island. Often practitioners of one religion may also follow or be initiated into more than one system (Ayorinde, 2004; Brandon, 2001; Garoutte & Wambaugh, 2007).

In Cuba today, there has been a resurgence of interest in *La Regla de Ocha* as the health care system falters and conditions for many Cubans continue to deteriorate. Furthermore, for decades *La Regla de Ocha* has had a wide following diasporically, and is a growing religion worldwide. In the diaspora *Santería* has been placed under scrutiny and restrictions based on a general misunderstanding and fear of the religion; for example, difficulty in acquiring the proper herbs due to restrictions, and prohibitions regarding animal sacrifice. A general lack of knowledgeable elders, institutional structure and licensing within the religion has also led to a number of problems, as the potential for exploitation, commercialization, and misrepresentation of the religion increases in a market economy (Hearn, 2004; Ramos, 2006).

In *La Regla de Ocha* the basis of belief includes many spiritual causes for misfortune, including illness. Often illness is read as a particular spiritual entity calling for attention and/or devotion from the affected person (Wedel, 2004). As well, the malintentions of other human beings (whether direct or indirect) are commonly attributed to cause illness. Healers will often suggest spiritual remedies along with a visit to the local medical practitioner.

There were many attempts to outlaw *La Regla de Ocha* in the 19th and early 20th centuries, for racist reasons. For example, "In 1922, legislation prohibited Afro-Cuban gatherings involving drumming and dance" (Ayorinde, 2004, p. 52). Because *La Regla de Ocha* was of African origin and practiced predominantly by poor people of African descent, it was seen by white Cubans to be primitive, barbaric, heathen, and linked to criminality (Ayorinde, 2004). The religion revolves around the veneration of the ancestors and several deities (*orichas*), therefore from a Eurocentric perspective its apparent polytheism was seen to be unevolved compared to Christianity[2] (Ayorinde, 2004; Lachatañeré, 2004). However, many white Cubans did secretly (and sometimes openly) participate in and become knowledgeable about *La Regla de Ocha*, largely through the influence and instruction of their black slaves or servants (Canizares, 1999; Sandoval, 1979). Furthermore, the lack of European doctors in the colonial days meant that "during the nineteenth century, medical treatment was partly administered by healers of African origin and their pharmacopoeias" (Wedel, 2004, p. 32). As Cuba developed, African practices took a back seat to European medicine, and "Afro-Cubans relied increasingly on orthodox health care for the treatment of infectious and organic diseases; while the religious system's strengths in solving problems of spiritual and emotional nature remained intact" (Sandoval, 1979, p. 142).

In post-Revolutionary Cuba, *La Regla de Ocha* was attacked as a cultural anachronism, not part of a new, modern, revolutionary Cuba. In regards to one of the main sources of pride for the revolutionary government—health care—it was

> thought to be that they (practitioners of *La Regla de Ocha*) promoted dependency on divination and traditional cures, which could lead people to imbibe harmful substances or to delay seeking medical advice. In spite of free health care, revolutionaries asserted, people were dying in the clutches of *babalawos*, healers and spiritists.
>
> *(Ayorinde, 2004, p. 118)*

Conversely, the Cuban revolution actually helped the religion to grow in Cuba: increased employment among the traditionally marginalized Afro-Cuban population meant more people could afford the expensive initiation ceremony, and the religion continued to grow.

After the *apertura* (political and cultural opening) in the 1990s, the state in Cuba co-opted many of the symbols of *La Regla de Ocha*, and began marketing the religion as an aspect of cultural tourism (Amores, 2010). In Cuba today, there has been a resurgence of interest in *La Regla de Ocha* as the health care system falters and conditions for many Cubans continue to deteriorate. Arguably, the promises of the Revolution have not materialized for many Cubans, particularly for a younger generation born in the 1970s and 1980s, and the religion is being regenerated by a young, multiracial population of initiates (Wedel, 2004). The increase in tourism in Cuba since the 1990s has exposed the religion to high numbers of foreign travelers, many who become interested in the religion and may become initiates themselves, thereby spreading it to their countries of origin (Amores, 2010).

This chapter examines some common beliefs about illness and well-being from the perspective of *Santería*, looks at a variety of healing methods employed and explores the healing practices of *La Regla de Ocha*. It begins by discussing the principles and practices. This is followed by an exploration of the healers and representations of illness. Subsequently, the chapter discusses *La Regla de Ocha* as an integrative approach to healing and, lastly, explores the implications for conventional health and mental health.

Principles and Practices of *Santería*

Central to the beliefs of *La Regla de Ocha* is the practice of divination. One must consult the diviner to ascertain problems and prescriptions, remedies which often include sacrifice (*ebbo*), to appease or gain the assistance of a particular *oricha*. Like many earth-based religions, *Santería* proposes the interconnectedness of all living things, that everything in nature is imbued with a spirit, and that the human condition expands beyond the material plane. Therefore, in *La Regla de Ocha* the basis of belief includes many spiritual causes for illness, which is "prevented and healing is achieved by creating and maintaining relations with these divine beings and spirits" (Wedel, 2004, p. 47). For adherents, "*iré ariku* – blessings of good health – (is) the most important iré of all, and it is the first blessing they ask the orishas for" (Nodal & Ramos, 2005, p. 181).

The main purpose of divination, ritual, and sacrifice in the religion is to re-establish harmony for those who are "off-path," or to "make firm" the blessings that the practitioner currently enjoys. Priests of the religion—the *santero/as* and *babalawos*—are the intermediaries who can communicate by divination between *Oludumare*, the *orichas*, and the client. There are many methods of divination, each involving varying levels of intricacy, detail, and accuracy. *Santeros/as*[3] (otherwise known in Yoruban as *babalochas* and *iyalochas*, literally "father" and "mother" of the *orichas,* or simply as *Olorichas*) generally perform consultations using 16 cowrie shells (a practice known in Cuba as *diloggun*). The priests of Ifá (*babalawos*), a somewhat separate yet interconnected aspect of *La Regla de Ocha* open only to men, use a chain to which four pieces of coconut shell are attached, known as an *opele*; as well they may use *ikin* (the seeds of the oil palm) with which to divine. Both systems of divination are performed in order to achieve a *letra* or *odu*, 1 of 16 bodies of knowledge contained in the entire corpus of Ifá, a compilation of verse and wisdom developed in the oral culture of the Yorubans centuries ago. Each *odu* contains a wealth of allegories, parables, advice, examples of correct conduct, *patakis* or moral fables, as well as the remedies for any potential *osogbo* or imbalance that may befall a client for whom this *letra* has fallen, or, alternatively, remedies to seal the *iré* (good luck, fortune) of a client who is being blessed by this particular *odu*. In these sometimes lengthy and detailed consultations with *santeros* or *babalawos*, it may be revealed that the client has a health issue that must be attended to. In addition, it is very common that *letras* will advise clients on how to conduct themselves in a variety of ways, for example avoiding certain foods, abstaining from alcohol and tobacco, being careful where they eat, etc., advice which may be read as preventative medicine.

In the case where a client is flagged as having a pertinent or even serious health issue, the first advice is usually that the client seeks immediate medical attention, after which several prescriptions are given by the diviner to restore health and spiritual alignment (Wedel, 2004). Prescriptions may include various forms of *ebbo* or sacrifice. Nodal and Ramos (2005) state that *ebbo* "is an indispensable element in Lukumi Orisha Worship. It serves as the means to various ends, all conducive to the mental and physical well-being of the devotee and the religious community in general" (p. 167). *Ebbo* is directed at specific *oricha* and sometimes marked for the dead (*egun* or ancestors).[4]

San Lázaro[5] holds much importance in the religion, and to Cubans in general, especially as he "is considered a miraculous healer" (Wedel, 2004, p. 85). San Lázaro is the Catholic saint syncretized with the *oricha Babalú-Ayé*, who in West Africa was the god of smallpox, leprosy, and infectious diseases, and in Cuba is associated with infectious diseases such as syphilis and AIDS, illnesses with which he can both punish and cure. The fact that San Lázaro is well loved and respected by so many Cubans, of all faiths, is significant in that he is believed to be a great healer, full of compassion for the afflicted.

Santería Healers

Most of the healers in the religion are initiated priests (*santeros* and *babalawos*) while others are devotees of *oricha* who may be at varying levels of initiation or affiliation with an *ile* (spiritual house). Most training is from elders in the religion through an oral transference of knowledge and through hands-on apprenticeship, attending various ceremonies, rituals, etc. *La Regla de Ocha* is traditionally a hierarchical religion that requires years of practice and involvement, and encompasses varying levels of initiation. An elder Cuban informant of Sandoval's (2006), Florencio Baró, recalls his experiences of *La Regla de Ocha* in Cuba in the 1940s and 1950s, in which he makes a distinction between Catholic priest and *santero*:

> the priest studies a lot to become a priest, while *santeros* are born with religious faculties. The priest advises according to his knowledge, with his

heart, and by invoking the saints and God, but he cannot divine. *Santeros,* however, are fortune-tellers who can predict and cure.

(p. 58)

Sandoval echoes this by stating that "In the past most believers were not initiated; the oracles generally did not advise devotees to go through initiation unless they showed particular signs of possessing faculties as a medium of other similar gifts" (2006, p. 93). Today people are not only initiating because of their inherent "gifts": some initiate for health reasons, others for the pursuit of power and of money, and others because they have been instructed to do so, either by the *orichas,* or by elders whose intentions may or may not be honorable. The expectations placed on priests today are therefore more based on knowledge of rituals rather than healing and/or divining abilities. The worldwide spread of the religion and the emphasis, particularly in North America, on "immediate" results, and a lack of competent, traditional elders in the diaspora have led to an erosion of the typical apprenticeship of days gone by. For this reason, there are priests in the diaspora who have not been properly trained or not trained at all.

Not all practitioners of *Santería* are initiates; Canizares (1999) identified varying levels of involvement in the religion, ranging from least to most involved: interested observers, occasional clients, habitual clients, amulet recipients, *Ellegua* initiates, *Guerreros* initiates, *Collares* initiates, *santeros,* and *babalawos* (in Newby, Riley, & Leal-Almeraz, 2006, p. 291). It is therefore the last two categories who would primarily be considered the healers in the religion. Sandoval (1979) states

> Santeria is characterized by its lack of homogeneity. It is not a religion governed by a narrow and strict orthodoxy. On the contrary, each *santero* subjectively interprets the beliefs and frequently introduces variations in the rituals and mythology according to his own knowledge, religious experience, convictions and needs of his followers.

(p. 138)

There are pros and cons to this lack of organizational structure—positively, it allows for re-adaptation to current circumstances and environment; more negatively it can result in charlatanism and corruption of important basic tenets of the religion, as well as "openness" of morality/ethics.

It must be noted that a great part of the divinatory process lies in the diviner's spiritual energy/power, known as *aché.* It therefore follows that initiatory status or years in the religion does not an effective healer make—part of this must come through the blessings of the *orichas* and one's own head (*Ori/eleda/Ángel de Guardia*). Without this, the diviner is just casting objects and following form. By the same token, someone relatively low in the religious hierarchy may have natural *aché* that imbues them with the ability to heal with very little effort. Interestingly, one can see a gendered component to this: in the early days of *Santería,* women held powerful positions as *oriates*, or "master of ceremonies," in initiation rituals and were highly accomplished diviners (Brown, 2003; Clark, 2005). Presently, as *La Regla de Ocha* has become a viable money making opportunity in Cuba, one sees less and less women acting in the role of *oriate*; furthermore, women in Cuba are prevented from becoming *babalawos*. These are the upper echelons of the religion (i.e., places where the most money is to be made), in which men now predominate. Consequently, women practitioners may find it more difficult to initiate, for economic reasons, yet they are followers of the faith and continue to practice, often without vestal authority. Many may find more powerful positions in the practice of *espiritismo* rather than *Santería* due to ongoing patriarchy in the latter (Brandon, 2001). However, Tracy (2005) argues that "healing through ritual for women in Santeria is made possible by gender based mythology, through the presence of powerful and complex female deities" (p. 4). In this instance, it is the presence of the female divine in this religion (in a multitude of forms) that is in and of itself healing for women, men, and societies.

Representation of Illness

Illness can sometimes be attributed to the punishment of an *oricha*, for wrongdoing or for lack of devotion. Each *oricha* has rulership over specific parts of the body, for example *Obatalá* rules the head, and punishment could therefore be mental illness, blindness, or addictions. Believers in *La Regla de Ocha* are frequently told to appease the *orichas*, to offer them specific foods, flowers, candles, or actions to ensure that one stays in their good graces. In general, followers of *La Regla de Ocha* believe that illness and bad luck are attributable to one or more of the following: anger or punishment of an *oricha*; the evil eye (*malojo*); witchcraft or sorcery (*brujería*); congenital "weakness" (such people are often referred to as *abiku* or "born to die"); spiritual attachment; a weakened head (*eleda, Ori*), or loss of one's soul, whereby sorcerers, paid by an enemy, buy the person's head (Sandoval, 1979; 2006; Wedel, 2004).

The physical manifestation of illness is but a cruder form of the spiritual/metaphysical manifestation: it is the invisible made visible. For this reason, clients are often sent to the physician to deal with the physical manifestation of illness, while *santeros* deal with the metaphysical or spiritual causes. Practitioners also believe that unless problems are dealt with in the spiritual realm first or in tandem with the physical, no genuine healing will take place. The prescriptions of *oricha*, *Ifá* or the spirits of the dead are meant to be heeded with all seriousness. Clients are advised to follow the advice and then return to the diviner to see if they are now "on path." However, *ebbó* can still be ineffective. This is often revealed beforehand through divination. When all else fails, the *orichas* will simply pronounce that there is nothing left that can be done. In Yoruban belief everyone has a predestined day of death; everything in life can be altered except for that.

According to Sandoval (1979), the bulk of white Cubans did not know about or visit healers in *La Regla de Ocha* prior to the Castro era as it was very much relegated to the Afro-Cuban, lower class population. However, in the revolutionary period, a time in Cuba of great upheaval, many Cubans of all backgrounds sought out religious support; similarly, those who migrated to the United States found themselves in upheaval again and, feeling a sense of powerlessness, turned to *La Regla de Ocha* to ground them (Brandon, 1997). In contemporary Cuba, many clients come to the *santera* to *resolver* or to fix the multitude of their everyday problems they face (finding food and money, trying to exit the country, etc.), problems which contribute to levels of extreme stress and anxiety. Both Sandoval (2006) and Wedel (2004) describe the difficulties and stresses Cubans face: "people often expressed how insecure they felt by saying 'I don't know what is going to happen to me', or 'I don't understand what is happening'" (Wedel, 2004, p. 41). Such conditions of uncertainty contribute to *nervios* or anxiety/ mental illness (Wedel, 2004), and Cubans often believe that this is the result of the *malpensimientos* (bad thoughts) of others, or other *maldiciones* (curses). Others come to the diviner for physical maladies that medical science has been unable to cure. The involvement of Cubans in the religion runs the gamut from those for whom the religion is a way of life and a lifetime commitment, to those for whom the religion is seen as a quick fix, a magical solution to their problems.

The versatility and openness of *La Regla de Ocha*, both historically and in contemporary times, allows for a fluidity of experience. Unlike fundamentalist forms of religion, there is no wrongdoing in seeking out other spiritual paths, or in practicing several at the same time. For this reason, many practitioners and believers in *La Regla de Ocha* will also consult a *palero* (*Palo Monte*) or *espiritista* (*espiritismo*), pray to Catholic saints, and perhaps also work with *voudouisants* (devotees of *Vodou*). Several initiates of *La Regla de Ocha* have been initiated in other Afro-Caribbean paths, and many practice *espiritismo* on a regular basis (Brandon, 2001; Dodson, 2008; Garoutte & Wambaugh, 2007). In many cases, suffering and ailment are seen to be the result of a negative spirit attachment. The remedy for this is a *misa* or spiritual mass for the dead, a central activity in *espiritismo*. Practitioners of *La Regla de Ocha* are often involved in *espiritismo*, and many maintain altars to both the dead and the *orichas*.

Santería and Mental Health Practices

Once a diviner has ascertained what kind of problem a client faces, the remedies for healing often include *ebbo* (sacrifice) and/or the use of herbs. *Ebbo* can be an offering (plant, animal, object, etc.) to the *egun* or *orichas*, or it can mean sacrificing (giving up) something such as a behavior or a particular food. Herbs can be used in a variety of ways—for baths, *limpiezas* (cleansings), infusions, or teas.

Healers will often suggest spiritual remedies along with a visit to the local medical practitioner. In Wedel's 2004 study of 100 client consultations with a *santero* in Matanzas, Cuba, he found that in 68% of the cases, clients were advised to visit a biomedical doctor. According to Wedel:

Today in Cuba, it is not uncommon that physicians and other health personnel practice, or have some common knowledge of santería. In Havana many physicians are also babalaos . . . When santeros and babalaos work as medical doctors, they frequently encourage patients to become involved in santería if religious healing is thought to be a more effective for of treatment than biomedicine.

(2004, p. 119)

Cuban *babalawo* Marcos Govarrubia states:

Hay personas no se sienten bien, que duermen mal, tienen algo de psicosis, hay personas que no saben movilizar situaciones en su vida, tan disorientada, entonces estan buscando un estimulo; entonces nosotros utilizamos en este religión a veces como un psicólogo.

There are people who don't feel well, that sleep badly, that have some type of psychosis, persons that don't know how to mobilize situations in their life, very disoriented, then they are looking for a stimulus; we function, then, at times like psychologists in this religion.

(Gonzalez, 1990, translation current author)

The *olorisha* or *babalawo* can therefore act as a doctor, psychologist, confidante, religious elder, and/or parent figure. Their role varies depending on the client, the client's situation, their own *aché*, and their own level of commitment to their godchilden (or *ahijados/as*—those who have been initiated by an *olorisha* or *babalawo*. This bond between the two is considered to be lifelong and sacred) and clients.

Ebbó and initiation into the religion are also used as forms of preventative and curative practice. *Ebbó*

is best understood as a religious act consisting of ritual procedures for establishing communication with spiritual and supernatural beings in order to modify the condition of the persons on whose behalf it is performed, or of objects with which they are concerned.

(Nodal & Ramos, 2005, p. 172)

For example, a *santero* will offer *ebbó* based on specific instructions provided through divination; this *ebbó* will commonly be to the *oricha* who spoke through divination to offer their assistance; to the guardian *oricha* of the person being seen; or to the *oricha* who "owns" the illness or body part afflicted by the client. An *ebbó* may be as simple as a bath or a cleansing using an animal that is then sacrificed to the *oricha* consulted, or it may involve more intense and costly endeavours. Sometimes *ebbó* requires a change of behaviour (e.g., constant arguing, or smoking); they "give up" or "sacrifice" this behaviour is order to achieve healing and *iré*. Initiation is perhaps the highest form of *ebbó*—literally sacrificing one's head to the *oricha*, after which the *oricha* becomes the lifelong guardian of that person's head. In all cases, healing "comes from within" in that "one gains a sense of agency over one's destiny as well as through the transference of energy" (Tracy, 2005, p. 32).

The use of herbs is central to healing practices of *La Regla de Ocha* (Cortez, 2000). *Santeros* and *babalawos* traditionally possessed a large body of knowledge of herbs for healing. Enslaved Africans had to find plants similar to the ones they had used in Africa; therefore many of the herbs used by the Yorubans have been substituted by those found in Cuba. Obviously, such use of fresh herbs can not always be transferred to other parts of the world; practitioners in Florida may be able to procure/grow the same herbs as those used in Cuba, but in the more temperate zones of North America, or other parts of the world, this is much more difficult. The unavailability of proper and fresh herbs in abundance can greatly hinder the efficacy of religious rituals and healing practices, a major problem for diasporic practitioners.

For *santeros*, a virtual bible of herbal lore is found in the book *El Monte* by Lydia Cabrera (1996). *El Monte* is an encyclopedia of herbal and spiritual knowledge as told to Cabrera, an ethnologist and anthropologist, by Afro-Cuban religious elders. Cabrera delineates the otherworldly connection between human and plant thusly: "*Curan, porque ellas mismas son brujas* [They (plants) cure, because they are the same as sorcerers]" (1996, p. 11, translation current author). It is the *aché* of the plants themselves, their mystical link with the *orichas* and with all spiritual forces, good and evil, that make them so powerful; this is why the use of them is so intrinsic to the religion. *El Monte* delineates how each plant is linked with different *orichas* and is attributed to have special powers, medicinal and spiritual. A good *santero* or *babalawo* has an extensive knowledge of herbs, knows how to procure them, and is familiar with their specific uses. They also know which *oricha* is the *dueño* or owner of each herb.

Some of the common healing techniques involving the use of herbs include *limpiezas* (cleansings), baths, infusions, and teas. A *limpieza* is effectively a transfer of (negative) energy from a person to an object (flowers, herbs, vegetables, fruits, grains, animals), after which the cleansing object is discarded and/or sacrificed. *Limpiezas* may also be effected with cigar smoke and/or spraying the person with alcohol (through the mouth of the *santera*). *Limpiezas* can be done to remove a troublesome or negative spirit. It is believed that even the negative thoughts and intentions of others can make you ill, therefore the necessity for constant cleansing of oneself and one's surroundings. Baths may be made with herbs alone, or sometimes additional ingredients are added (Cortez, 2000), and are often taken for a set period of days. Clients may also consume herbs in teas or by eating them.

Scholarly research on *La Regla de Ocha* began in Cuba early in the 20th century (1900s–1950s) through the works of ethnologist Fernando Ortiz, anthropologist Lydia Cabrera, and ethnographer Rómulo Lachatañeré. In later years, Cuban and international scholars have continued to research the religion and expose many formerly secret practices to a worldwide audience. Ortiz graduate Miguel Barnet (2001) continues to document the practices and history of Afro-Cuban religions from inside Cuba, while others, such as cultural anthropologist Migene González-Wippler, of Puerto Rican origin, can be credited with popularizing and demystifying *Santería* diasporically outside of the Cuban and Spanish-speaking communities with a number of books she published in the 1970s. Given the extreme popularity of González-Wippler's books, many publishers became interested in the topic of *Santería*, and a new body of literature on the subject evolved. Nodal and Ramos (2005) note that:

> . . . in the last few years more and more medical personnel and people in such professions as therapy, social work, and counselling are beginning to realize the importance of Lukumí religion in Hispanic communities in the United States: the therapeutic value of its magical and spiritual practices in treating different kinds of illnesses, as well as dealing with certain kinds of social and adaptational problems. Gonzalez-Wippler reports that Belleview Hospital in New York City has an Olorisha on the counselling staff for those who seek such assistance.
>
> *(p. 181)*

Some of these authors are initiates of *La Regla de Ocha*; this is of note because within the *Regla de Ocha* community the importance of guarding ritual secrets and protecting sacred knowledge is still practiced. For this reason, some of these researchers have come under criticism for making public that which, in the eyes of many elders in the religion, is not meant for everyone.

Despite its growing popularity and visibility, in the diaspora *La Regla de Ocha* is often under scrutiny and restrictions based on a general misunderstanding and fear of the religion (Murphy, 1993). Difficulty in acquiring the proper herbs, ordinances prohibiting animal sacrifice, and a general lack of knowledgeable elders, institutional structure, and licensing within the religion itself has led to numerous problems, as the potential for exploitation, commercialization, and misrepresentation of the religion increases. Diasporic practitioners frequently face discrimination, particularly in areas where ordinances banning animal sacrifice, noise (drumming is an important part of ritual work), certain herbs, and the use of mercury (Newby et al., 2006) exist. Furthermore, debates internal to the religion ensue over issues such as exposure to blood and the necessity of practicing proper precautions against the spread of HIV and other infectious diseases (some rituals involve cutting, shaving, or scratching of the body).

In terms of health care, *La Regla de Ocha* in the diaspora has become a "viable mental health delivery system, which offers support, counselling, and socialization opportunities to many people who are suffering from the tensions that characterize acculturation and deculturation processes" (Sandoval, 2006, p. 333). This is certainly the case in major American urban centres with large Cuban populations (notably the greater Miami and New York areas).

> For Cubans in the United States who adopted the religion here, Lukumí religion has had a major healing function, since it served a purpose for them that it did not serve in Cuba. It has become a system through which adjustments to a foreign land and an alien culture may be mediated . . . They use rituals like ebó to help them cope with illness, isolation, unemployment, mental problems, discrimination, social and personal difficulties, and many other conflicts that may arise.
>
> *(Nodal & Ramos, 2005, p. 184)*

The same can be said for other Latino, Caribbean, and African American groups for whom it may offer important alternatives in a racist and discriminatory society.

Conclusion

One can only hope that the growth in *La Regla de Ocha* will be positive, with an adherence to ethical practices and accountability. Furthermore, it is hoped that in the diaspora *Santería* will be recognized, respected, and accommodated as a legitimate religion. The *orichas* have survived the Middle Passage, slavery, colonialism, prohibition, and outlawing. This is a testament to the strength of the *orichas* and to their believers, a strength that can surely be utilized and respected in the ongoing healing of humanity that is taking place in the 21st century.

Notes

1. I have chosen to preference the term *Regla de Ocha* (rule of Oricha) for the religion rather than the more commonly known term *Santería* as the latter is "a derogatory creation imposed on the religion by white Cuban Catholic clergy to ensure it is distanced from their Christian faith" (Murrell, 2010).
2. Adherents do believe in a supreme omniscient being—*Olodumare/Olorun/Olofin*.
3. *Santero* (male) and *santera* (female) are the Spanish names given to *oricha* priests in Cuba. Here I use them interchangeably.
4. An *ebbo* may be very elaborate or very simple, ranging from *omi tutu* or cool water offered to an *oricha*, to various *limpiezas* or cleansings utilizing herbal baths, grains, or cigar smoke, to animal sacrifices that may require a significant investment of work, time, and money. Sometimes the *orichas* insist that the person who has come for divination must be "crowned" or initiated into the religion, and that only this will appease the *oricha* and perhaps save that person's life.
5. Pilgrimages to San Lázaro are made by the faithful to El Santuario de San Lázaro, a leprosarium and chapel in the town of El Ríncon , just outside of Havana, especially on his feast day December 17. Each year, Cubans fulfill promises to the saint/*oricha* in gratitude for health restored, some crawling on their knees for miles, or dragging heavy bricks, many dressed in the sackcloth with which this saint/*oricha* is associated.

References

Amores, G. P. (2010). Orishas, turistas y practicantes. La comercialización del patrimonio religioso en Cuba: Un ejemplo de estrategia de revitalización identitaria y económica. *Pasos: Revista de Turismo y Patrimonio Cultural, 8*(1), 167–184.

Ayorinde, C. (2004). *Afro-Cuban religiosity: Revolution, and national identity.* Gainesville, FL: University Press of Florida.

Barnet, M. (2001). *Afro-Cuban religions.* Princeton, NJ: Markus Wiener Publications.

Brandon, G. (1997). *Santeria from Africa to the New World: The dead sell memories.* Bloomington, IN: Indiana University Press.

Brandon, G. (2001). Ochun in the Bronx. In J. Murphy and M. Sanford (Eds.), *Òsun across the waters: A Yoruba goddess in Africa and the Americas* (pp. 155–164). Bloomington, IN: Indiana University Press.

Brown, D. H. (2003). *Santería enthroned: Art, ritual, and innovation in an Afro-Cuban religion.* Chicago, IL: University of Chicago Press.

Cabrera, L. (1996). *El Monte.* Ciudad de la Habana, Cuba: Editorial SI-MAR.

Canizares, R. (1999). *Cuban Santería: Walking with the night.* Rochester, VT: Destiny Books.

Clark, M. (2005).*Where men are wives and mothers rule: Santería ritual practices and their gender implications.* Gainesville, FL: University Press of Florida.

Cortez, J. (2000). *The Osha: Secrets of the Yoruba-Lucumi-Santeria religion in the United States and the Americas.* Brooklyn, NY: Athelia Henrietta Press Inc.

Dodson, J. (2008). *Sacred spaces and religious traditions in Oriente Cuba.* Albuquerque, NM: University of New Mexico Press.

Garoutte, C., & Wambaugh, A. (2007). *Crossing the water: A photographic path to the Afro-Cuban spirit world.* Durham, NC: Duke University Press.

Gonzalez Gallardo, C. (1990). *Ache Moyuba Orisha: Sobre la santería cubana.* Video. TVL Television Latina.

Hearn, A. (2004). Afro-Cuban religions and social welfare: Consequences of commercial development in Havana. *Human Organization, 63*(1), 78–88.

Lachatañeré, R. (2004). *El Sistema Religioso de los Afrocubanos.* Habana, Cuba: Editorial de Ciencias Sociales.

Murphy, J. (1993). *Santería: African spirits in America.* Boston, MA: Beacon Press.

Murrell, N. S. (2010). *Afro-Caribbean religions: An introduction to their historical, cultural and sacred traditions.* Philadelphia, PA: Temple University Press.

Newby, A. C., Riley, D. M., & Leal-Almeraz, T.O. (2006). Mercury use and exposure among Santeria practitioners: Religious versus folk practice in northern New Jersey, USA. *Ethnicity and Health, 11*(3), 287–306.

Nodal, R., & Ramos, M. (2005). Let the power flow: Ebó as a healing mechanism in Lukumí Orisha worship. In P. Bellegarde-Smith (Ed.), *Fragments of bone: Neo-African religions in a New World.* Chicago, IL: University of Illinois Press.

Ramos, M. (2006). Diplo *Santería* and pseudo-Orishas. *Eleda.org.* Retrieved April 10, 2006, from http://ilarioba.tripod.com/articlesmine/diplororishas.htm

Sandoval, M. (1979). Santeria as a mental health care system: An historical overview. *Social Science and Medicine, 13B,* 137–151.

Sandoval, M. (2006). *Worldview, the Orichas, and Santería.* Gainesville, FL: University Press of Florida.

Tracy, E. A. (2005). Divine women in Santeria: Healing with a gendered self (master's thesis). Florida State University.

Wedel, J. (2004). *Santería healing: A journey into the Afro-Cuban world of divinities, spirits, and sorcery.* Gainesville, FL: University Press of Florida.

9

PUERTO RICAN SPIRITISM (*ESPIRITISMO*)

Social Context, Healing Process, and Mental Health

Jesus Soto Espinosa and Joan D. Koss-Chioino

Introduction

Spiritism is a philosophical and "scientific" movement codified by a French scholar in Paris in the mid-19th century. *Espiritismo* (Spiritism) developed from a "scientific exploration" of disincarnate, eternal spirits that survive the death of human beings, using records of the experiences of young mediums in séances, and later collecting similar data from many groups across the world (Kardec, 1994). The scholar, Allan Kardec (1804–1869), a pseudonym chosen by Leon Hippolyte Denizarth Rivail, published six books and a review organ, which were translated and republished throughout many countries. These works codified the practices and philosophy of Spiritism. The movement spread first to Spain and then to Latin America, carried by scholars who studied in France or Spain. The ideas and moral philosophy of Kardec lead to Latin American elites' view of Spiritism as a special psychological science. Moreira-Almeida and Klaus Chaves (2011) note:

> Allan Kardec was a pioneer in proposing scientific investigation of psychical phenomena. Kardec was an influential scholar in Europe during the second half of the 19th Century (Sharp, 2006, p. xvi). According to Monroe (2008, p. 96), he was one of the most widely read philosophers of the period; his first book on Spiritism, *Le Livre des Esprits* (The Spirits' Book), was a best seller, with 22 editions in 17 years. Despite his historical relevance and the fact that Kardec's books were translated into several languages, and continue to be quite popular selling millions of copies,[1] his research work and methods are still poorly known by historians, Spiritists, and parapsychologists.
>
> (p. 136)

This is still the view of many educated Spiritists in the 21st century; however, less educated people in the rural and urban barrios in Puerto Rico, Latin America and the Latin Caribbean syncretized Spiritism with their indigenous systems of healing, consisting of folk, Catholic and Afro-Caribbean beliefs and practices (Nuñez Molina, 1991) This movement includes ethical and moral regulations about spirit behavior (both incarnate and disincarnate), and an ontological epistemology that specifies a cycle of disincarnation and reincarnation with a goal of the inevitable evolution of the individual spirit. Disincarnated spirits reside in a dimension apart from incarnated beings, but they contact that world mainly through mediums who have developed their faculties (Kardec, 1998).

This chapter first offers an overview of the principles of Spiritism, its history, philosophy, and belief system. It then offers a discussion of the impact of Puerto Rico's colonial status vis-à-vis Spain and then the United States on the acceptance of Spiritist healing. It then reviews the principles and belief system of Spiritists. It describes healing practices and the processes by which one becomes a healer and how it is viewed by the mental health profession. We then consider the current sociocultural perspective towards spirituality as significant for well-being among Puerto Ricans. Finally, we briefly describe the implications of spirit healing for mental health, and for broadening an understanding of spirituality. We propose that this understanding is important to training mental health professionals who treat both Puerto Ricans and other Latin Americans. A brief description of a training project in Puerto Rico in the late 1970s is included. The project aimed to create a bridge among community mental health workers, medical residents and Spiritist healers over three years in three large mental health catchment areas.

Spiritism under Spanish and American Colonial Influence

Allan Kardec established Spiritism in France during the year 1857 with the publication of *The Spirits' Book*. This was just after the foundation of the Spiritualist movement by Emanuel Swedenburg in England (in 1840), and the Fox sisters' phenomena in the United States in 1848. Spiritualism was accepted by many in the United States, while Spiritism spread to Latin America and the Hispanic Caribbean. *Espiritismo* was introduced into Puerto Rico during the second half of the 19th century. Puerto Rico was then a Spanish colony and, therefore, Puerto Ricans went to Spain to obtain university degrees. Consequently, the educated islanders were influenced by Spiritist ideology and brought it back to the Island. Officially the first Spiritist group was instituted in the year 1881—"Centro Union," known today as "Centro Renacimiento." Nevertheless, informal Spiritist activities took place many years before 1881, as recorded by some Puerto Rican philosophers' writings (Ramos-Perea, 2011). By 1889 Spiritists founded their first charity hospital, open to persons of all socioeconomic and religious backgrounds (Rodriguez-Escudero, 1991).

The first reference to Spiritualism in Puerto Rico was in 1856 in *La Guirnalda*, a popular Spanish magazine that reported an abundance of séance activity in San Juan. However, under Spanish political influence all Spiritist activities were suppressed, both by the government, the Catholic Church, and the proto-medicates. These last two basically were one social body. However, a number of Puerto Rican patriots acted to develop progressive legislative reform and spread Spiritism throughout the community. In 1873, Don Manual Conchado Juarbe, a deputy from Puerto Rico, presented to the Spanish Cortes a revision of a bill for educational reform in which Spiritism should be substituted for the teaching of metaphysics in secondary schools (Rodriguez-Escudero, 1991). In sum, the Spanish period was characterized by social–political intolerance towards the Spiritist movement—and sporadic, active repression.

Under the American influence, however, repression was released to a large extent, giving way to the development of a significant presence of the Spiritist movement in the early 20th century. An example of this is that, mainly due to the Spiritist Federation campaign, the death penalty was eliminated as a corrective option of the Puerto Rican penal code (Rodriguez-Escudero, 1991).

The North American Spiritualists' movement influenced the Island's belief system towards accepting *Espiritismo*. Overall, America presented a sort of religious and spiritual crisis; the romanticist and rationalist values, together with new perspectives of science and the need for a more personal encounter with the spiritual, made Spiritism a perfect vehicle for the nourishment of its movement (Herzig, 2001). Spiritism, in Puerto Rico, is also associated with a nationalist ideology. Spiritism teaches independence as a natural consequence of the spirit's evolution. Therefore, many Puerto Ricans adapted this knowledge, from a sociological perspective, as a way to appraise the Island's social–political reality. But, such ideas made Spiritism fall under prejudice and suspicion from the Spanish colonial government. Religious freedom and tolerance was truly practiced after the American invasion in 1898. North American's political dominance gave way to the progressive movements of modernization and classical liberalism. Kardec's work advocated that the State facilitate the expressions of fundamental civil rights—free from harassment, censorship, and repression (Garcia-Leduc, 2009). Under the new flag of U.S. colonialism, the Spiritist Federation was established in 1903. It campaigned to optimize civic democracy, separation between the church and state, literacy, feminism, the abolition of the death penalty, and the right to vote (Herzig, 2001).

Under this new air of social tolerance, by the last half of the century, behavioral health professionals began to explore Spiritist healing procedures and their health relevance in a systematic manner (for example, Koss, 1975; Rogler & Hollingshead, 1965). As the Puerto Rican migration made Puerto Ricans more visible on the mainland, the American health system needed to better understand Puerto Ricans' attitudes towards the health system. It had to find ways to encourage this group of Latinos to engage with it.

The Social and Political Context of Popular Healing in Puerto Rico

Puerto Ricans are heirs to two equally popular but competing worldviews from the 19th century: the "scientific" and the "spiritual." Examples of this conundrum are the persistence, since the late 19th century, of the widespread philosophy of "Spiritism" (*Espiritismo*) and the ready reception of the Cuban cult, *Santería*, since the mid-20th century. There are actually three main types of Spiritism in Puerto Rico: "Popular," "Christian oriented," and "Kardecian." Popular Spiritist healing rituals are focused on "working" with spirits in small home-based *centros* staffed by four to six mediums, most of whom are usually women. These centers hold two or more weekly sessions with as many as 25 to 40 attendees. The mediums may incorporate spirits and/or experience visions in order to heal (*sanar*) supplicants, who bring a wide diversity of health and social problems (Garrison, 1977; Harwood, 1977; Koss, 1975; 1977; Rogler & Hollingshead, 1965). Christian oriented Spiritism is known as the Consejo Moral movement, which is even more popular in Latin American countries such as Brazil, Colombia, and Mexico. Although healing is practiced, this religious movement focuses more on the study of moral and philosophical implications of individual distress as communicated by spirits (Saavedra, 1969). The Kardecian movement has centers in most towns and cities in Puerto Rico. It values all of the above mentioned practices, including healing. However, it also focuses on philosophical and scientific study of the spirit world as "free thinkers," constantly seeking knowledge of the dual worlds of incarnate and disincarnate spirits (Aizpurua, 2000).

Spiritist adherents and those who utilize healing rituals in Puerto Rico range in social–economic strata from lesser educated rural persons, to relatively rich upper class persons, some of whom are politically influential. There is a wide range of reasons for utilization of Spiritist healing as detailed below.

The popular acceptance and practice of Spiritist healing appears to be the result of widespread social conflicts within a difficult island economy (Hohmann et al., 1990). These situations are generated by a continuing quasi-colonial status which creates numerous acculturative stresses. Variations on this form of popular ritual healing have developed over the last three decades; *Santería*, a Cuban import, based on mostly West African religious beliefs and rituals, has gained in popularity since the mid-20th century (Fernandez Olmos & Paravisini-Gebert, 2003). It has been syncretized with Spiritism, mainly in the United States (often referred to as Mesa Blanca), but may now be waning in Puerto Rico. There are also other religious groups with healing practices that have steadily increased in popularity, such as hundreds of Evangelical and Pentecostal churches. What we now call "comprehensive and alternative medicine" (CAM) has been increasingly accepted in this mix of popular healing systems over the last three decades, and includes some spiritually based healing disciplines (Koss-Chioino & Soto Espinosa, 2013).

Early observers of spirit healing among the less educated noted that popular Spiritism was a resource for the less educated and lower socioeconomic classes to use to manage emotional and behavioral problems. Popular healing is used as a strategy to overcome the despair of chronic illness, difficult family problems, and existential discomfort—all of the persistent ills that plague human beings. Although the community mental health system was established in Puerto Rico beginning in 1963, mandated to deal with severe behavioral problems, such as addictions and mental illness for all Puerto Ricans, nevertheless persons from all socioeconomic classes in Puerto Rico take recourse to Spiritist healers in times of emotional distress. This is the case whether they are being treated by mental health professionals in the public health system or privately seeing a pastoral counselor, psychiatrist, or priest. Theirs is a pragmatic approach to dealing with emotional problems, whether caused by stress or physical illness.

Principles of *Espiritismo*: History, Philosophy, and Belief System

Spiritism's basic principles have been borrowed from different philosophical, cultural, and religious traditions. Its ideas about the Supreme Being, life as eternal and spiritual and as an evolutionary experience, the immortality of the soul, spirit communication, the Law of Cause and Effect, and reincarnation are not new. However, Spiritism contributes a new theoretical approach and an understanding of these ideas from rationalist, naturalist, humanistic, non-dogmatic, and free thinker perspectives. The idea of a Supreme Being or God is, in Spiritism, the acknowledgment of the existence of a greater intelligence that organized life. Life is inexorably without end, where the spirit continuously progresses through different experiential stages of existence that guide it toward greater levels of spiritual maturity, individuality, and humanism (Denis, 1909; Novich-Hernandez, 1999). Therefore, the spirit/Self or consciousness, which is an emotional and intellectual entity, develops from being unconscious to conscious of its self individuality and independent decision making processes (Geley, 1995; Guimares-Andrade, 1992). The dynamics of this process is guided by free-willed decisions which generate positive and negative outcomes that influence the souls' evolutionary process. The spirit utilizes reincarnation as a method to access corporal life experiences, beyond those of non-corporal nature, as well. Each entity, while in the spirit dimension, assesses its moral and intellectual evolutionary necessities to then select an appropriate physical life environment that cultivates and complements the continuous formation of the Self. In sum, life is viewed essentially as one, where sometimes the spirit acquires schooling through corporal bodies, and, at other times without a body.

It is the reincarnation principal that mainly distances *Espiritismo* (Spiritism) from Spiritualism; reincarnation is not accepted by spiritualists (Moreira & Lotuf Neto, 2005a). Nevertheless, Spiritists, through the use of the reincarnation factor, consider themselves to be better equipped to theorize upon concerns associated with natural differences among individuals, societies, justice, and ethical/moral inequities at large. Although Kardec considered *Espiritismo* a science, it is equally viewed by him as a philosophy. Science is the instrument that facilitates the exploration and validation of the spirit's world (Delanne, 1990; Grosvater, 1974).

The core Spiritist belief is that after a person's corporal death there is life after life. This means that the disincarnated person's spirit can communicate with incarnated spirits after the disposal of its body. The return of a spirit or its consciousness may present positive or negative effects over the environment where such intelligent energy communicates. Communication will be dependent upon the level of spiritualization to which each spirit has evolved within the spiritual levels. Materialistic spirits tend to focus their psychological necessities towards the material world; these tend to deny their new spiritual reality, therefore, insisting on reenacting activities they performed while incarnated. On the other hand, spiritualized beings may reappear among the incarnated, limited to the purpose of sharing some idea that may inspire the observed to evolve on intellectual and moral terms. Therefore, Spiritist sessions continuously assess each of their participants' spiritual needs. And, if a spirit is detected that insists on being intrusive, persistent, and recurrent over the free will of another person, using the Spiritist diagnostic condition, "spirit obsession," mediums act to correct this situation.

Spirit obsession differs from Christian possession in that Spiritism does not acknowledge that a spiritual being was created with the only purpose of developing destructive behaviors. Spiritism postulates that neither demons nor evil exists; instead that life is surrounded by independent self-evolutionary decision-making processes that develop positive and negative effects towards the self and its environment. People and spirits are neither good, nor bad; their moral character is dependent upon their spiritual, intellectual, and moral self-evolution. Therefore, the Spiritist psycho-spiritual therapy to treat spiritual obsession is known as "dis-obsession" therapy. Here mediums basically first educate the incarnated participants about the existence of spirits and their possibilities of action. Then, the mediumistic therapeutic team (mediums with clairvoyance, incorporation, telepathy, magnetism, automatic writing—among other faculties) works to detach the spirit obsessor, and educate it. The incarnated person affected is informed about the ties that attach them, and about the mutual benefits for the spirit's retreat and spiritualization. Another general core treatment issue, treated many times during mediumistic sessions, is the identification of persons who are suffering due to their misunderstanding of spiritual experiences, once mainstream medicine has been exhausted. For example, some persons begin to hear voices that are logical, coherent, relevant, intelligent, and able to offer details that are verifiable. Nonetheless, these experiences are usually taken by psychiatrists for psychotic symptoms that in spite of psychiatric treatment do not end. These participants in the sessions are often viewed as mediums who are beginning their mediumistic development. Consequently, if the participant agrees, he/she is trained to carry out mediumistic work. Hence, what once was interpreted as psychopathology, now, through knowledge of Spiritist work, is understood as an opportunity to spiritually develop and engage within a community healing network (Koss-Chioino, 2012; Moriera-Almeida & Lotufo, 2005b).

Spiritism and the Healing Process

In the early 70s, at the request of the Department of Health of Puerto Rico, the second author applied to the National Institute of Mental Health (NIMH) for a grant to develop an interface between Spiritist healers and the public (mental) health system (Koss-Chioino, 2008). The Puerto Rican Department of Health proposed that encounters of traditional spirit healers with mental health professionals might facilitate the health department's mandate to deliver community care to the mentally ill, because popular healers saw more troubled persons than did mental health care professionals. The NIMH division that received the application sponsored a site visit of one of its project officers. At the San Juan airport at the specified time Koss-Chioino and students met a distinguished older man. He was somewhat distressed, claiming that our typical Puerto Rican hospitality was excessive, that we should not have met him at the airport, or arranged for his accommodations. That evening he was taken to a Spiritist healing session. Halfway through the three-hour session the spirits called him to the table to be treated. In good grace he went to the table where the mediums were seated and afterwards demanded that we translate what they (actually the spirits) had said. In considerable discomfort, we softened the spirits' words: he would suffer from cancer in the next several years! Despite his open disbelief in their prediction and our fears, he recommended that the project be funded. Three years into the project we received word from the NIMH that he was no longer there, having succumbed to cancer!

This sort of revelation occurred many times in the course of research in Puerto Rico. It was especially startling when a consultant or friend attending a healing session for the first time would be told by the spirits about a serious illness that the friend had never discussed. How could the spirit mediums divine problems so accurately when these visitors had never attended a Spiritist session?

Although educated Spiritists study and discuss Kardec's writings, and some channel the spirits' advice and predictions, most adherents' contact with Spiritism in Puerto Rico is in healing rituals at a *centro* as a medium or supplicant. Explanations in the literature do not adequately account for Spiritist healers' work, the spirits' diagnoses and predictions, or the affects of both healers and supplicants, both positive and negative. Here we describe a model of ritual healing process related to becoming a medium for most healers. There are three foundational components: spiritual transformation, relation, and radical empathy. In this model of the core elements of ritual healing process, spiritual transformation is both the entry event in healer development and an ongoing personal experience of healers—often begun when they undergo their initiatory experience (see, for example, Csordas & Lewton, 1998; Katz, 1993; Katz & Wexler, 1990; Peters,

1981). Sufferers in many healing traditions also undergo spiritual transformation as a result of their contact with a tradition that recognizes its importance in healing practices.[2] Among the Puerto Rican Spiritist healers studied, some sufferers were diagnosed as "in development" as a healer when they showed signs, such as vivid visions or communication with spirits during or following severe illness, which indicated that an spiritual awakening and/or transformation was taking place (Pargament, 2006).

Koss proposes a model supported by the assumption that cultural variations in ritual healing—very different mythic worlds, including different schemas to identify illness and disorder and variations in many ritual procedures—are elaborations of content and context rather than process (Koss-Chioino, 2006). This parallels Hufford's (2005) notion of "core spiritual experiences (CSE)" that "show complex and consistent subjective patterns independent of cultural context" (p. 33). Hufford proposes that core spiritual experiences form a "distinct class of experience with a stable perceptual pattern" (2005, p. 33). This is also characteristic of spiritual transformation, which could be considered a special variant of CSE. Spiritual transformation appears to be particularly associated with rituals that heal with spirits, which have very similar forms across diverse cultures and regions of the world.

We note that some healers do not undergo a painful wounding and transformation. Instead, they experience deepening knowledge of the spirit world that becomes inspirational and spiritually redirects their lives. Observations show that they are no less effective as mediums who undergo transformative experiences; they also serve to anchor a therapeutic space on behalf of sufferers. Whatever the path to mediumship, mediums may employ or specialize in the use of clairvoyance, automatic writing, intuition, healing at a distance, telepathy, and incorporation of spirits.

Relationship of Healers to the "Sacred"

In most cultures living beings and spirit/god beings are commonly believed to occupy separate realms. In Spiritism spirits are visible under special ritual circumstances but may also appear to persons outside of the ritual context who have developed the faculties to see into or communicate with the spirit world (Koss-Chioino, 2006). Actual contact with what is deemed sacred is often achieved when living beings and spirit/god realms interpenetrate. Sacred space is created anew at each ritual session through communion with spirits/gods. Communion (defined this way) may take three main forms: visions of the spirit world; journeys to that world; and voluntary (but also involuntary for persons who are not "developed") intimate contact (i.e., embodiment,) with spirit beings. In Spiritism for example, embodiment both by a protector/guide spirit or by an intrusive, often harmful spirit takes place (the latter resulting in displacement of one's own spirit). Healers learn how to control communication with spirits or gods through the tutelage and/or observation of other healers. The most important aspect is that they experience spirits in ways that are both personally and cosmically meaningful (Koss-Chioino, 2006). In fact, all of the spirit-medium healers worked with (over 100) did not identify themselves as "healers," but rather as the vessels through which healing forces are summoned and transmitted to and from supplicants. Spiritist healers say that they "lend their bodies" to spirits, high or low, good or misguided, who are agents of both distress and removal of distress.

Given widespread belief in the special qualities of extraordinary beings across many cultures, experience of these beings during a life-threatening illness can make a significant impression on the sufferer (who is in a state of high emotional arousal—confused, fearful, desperate, and socially withdrawn). As Frankl (1959) observed long ago (and many writers since), there are many reports of transcendence in the context of suffering, facilitated by both psychological and physical factors. If a healer is present who establishes a meaningful association between a spiritual entity and the hope of, or actual relief from, danger and /or suffering, the spirit can take on significant personal meaning for the sufferer. This then appears to reinforce or establish belief in the power of extraordinary beings (spirits, God, gods), as has been noted throughout years of anthropological writings on illness and healing. One might say, following Csordas (1994), for those who hold a worldview centered on the self, that the spirit-other becomes "embodied" within the self. In Spiritism and numerous other spirit-healing cults, embodiment of spirit can be experienced as the continual, often lifelong, presence of one or more spirit alters with whom a special relationship is maintained. A personal spirit protector/ guide (or several) in Spiritism makes healing work not only possible but also safe from contagion, that is, free of being affected by distress-causing spirit beings brought to the healing session on behalf of suffering clients.

Spiritist healers described vivid, dissociated states during their initiation illness: they saw themselves as "doubled," "suspended from the ceiling looking down on themselves lying in bed," and said they "knew" they were dead and their soul had separated from their body. A strong emotional impact lingers after their return to the daily world; familiar landmarks of adaptive feeling and thinking appear to lose their meaning. Marking of the internal passage of time is either distorted or missing during the crisis phase of the illness. In this state of consciousness the novitiate healer acquires the capacity to see into and then directly experience the spirit/ God/gods realm. The affects in this experience of the sacred are deep fear, awe, and fascination. Later, the novitiate gradually learns how to interact with beings in this realm and loses some of the fear and awe, but never all of it. These experiences seem to have a strong effect on the sufferer's view of their life world and their role in it. What the recovering person reports is a sea change, a transformation that includes the realization of a mission on which they feel compelled to embark, albeit with the aid of the extraordinary being(s) encountered during their illness. Heightened social bonding is also a common outcome. And there is fear and awe, as well as fascination, much as Otto (1923) describes. These changes are not always or immediately acted upon, however.[3]

Facility at visual imagery, as the beginning and most common form of communion with the spirit realm, seems to emerge from the initial crisis event when the novitiate healer begins to interpret, concretize, and integrate belief in what she/he has "seen" while in an altered state. In Spiritism, as in other shamanic healing practices, this ability is cultivated and expanded through the tutelage of healer-adepts, but it also seems to be cultivated by the healer herself/himself. Many ascribe this ability to the teaching of a spirit.

Although largely speculative, we will attempt to briefly describe the current extent of popularity of Spiritism in Puerto Rico and the United States. In general, in both places, spirituality as an interest and experience among Latinos is more widespread now than it was in the 20th century, both within and without religious institutions. In Puerto Rico, many Catholics attend mass and observe the sacraments but also may take recourse to Spiritist rituals when they or family members are in distress. This is not the case, however, for those involved in evangelical churches, such as Baptist or Pentecostal. More Puerto Ricans and North Americans now enjoy a college education, and many exercise an intellectual interest in spirituality. In Puerto Rico this is aided by visiting lecturers from the US and from some Latin American countries, such as Brazil and Venezuela. Small town folks, outside of the large metropolitan areas, continue to practice spirit healing in their home-based centers as they have since the early 20th century.

In Puerto Rico we are now documenting how conventional medical doctors who experienced Spiritism as part of early family life, or have been spiritually transformed by traumatic events, incorporate their beliefs in spirits, or their ability to be psychic, into their, mainly allopathic, clinical work.

A group of Brazilian Spiritists have been establishing *centros* across the United States, in addition to several of Puerto Rican origin dating back to the 1950s and 1960s. There is a Brazilian Spiritist Medical Association that has held two annual meetings in the Washington, DC area and also one in Florida. This is one aspect of a series of conferences that aim to link Spiritist principles and healing techniques with mainstream medicine in the United States, according to the model of psychiatric hospitals in Brazil (Bragdon, 2012). Given this growing popularity, the future of Spiritism looks quite promising, even though belief in and experience of spirits is still suspected of heresy and superstition in many formal religious settings, and of pathology in many conventional psychiatric institutions.

Espiritismo and Mental Health Care Practices

As referred to above, Koss-Chioino was invited by the NIMH to submit a proposal for a project in Puerto Rico that would incorporate Spiritist healing practices as a community mental health resource. The Division of Mental Health of the Department of Health of Puerto Rico had been reorganized as a community mental health program in accordance with the U.S. Community Mental Health Act (1963), and its chief agreed to sponsor the project as part of its community mandate. Moreover, Spiritist practitioners were perceived as seeing more persons in emotional distress than did the community mental health clinics. The general goals of the Therapist-Spiritist Training Project as conceived in 1975 were: 1) to establish a forum for the meaningful mutual exchange of information between Spiritist mediums and mental health professionals (primary care medical doctors in training were later added); 2) to offer a training curriculum to transfer knowledge and skills across the two healing systems; and 3) to develop new psychotherapeutic approaches from a synthesis of the most relevant and effective healing techniques in both systems. It was decided to run the same program in three different communities for three years, in order to explore possible differences in community response and conditions for replication.

Data from the Spiritist-Therapist Training Project documented the types of complaints taken to the Spiritists compared with those brought to the mental health system (Koss-Chioino, 1992; 1995; Moreira-Almeida & Koss-Chioino, 2009). Forty-nine medium healers were the focus of several studies that included: interviews in which they told their life stories, especially their development as spirit healers; videotaped observations of them at work in their *centros* (portrayed in four video-shows that are still available); and interviews with a sample of new clients they treated at *centro* sessions. Participants who contributed their life stories and samples of patients also included 38 mental health professionals and 17 medical residents. These data showed a clear division of labor: non-serious emotional and bodily distresses were more often brought to the Spiritists, and severe emotional distress (diagnosable as mental illness) was most often seen by mental health professionals. However, many persons used the two systems consecutively according to the amount of relief each was expected to provide, or due to dissatisfaction with any of the interventions.

The most salient outcome was that Spiritists and therapists began to refer themselves to the other healing system for help; they later began referring a few patients. The possibility of formalizing referrals was realized when a mental health technician participating in the project, who had experience with Spiritism through seeking help for her schizophrenic mother, made a suicidal gesture. She was found by a boyfriend who took her to a health center in a town they were visiting. The attending physician had been at the project seminars and agreed with her plea that she not be referred to mental health services. Instead she self-referred to a well-known Spiritist medium who participated in the project. She told the physician that she was afraid she would lose her job if treated in a mental health setting. He also felt that she might get better care (i.e., protection against another attempt) from the Spiritists, since he was dissatisfied with the lack of attention given another of his patients at the Community Mental Health Center (CMHC) emergency service. When the crisis had passed the therapist called a meeting of her colleagues and her supervisor at the home of the Spiritist who had cared for her and whose sessions she was still attending. Under the thin disguise of an anonymous recording as a "training" vehicle, she told the story of her psychological crisis. Since the Spiritists had diagnosed her as "obsessed" (i.e., taken over by a spirit), she could claim lack of awareness of her actions and lack of responsibility; therefore, she did not expect negative sanctions. Her plan worked. It illuminated the dilemma faced by mental health professionals who feel they cannot seek help for emotional crises from their colleagues. This lead to the establishment of a referral unit at the CMHC where we held the program during the second year.

The referral unit had its beginnings in the very first year of the Project's programs when four therapists and eight other CMHC staff participants consulted Spiritists about their anonymous patients. In years 2 and 3 a few referrals by Spiritist participants, of their relatives or themselves, to mental health professionals, and referrals by therapists to Spiritists also occurred. We documented this process for four mental health workers and six medical doctors; in addition, four Spiritists consulted mental health professionals for their own problems. Once they acquired more knowledge about mental illness the Spiritists developed a new etiological category, "psychic cause," an addition to the usual dichotomy into material and spiritual causes, and a label that pointed to the need for psychological or psychiatric treatment.

Conclusion

Research into Spiritism as an ethnomedical practice continues to be important since distressed persons of various social strata and ethnicity in Puerto Rico and elsewhere seek help and solace from Spiritist mediums, as well as from complementary and conventional medicine. One attraction of Spiritist healing is that it avoids the stigma of psychiatric illness; it is also person-centered and empathic. It deals with spiritual crises without being dogmatic; supplicants feel supported and understood. Study of Spiritism as an ethnomedical system illuminates one kind of spirituality that is a model for health and mental health clinicians.

Notes

1. In Brazil alone, the three main publishing houses of the Spirits' Book (Federação Espírita Brasileira, Instituto de Difusão Espírita, and LAKE) have sold more than 4.5 million copies and new editions have been continuously printed.
2. What is healing? There are many versions of what healing means; a common explanation of the English term translates the word as "wholeness," with all of its many implications. Barasch (1993) provides a useful list of five healing outcomes (apart from curing a disease or injury): 1) sensitization, in which healing restores communication within oneself; 2) acceptance of pain; 3) finding meaning; 4) restoration of balance (physical, social, emotional, spiritual, etc.); and 5) willingness to change one's behavior and life style, to adapt to new circumstances. The model implicates all of these aspects of healing and is also inclusive enough to chart how each type is facilitated for both healers and clients. However, that exercise is beyond the scope of this chapter.

3. Highly significant mystical or transcendent experiences are reported to be associated with extensive change in the person's life in Puerto Rico, apart from development as a spirit healer or *santero*. It might also be noted that spontaneous visions of deceased persons are frequently reported by non-healers and nonbelievers in Spiritism, but they often involve personal meanings rather than cosmic or mystical associations.

References

Aizpurua, J. (2000). *Los fundamentos del Espiritismo*. Caracas, Venezuela: Ediciones CIMA.

Barasch, M. I. (1993). *The healing path: A soul approach to illness*. New York: G. P. Putnam's Sons.

Bragdon, E. (Ed.) (2012). *Spiritism and mental health*. London and Philadelphia, PA: Singing Dragon.

Csordas, T. (1994). *The sacred self: A cultural phenomenology of charismatic healing*. Berkeley, CA: University of California Press.

Csordas, T., & Lewton, E. (1998). Practice, performance and experience in ritual healing. *Transcultural Psychiatry, 35*, 435–512.

Delanne, G. (1990). *El Alma es inmortal* [*The inmortal soul*]. Barcelona: Editora Amelia Boudet.

Denis, L. (1909). *Here and hereafter: Being a treatise on spiritual philosophy*. New York: Brentano's.

Fernandez Olmos, M., & Paravisini-Gebert, L. (2003). *Creole religions of the Caribbean: An introduction*. New York and London: New York University.

Frankl, V. E. (1959). *Man's search for meaning*. Boston, MA: Beacon Press.

Garcia-Leduc, J. M. (2009). *Intolerancia y heterodoxias en Puerto Rico* [*Intolerance and heterodoxy in Puerto Rico*]. San Juan, Puerto Rico: Editorial Isla Negra.

Garrison, V. (1977). Doctor, espiritista or psychiatrist?: Health-seeking behavior in a Puerto Rican neighborhood of New York City. *Medical Anthropology, 1*, 64–185.

Geley, G. (1995). *Del inconsciente al consciente* [*Unconscious to the conscious*]. Caracas, Venezuela: Ediciones CIMA.

Grosvater, D. (1974). *Espiritismo laico* [*Laical Spiritism*]. Mexico City: Editores Mexicanos Unidos, S.A.

Guimares-Andrade, H. (1992). *Muerte, renacimiento, evolution* [*Death, rebirth, evolution*]. Caracas, Venezuela: Ediciones CIMA.

Harwood, A. (1977). *Rx: Spiritist as needed*. New York: John Wiley & Sons.

Herzig, N. (2001). *El Iris de Paz* [*Rainbow of peace*]. Rio Piedras, Puerto Rico: Ediciones Huracán.

Hohmann, A. A., Richeport, M., Marriott, B. M., Canino, G. J., Rubio Stipec, M., & Bird, H. (1990). Spiritism in Puerto Rico: Results of an island-wide community study. *British Journal of Psychiatry, 156*, 328–335.

Hufford, D. J. (2005). Sleep paralysis as spiritual experience. *Transcultural Psychiatry, 42*, 11–45.

Kardec, A. (1998). *El libro de los espiritus* [*The spirits' book*]. Buenos Aires, Argentina: Kier S. A. (Original work published 1857).

Kardec, A. (1994). *El libro de los médiums* [*The mediums' book*]. Caracas, Venezuela: Editora Cultural Espirita Leon Denis C.A.

Katz, R. (1993). *The straight path: A story of healing and transformation in Fiji*. Reading, MA: Addison-Wesley.

Katz, R., & Wexler, A. (1990). Healing: A transformational model. In K. Peltzer & P. Endigbe (Eds.), *Clinical psychology in Africa*. Eschborn, Germany: Fachbuchhandlung für Psychologie.

Koss, J. D. (1975). Therapeutic aspects of Puerto Rican cult practices. *Psychiatry, 38*, 160–170.

Koss, J. D. (1977). Social process, healing and self-defeat among Puerto Rican spiritists. *The American Ethnologist, 4*(3), 453–469.

Koss-Chioino, J. D. (1992). *Women as healers, women as patients: Mental health care and traditional healing in Puerto Rico*. Boulder, CO: Westview Press.

Koss-Chioino, J. D. (1995). Traditional and folk approaches among ethnic minorities. In J. F. Aponte, R. R. Rivers, & J. Wohl (Eds.), *Psychological intervention and treatment of ethnic minorities: Concepts, issues, and methods* (pp. 145–163). Needham Heights, MA: Allyn and Bacon.

Koss-Chioino, J. D. (2006). Spiritual transformation, relation and radical empathy: Core components of ritual healing process. *Transcultural Psychiatry, Special Issue dedicated to Dr. Raymond Prince, 43*(4), 652–670.

Koss-Chioino, J. D. (2008). Bridges between mental health care and religious healing in Puerto Rico. In R. A. Hahn & M. C. Inhorn (Eds.), *Anthropology and public health: Bridging differences in culture and society* (pp. 221–244). New York: Oxford University Press.

Koss-Chioino, J. D. (2012). Jung, spirits and madness. In E. Bragdon (Ed.), *Spiritism and mental health* (pp.126–139). London and Philadelphia, PA: Singing Dragon.

Koss-Chioino, J., & Soto Espinosa, J. (2013). Science and spirituality in the clinic: Medical doctors in Puerto Rico. MS in process.

Monroe, J. W. (2008). *Laboratories of faith: Mesmerism, Spiritism, and occultism in modern France*. Ithaca, NY: Cornell University Press.

Moreira-Almeida, A., & Klaus Chaves, A. (2011). Allan Kardec e o desenvolvimento de um programa de pesquisa em experiências psíquicas. In Jader dos Reis Sampaio. (Org.). *A Temática espírita na pesquisa contemporânea* (pp. 132–158). São Paulo: Centro de Cultura, Documentação e Pesquisa do Espiritismo.

Moreira-Almeida, A., & Koss-Chioino, J. D. (2009). Recognition and treatment of psychotic symptoms: Spiritists compared to mental health professionals in Brazil and Puerto Rico. *Psychiatry, 72*(3), 268–283.

Moreira-Almeida, A., & Lotufo Neto, F. (2005a). History of spiritist madness in Brazil. *History of Psychiatry, 16*, 5–25.

Moreira-Almeida, A., & Lotufo Neto, F. (2005b). Spiritist views of mental disorders in Brazil. *Transcultural Psychiatry, 42*(4), 570–594.

Novich-Hernandez, H. (1999). *Salud, enfermedad y muerte [Health, illness and death]*. Caracas, Venezuela: Ediciones CIMA.

Nuñez Molina, M. (1991). Reflexiones sobre posibles elementos anti-terapéuticas de las practicas espiritistas [Thoughts about possible anti-therapeutic Spiritist practics]. *Revista Puertorriqueña de Psicología, 7*, 13–22.

Otto, R. (1923). *The idea of the holy*. London: Oxford University Press.

Pargament, K. (2006). The meaning of spiritual transformation. In J. D. Koss-Chioino & P. Hefner (Eds.), *Spiritual transformation and healing: Anthropological, theological, neuroscience and clinical perspectives* (pp. 10–24). Walnut Creek, CA: Altamira Press.

Peters, L. (1981). An experiential study of Nepalese shamanism. *The Journal of Transpersonal Psychology, 13*, 1–26.

Ramos-Perea, R. (2011). *Literatura puertorriqueña del siglo XIX escrita por negros* [*Puerto Rican 19th century literature written by blacks*]. San Juan, Puerto Rico: Publicaciones Gaviota.

Rodriguez-Escudero, N. A. (1991) *Historia del Espiritismo en Puerto Rico.* Quebradillas, PR: Imprenta San Rafael.

Rogler, L. H., & Hollingshead, A. B. (1965). *Trapped: Families and schizophrenia.* New York: John Wiley & Sons.

Saavedra, A. (1969). *El Espiritismo como una religión: Observaciones sociologías de un grupo religioso en Puerto Rico.* Centro de Investigaciones Sociales: Universidad de Puerto Rico.

Sharp, L. L. (2006). *Secular spirituality: Reincarnation and Spiritism in nineteenth-century France.* Lanham, MD: Lexington Books.

10

REVIVAL

An Indigenous Religion and Spiritual Healing Practice in Jamaica

William Wedenoja and Claudette A. Anderson

Introduction

Revival is an indigenous Jamaican religion, with roots in West and Central African religious traditions and a slave religion known as *Obeah*. It took shape under the influence of Christian missionaries in the 19th century. Although a unique product of Jamaican history, Revival, which is also known as Zion or Revival Zion and as *Pocomania*, has much in common with other African-derived religions of the Caribbean. It is fundamentally African in the centrality of spirit possession and spiritual healing, as well as spiritual warfare, but it has also made significant accommodations to European Christianity.

Revival healing or Balm generally occurs in places called "balmyards" as well as in Revival healing services, worship services, and various "duties," "tables," and feast services. Practitioners—known variously as Spiritualists, Mothers or "Moddas", Bishops, Pastors, and Physicians—specialize in the relief of suffering, including mental illnesses, seen as spiritual illnesses. Although marginalized and criminalized, Revival healing is practiced widely and, in our view, is an effective and indispensable complement to the Jamaican biomedical system.

Indigenous religion and healing were demonized during the colonial period, which formally ended with independence in 1962, but they have gradually gained respect in the postcolonial period, beginning with a famous report on the Rastafari movement (Smith, Augier, and Nettleford, 1960) that paved the way to its acceptance by society. Since then Kumina, Revival, and even Obeah have been subjects of research by prominent Jamaican scholars such as Seaga (1969), Brathwaite (1978), and Chevannes (1995); articles in the popular periodical *Jamaica Journal* issued by the Institute of Jamaica; and exhibits produced by the African Caribbean Institute of Jamaica, including one on Obeah in 2011.

The public is generally supportive of traditional healing, particularly the use of herbs or "bush," so the practice of Balm is likely to persist for some time, even if the Revival religion itself does not. The medical profession, on the other hand, takes a dim view of it, believing that healers are guilty of practicing medicine without a license. From the perspective of the law, healers are also engaging in sorcery or Obeah, which is prohibited by Acts passed in 1760, 1810, 1817, 1833, and 1898 and renewed in 1973. Therefore, healing must be practiced clandestinely, although police and government will "look the other way" so long as healers keep a low profile or operate within the setting of a church.

Spiritual healing is not a dangerous activity. Nothing in our long association with Revival healers gives us reason to be concerned about them. Indeed, we have found Moddas to be generally wise, caring, trustworthy, and sincere people who are skilled in human relationships. Nor is spiritual healing antagonistic to medicine. In fact, healers themselves seek medical attention when necessary, and they refer their patients as well. Healers and doctors are not competitors but complementary parts of a single overall system of health care that have coexisted for centuries (Vom Eigen, 1992). Although biomedical and ethnomedical systems are based on different epistemologies, and serve different needs, patients demand both. They go to the medical doctor with natural illnesses and injuries, and seek herbal medicines as well as spiritual counseling and emotional support from spiritual healers. Healers are not practicing medicine in the biomedical sense; nor are they practicing sorcery. They are carrying on a cultural tradition with African roots, a tradition of problem solving that relies on spiritual experience and knowledge. According to this tradition, spirits influence our lives, for better or worse, and we must therefore attend to them. Those of us who cannot believe in spirits can at least concede that healing is a form of psychotherapy (Frank, 1974; Torrey, 1972) or "folk psychiatry" (Kiev, 1964) in which spirits symbolically represent subjective or mental realities. Healers are more like counselors or psychotherapists than doctors. But professional counseling and clinical psychology are not well established in Jamaica. And even if they were, healers would still be in demand because of their spirituality, which is immensely popular and something that counselors, psychologists, and doctors generally do not provide (Griffith, 1983).

Traditional healers should be allowed to practice publically, perhaps as "spiritual counselors." But some regulation would be necessary to protect the public, as is the case with other professional services. The distinction between Revival and Obeah is fuzzy. The Obeah Worker has the reputation of being a charlatan who takes advantage of desperate people. In addition, herbal remedies, like medicines, can be harmful. Government should therefore set standards and license and regulate healers. It is too easy for government to be repressive, or at least to be perceived as such, particularly by a profession that has always been marginalized. Therefore, healers need to regulate themselves as much as possible, by forming an association. One possible solution could be to create an advisory or regulatory board comprised of representatives from the biomedical community, the healing community, and researchers.

One of the main advantages of licensing is that healing would come under public scrutiny. Healers could be made to pay licensing fees and taxes and maintain proper accounting standards and hygiene. They would have to adhere to a professional code of ethics. Government could provide training in health care to licensed healers and facilitate referrals to biomedical practitioners. Surely these measures would lead healers to a higher standard of practice while reducing the stigma of traditional healing practices and mental illness and meeting the needs of the poor in particular.

The first step is to repeal the Obeah Act,[1] which defines Obeah so broadly that it could encompass any form of religious activity, if not the study of it. The law proscribes 1) consulting an Obeah Man, 2) being in possession of instruments of Obeah, and 3) composing, printing, selling, or distributing printed matter promoting "the superstition of Obeah," the punishment being imprisonment and/or flogging. Obeah laws were originally passed to deter resistance to slavery; hence, they are unnecessary today and only serve to marginalize African culture and privilege European culture, which "has left very deep scars" on the Jamaican psyche, according to the psychologist Madeline Kerr in her classic and incisive book *Personality and Conflict in Jamaica* (1952, p. x).

Additionally, government can and should promote research on healers. This can be accomplished via grants to the Institute of Jamaica, the African Caribbean Institute of Jamaica, and the universities, all of which have a mandate to investigate and promote the cultural heritage of Jamaica. The results of this research should be disseminated to the public. Healers would be encouraged to dialogue with researchers and with each other in conferences and workshops. A systematic study of balmyards and healers would be necessary to assess the income potential and health benefits of integrating folk psychiatry and psychotherapy into Jamaica's biomedical system. Repealing the Obeah Act and permitting healers to practice openly are vital first steps in healing the mental dis-ease of a postcolonial, post-slavery society that has long been forced to reject its own roots (Wedenoja, 2012).

The Emergence of Revival

Religion is a central facet of Jamaican life, and it seems to have three forms: 1) European denominations, including Anglicans, Moravians, Baptists, Methodists, Congregationalists, and Presbyterians (now merged in the United Church), Quakers, and the Salvation Army, which are waning; 2) American evangelical and Pentecostal churches such as the Adventists and several branches of the Church of God, which are very popular; and 3) religions that are indigenous to Jamaica, including *Kromanti* or *Maroon* religion, *Myalism*, the Native Baptists, *Kumina*, Revival, *Pocomania*, "Science," and *Jah Rastafari*, which emanate, to varying degrees, from *Obia* or African spiritualism (Anderson, 2010).

Revival is built on a syncretic foundation that includes Central and West African religion and European missionary Protestantism. It is fundamentally African in its emphasis on ritual possession by a pantheon of intermediary spirits that bear messages from God; a pattern of worship based on polyrhythmic drumming, dancing, and polyphonic song; elaborate mortuary rites to satisfy departed ancestors; healing practices that extend to all problems in living; and spiritual combat with *duppies*, restless souls that linger near the roots of silk cotton trees and can be captured and set on the living (Wedenoja, 1988, p.106).

The first recorded indigenous religion and medical practice was known as Obeah. Obeah Doctors interceded with spirits, to practical ends; healing the sick, protecting crops from thieves, finding lost or stolen property, gaining revenge, predicting the future, and offering protection from sorcery (Edwards, 1794). But Obeah acquired a sinister reputation. Obeah Doctors were feared for their skill in poisons, and they led numerous revolts, such as Tacky's Revolution in 1760, which led the Jamaica Assembly to pass the first of several laws criminalizing Obeah.

Obeah Men allegedly performed a ceremony called the "Myal Dance" to bring people back from death by administering a tonic and dancing around a subject "in a circle, stamping the ground loudly with their feet" (Lewis, 1834, p. 354), as in the "shouting" or "laboring" ritual practiced by Revival groups today. This practice became the core of an indigenous slave religion called Myalism. Myalists were also skilled at herbal remedies and often employed in the "hot houses" or slave infirmaries on plantations during the latter years of the 18th century (Sheridan, 1985).

A freed slave and ordained Baptist minister named George Lisle emigrated to Jamaica from America and established the Jamaica Baptist Free Church or "Black Baptists" in Kingston in 1784 (Brown, 1975). His church grew rapidly, but some of his leaders deviated from his teachings, apparently drawing on Myalism as they emphasized visions, dreams, and spirit possession and formed independent "Native Baptist" groups (Schuler, 1979). Lisle sought assistance from the British Baptist Society, which sent a missionary in 1814, and the Baptists quickly grew to be the most popular mission (Phillippo, 1843). A major insurrection known as "the Baptist War" occurred over the Christmas holiday of 1831 in northwest Jamaica. The revolt was organized by a slave and Baptist deacon by the name of Sam or "Daddy" Sharpe (Reckord, 1969). The seriousness of this revolt, which the planters blamed on missionaries, particularly the Baptists, and the severe reprisals inflicted by planters on slaves and missionaries, led Parliament to pass an Act of Emancipation in 1833 ending slavery in the British Empire.

A peasant society emerged after Emancipation with assistance from missionaries. But there was great hardship, due to the abrupt shift to free labor, demands for rent, wage disputes, severe drought, and a cholera epidemic, which was blamed on *duppies* and Obeah. Myalist "angel men" searched for Obeah substances using a talisman called the "amber," hunted down Obeah Men, and recovered lost "shadows" (souls) in the "Great Myal Procession" of 1841–1842, with similar incidents in 1845, 1848, 1849, and 1852 (Buchner, 1854). Membership in the Christian denominations declined dramatically (Patterson, 1967, pp. 214–215).

Missionaries sought to counter their decline by initiating a revival campaign in 1860, which spread rapidly across the island, as thousands sought redemption from sin. This "Great Revival" took on an ecstatic form in 1861 under the influence of Native Baptists and Myalists, who led processions from village to village, singing, drumming, becoming possessed by "angels," and gaining powers such as divination and healing (Gardner, 1909; Henderson, 1931). A new indigenous religion emerged, known simply as "Revival," which persists to this day. Revival became the spiritual backbone of the emerging peasant culture, in a society increasingly divided into what the historian Philip Curtin (1955) called "Two Jamaicas," black and white, indigenous and European.

Revival flourished for several decades after the Great Revival, with healing becoming increasingly prominent (Elkins, 1977) due to chronic distress, rampant disease, and lack of medical care. The religion also continued to evolve, being influenced by the arrival of the Salvation Army from England and Holiness churches from the United States. The culmination of the Revival tradition was the millenarian movement of Alexander Bedward, a healer who blessed the waters of the Hope River, near Kingston, and invited crowds numbering as many as 12,000 to be cured by it. Bedward was arrested and committed to an asylum in 1921 (Beckwith, 1929). Revival was eclipsed by the Adventist and Pentecostal movements during the 20th century (Wedenoja, 1980, 2002) and came to command a very small following as a religion, although remaining popular as a healing practice. Today, however, the religion seems to be enjoying a resurgence.

The Revival Healer

Revival healers are almost always women, commonly called "Mothers" or "Moddas," who define themselves as spiritualists or spiritual healers. Revival healers may also refer to themselves as "physicians," and say they are doing "physician work" (in the esoteric sense). Healing is understood to be a "gift" of the Holy Spirit, bestowed by a "messenger," an angel of God that teaches one how to heal and guides the practice. The messenger may take one on a journey in the spirit world, to gain knowledge and power. In return, the healer is obliged to "feed" the spirit. Healing is also a duty or obligation incurred in a "vision," typically during a severe illness, as a condition for getting well. Therefore, one cannot refuse this calling. People who become healers typically say they had strange dreams and visions as a child and were often sickly or otherwise different. These episodes are interpreted as a calling, which is often resisted but finally accepted.

A healer has at least two major powers. In addition to healing, there is the gift of discernment; that is, healers can see and identify spirits others cannot, and interpret messages from the spirit world. Discernment also allows the healer to "read" the condition of a client, as well as their past and future. Some claim to even feel the condition of the patient in their body and "draw" their pain. Revival leaders commonly have the gift of prophecy, to see into the future, and often issue "warnings" of "Judgment." Leaders and healers have mastery over the experience of trance, and can enter and exit the state seemingly at will, to consult their messengers.

The charismatic authority of a spiritual calling and spiritual gifts are foundations for healing, but certain personality characteristics are important too. Healers are often strict, authoritarian figures, who command respect. They have to show self-confidence to retain a following and clientele. They may be confrontational, using the force of their personality to change the direction of people's lives. At the same time, they must be caring and empathetic too. Hence, as Wedenoja (1989) has argued, a healer is a strong mother-figure, and mothers are revered in Jamaica. Most Moddas are associated with a Revival church. Revival provides the theological rationale for their work, which is always defined as spiritual healing. Typically, the founder and leader of a church is a healer.

The Revival Church and Balmyard

Revival is a pragmatic, this-worldly religion based on dramatic rituals and an unshakable belief in the power of The Spirit to affect human affairs. Virtually every Revival congregation is an autonomous group, formed by an inspired leader, typically in response to a vision or dream. Congregations are normally small, ranging from 10 to 50 in number. The membership is generally poor, although some Revival churches are now attracting middle-class followers. Members form a close-knit, supportive community and worship together several times a week. The place of worship could be as simple as a bamboo "booth" or a board shack with a tin roof, but some older and more successful groups have built substantial concrete buildings. The leader typically lives in a house next to the church.

Some Revival leaders receive a special "gift" of healing from God and operate a balmyard or healing center, where healing is performed regularly, both in public services and in private sessions. Healing is an important source of income for the leader and for the church. Private healing sessions are particularly remunerative. A balmyard is generally associated with a Revival church, but some do not have congregations, although they usually hold a short service before seeing clients. In either case, the Jamaican balmyard is understood to be a holy place where people are "working The Spirit" to effect healing.

A common sign of a Revival church and/or balmyard is one or more tall poles with colorful banners, erected to attract spirits as well as "pilgrims," particularly those in search of healing. Outside every church there will be a circular clearing with a pillar in the center and a glass of water with "leaf-of-life" in it and various fruits on top. This is a sacred place called the "seal" or "seal ground" where "angels" (Biblical spirits) dwell. Services include announcements, invocations, prayers, readings from the Bible, fasting, "testimonies," sermons, and hymns and "lively choruses" sung to musical accompaniment during which people stand and often dance.

Every effort is made to attract spirits to a service, using banners, altars, candles, uniforms, specific colors, flowers, oils, scents, drumming, singing, and the like. The spirits are called "angels" but they include Old Testament prophets and archangels (particularly Michael, Gabriel, Jeremiah, and Miriam), New Testament apostles, and sometimes a dove spirit, an Indian spirit, a fish spirit or an African spirit. Spirits are "messengers," conveying "warnings" from God and empowering participants in *myal* or possession, commonly known as "being in The Spirit." Possession is facilitated by a joyful state encouraged by lively singing and dancing, formerly to the tune of two goatskin drums and tambourines but now commonly to an electric guitar, keyboard, and trap set. Revival services have a structure, but there is much room for improvisation or spontaneity as The Spirit manifests itself. In addition, services are highly participatory events; everyone is encouraged to get directly involved.

Revival churches typically set aside at least one day a week for a public healing service. Each patient is commonly given a glass of "consecrated water" to drink in the service and then escorted individually to a private room where a bather rubs them, naked, with a wet cloth soaked in a basin of water in which herbs have been boiled, to cleanse their spirit (Barrett, 1976). Then the patient will have a private consultation with the healer in her "office." Healers also see clients privately throughout the week (Wedenoja, 1989). People with serious problems, as well as those of higher social status, generally prefer a private consultation, not wanting their condition to be public knowledge.

A private consultation with a healer begins with a "reading" or diagnostic exam, which can be done in various ways. According to Joseph Long (1973), Mother Rita read a patient's tongue, whereas Leonard Barrett (1976) said she read the palms of the client's hands. Steve Weaver (2003) reported that a healer selected passages at random from a Bible. Edward Seaga (1955) mentioned card-cutting and reading a leaf or the flames of a candle or a glass of water with a coin in it. Whatever the means, the healer is able to "see" a client's problem and prescribe a cure for it, with the assistance of her messenger, who may speak to her or put a thought in her head.

In a study by Long (1973), which compared the patients of doctors' and healers', patients preferred healers. As Keith Vom Eigen (1992) noted, healers spend more time with patients than do doctors. They conduct a more thorough diagnostic exam and provide a more detailed explanation of the problem. Healers and their clients are typically from the same social class and share a common worldview, whereas doctors are much better educated and of higher standing than the majority of patients. Therefore, healers usually have better communication and rapport with their clients (Wedenoja, 1989). Lower-class patients are generally submissive and deferential to a doctor because of their social standing, and are often reluctant or embarrassed to speak freely, particularly concerning spiritual matters. Healers are more attuned to interpersonal relationships and the psychosocial matrix of illness experiences, and they engage in much more counseling than doctors. The medical doctor sees illness in material and impersonal terms, as a natural condition, whereas the healer, and usually the client, sees it in a more personalistic and moral light, as something done to the client by another person, in which case it is an act of aggression. Healers are not just dealing with sickness, they are often confronting evil.

Conceptualizations of Illness and Health

Like the rest of Caribbean, Jamaicans are very health-conscious, and pursue a variety of natural and spiritual strategies to maintain health and well-being, such as: 1) eating good, clean, carefully prepared, and preferably natural, fresh, and hot foods; 2) keeping the body clean, not just externally but more importantly internally, including a periodic "washout" or purging of the colon; 3) avoiding imbalances created by mixing "hot" and "cold" matter; 4) drinking "bush teas" for preventive purposes and "roots tonics" to build potency, vitality, and nerves; 5) being careful not to strain one's "nerves," which is to say avoiding stress and overwork; 6) going to church, fasting and praying regularly, and getting baptized to build The Spirit; 7) refraining from evil ways and living "good" by avoiding offense to others or giving cause for envy; and 8) burning frankincense and myrrh in the house and keeping a Bible handy to ward off demons.

Two kinds of illness are generally recognized, "temporal" or natural and "spiritual" or unnatural (Wedenoja, 1989, p. 79). Natural illnesses are due to cold, gas, heat, bile, blood imbalances, and germs (Mitchell, 1983). Caribbean culture follows the humoral theory of illness of 18th century European medicine, which classified substances as hot or cold and strived to maintain a balance, often using bitter and sweet substances (Payne-Jackson & Alleyne, 2004, p. 39; Vom Eigen, 1992, p. 431). Spiritual illness could be a "chastisement" from God or an ancestor, but it is usually ascribed to a supernatural "trick" or "blow," employed through the medium of Obeah and motivated by envy, jealousy, or hatred.

Self-medication is the first course of action when illness appears (Wedenoja, 1989). One of the easiest, cheapest, and most popular remedies is "bush" or herbal medicine. If an illness does not respond to self-medication, then it is time to see a medical doctor. A sick person will generally visit a healer under three conditions: 1) in cases where biomedical practice has failed to provide relief, 2) upon experiencing vague symptoms that lead to feelings of disquiet and unease known as "bad feeling" or "funny feeling," and 3) on the occasion of prolonged or sudden and catastrophic misfortune. Mental illness may fall into any one of the foregoing categories. However, because of the stigma attached to mental illness and to treatment in a mental institution, many people take their mentally ill to the Revival practitioner as a first resort, even in extreme cases.

Mental illness is conspicuously public in Jamaica, and one of the main illnesses treated by Revival healers (Wedenoja, 1995). It is generally attributed to 1) natural causes, 2) supernatural causes or malevolent spirits, or 3) a spiritual calling to the healing profession. In the capital city of Kingston and surrounding parishes many balmyards can be recognized not by the usual multicolored flags, but by numerous "mad" persons milling about. In many cases, Revival healers assume the role of caretaker, often feeding them, taking them to hospital, and ensuring they are medicated by a medical doctor. Accordingly, although marginalized, the Jamaican Revival Church and its healing mission or balmyard may be seen as the preferred form of mental health care for many Jamaicans.

Revival and Mental Health Practices

Signs of mental illness are sometimes interpreted as a divine call to become a spiritualist. After a diagnosis is made, clients are usually "put on the ground" to "journey," so they may receive various "gifts" and begin to heal others. In this way, illness is normalized and the client assumes an elevated position of prestige and authority as well as a new role. However, if the patient is an "unwilling spiritualist," illness may persist so long as the individual refuses her divine vocation. This could mean a somewhat normal life with acute episodes, or an extended period of chronic illness. Hearing voices and seeing "visions," as well as vivid dreaming, are seen as "gifts of The Spirit," to be employed in the practice of healing. The client's ability to perfect these gifts under proper tutelage leads to unquestionable spiritual authority and makes for a successful and reputable healing practice.

Agitation and confusion resulting from stressful situations are often treated with counseling, bush teas, and bush baths. Recitation of verses from the Bible, chanting and the singing of hymns are also employed, along with head, foot, and hand massages. Revival healers are skilled at working with The Spirit, conceived as a form of spiritual energy, and energy work is one of the hallmarks of their trade. This is particularly true of healers whose balmyards or churches are located near rivers and ponds or where working with water is one of the healer's gifts. In such cases, people congregate at these places simply because being in the space makes them "feel better." Individuals are often obsessively concerned with maintaining their jobs, marriages, and relationships; securing the welfare of their children; and preserving their health, status, and possessions. Very often small misfortunes are seen as preludes to major disasters. One must be constantly on guard to protect hard-won respect and material possessions. Therefore, clients seek out healers for spiritual control and protection.

The use of spiritual techniques for personal retribution is widespread. "Madness" is sometimes said to result from a "spiritual blow" or "spiritual lick," which requires an involved and extensive treatment as well as protection from future attacks. In some cases people are said to be "set fi mad" for a specific number of days, after which they will return to full health. In such cases, where the period responds to a major event such as an exam or promotion, the Revival healer's job is simply to see that the patient comes through the period without undue harm to self. These acute cases contrast with the more chronic ones where individuals are said to be made to eat garbage, roam the streets naked, and inflict violence on themselves and others. If the patient can be taken to a healer then they generally remain with her until they have been cured. In cases where a patient has to be hospitalized, the healer may visit them in hospital or work on the case from a distance. Healers often counsel clients on the importance of good living, and try to steer them away from destructive behaviors and relationships.

Conclusion

As we have seen, Revival is a pragmatic, this-worldly, indigenous religion of Jamaica that is intimately associated with healing. Revival healing takes place in church services, healing places called balmyards, and in the offices of Revival healers. Revival healers are spiritual counselors who rely on trance or possession and spiritual insight to help clients, and their spiritual charisma gives them their authority and influence. They address the fears and anxieties of people, particularly the poor, in culturally appropriate ways that seem to be generally effective. Revival has its foundation in African beliefs and practices that were transformed under slavery, colonialism, and Christian missionization. It was marginalized and criminalized by a Eurocentric power structure and has to be practiced surreptitiously today, under the guise of religion, because of the Obeah Acts. Nonetheless, Revival is an essential part of the Jamaican heritage that should be embraced rather than disparaged. It has been healing the sick and comforting the distressed for centuries and should be allowed to do so publicly, ideally in conjunction with the biomedical system.

Note

1. "The Obeah Act," in *The Revised Laws of Jamaica*, Ministry of Justice. Retrieved February 2, 2011, from http://www.moj.gov.jm/law

References

Anderson, C. (2010). *Gnostic Obia from Chukwu Abiama to Jah Rastafari: A theology of the JamAfrican Obia Catholic Church* (Ph.D. dissertation). Interdisciplinary Studies, Emory University.

Barrett, L. (1976). Healing in a balmyard: The practice of folk healing in Jamaica, W.I. In W. D. Hand (Ed.), *American folk medicine* (pp. 285–300). Berkeley, CA: University of California Press.

Beckwith, M. W. (1929). *Black roadways: A study of Jamaican folk life.* Reprinted in 1969 by Negro Universities Press, New York.

Brathwaite, E. K. (1978). Kumina. The spirit of African survival in Jamaica. *Jamaica Journal*, *42*, 44–63.

Brown, B. (1975). George Liele: Black Baptist and Pan-Africanist 1750–1826. *Savacou*, *11/12*, 58–67.

Buchner, J. H. (1854). *The Moravians in Jamaica*. Reprinted in 1971 by Books for Libraries Press, Freeport, New York.

Chevannes, B. (Ed.) (1995). *Rastafari and other African-Caribbean worldviews*. New Brunswick, NJ: Rutgers University Press.

Curtin, P. D. (1955). *Two Jamaicas: The role of ideas in a tropical colony 1830–1865*. Cambridge, MA: Harvard University Press.

Edwards, B. (1794). African religions in colonial Jamaica. Reprinted in M. C. Sernett (Ed.), *Afro-American religious history* (pp. 19–23). Durham, NC: Duke University Press, 1985.

Elkins, W. F. (1977). *Street preachers, faith healers, and herb doctors in Jamaica*. New York: Revisionist Press.

Frank, J. D. (1974). *Persuasion and healing: A comparative study of psychotherapy*, revised edition. New York: Schocken.

Gardner, W. J. (1909). *A history of Jamaica from its discovery by Christopher Columbus to the year 1872 . . .* London: T. F. Unwin.

Griffith, E. E. H. (1983). The significance of ritual in a church-based healing model. *American Journal of Psychiatry*, *140*, 568–572.

Henderson, G. E. (1931). *Goodness and mercy: A tale of a hundred years*. Kingston: The Gleaner Company.

Kerr, M. (1952). *Personality and conflict in Jamaica*. Reprinted by Collins of London in 1963.

Kiev, A. (1964). The study of folk psychiatry. In A. Kiev (Ed.), *Magic, faith, and healing* (pp. 3–35). New York: The Free Press.

Lewis, M. G. (1834). *Journal of a West India proprietor, kept during a residence in the island of Jamaica*. Reprinted by Greenwood Press, Westport, CT, in 1970.

Long, J. K. (1973). *Jamaican healing: Choices between folk healing and modern medicine* (Ph.D. dissertation). Anthropology, University of North Carolina, Chapel Hill.

Mitchell, M. F. (1983). Popular medical concepts in Jamaica and their impact on drug use. *The Western Journal of Medicine*, *139*, 841–847.

Patterson, O. (1967). *The sociology of slavery*. Reprinted by Granada Publishing, London, for Sangster's Bookstores Limited, Jamaica, 1973.

Payne-Jackson, A., & Alleyne, M. C. (2004). *Jamaican folk medicine: A source of healing*. Kingston, Jamaica: University of the West Indies Press.

Phillippo, J. M. (1843). *Jamaica: Its past and present state*. London. Reprinted by Dawsons of Pall Mall, London, 1969.

Reckford, M. (1969). The slave rebellion of 1831. *Jamaica Journal*, *3*, 25–31.

Schuler, M. (1979). Myalism and the African religious tradition in Jamaica. In M. E. Crahan & F. W. Knight (Eds.), *Africa and the Caribbean: The legacies of a link* (pp. 65–79). Baltimore, MD: The Johns Hopkins University Press.

Seaga, E. (1955). Jamaica's primitive medicine. *Tomorrow* (Spring), 70–78. Reprinted in 1968 as Healing in Jamaica. In M. Ebon (Ed.), *True experiences in exotic ESP* (pp. 98–108). New York: Signet Mystic Books, The New American Library.

Seaga, E. (1969). Revival cults in Jamaica: Notes towards a sociology of religion. *Jamaica Journal*, *3*, 3–15.

Sheridan, R. B. (1985). African and Afro-West Indian medicine. In R. B. Sheridan (Ed.), *Doctors and slaves* (pp. 72–97). New York: Cambridge University Press.

Smith, M. G., Augier, R., & Nettleford, R. (1960). *The Ras Tafari movement in Kingston, Jamaica*. Mona, Jamaica: Institute of Social and Economic Research, University College of the West Indies.

Torrey, E. F. (1972). *The mind game*. New York: Bantam.

Vom Eigen, K. A. (1992). *Science and spirit: Health care utilization in rural Jamaica* (Ph.D. dissertation). Anthropology, Columbia University.

Weaver, S. R. (2003). *Health and illness in a rural community: A study of traditional health care practices in the Parish of St. Thomas, Jamaica* (Ph.D. thesis). Sociology, University of the West Indies, Mona, Jamaica.

Wedenoja, W. (1980). Modernization and the Pentecostal Movement in Jamaica. In S. D. Glazier (Ed.), *Perspectives on Pentecostalism: Case studies from the Caribbean and Latin America* (pp. 27–48). Washington, DC: University Press of America.

Wedenoja, W. (1988). The origins of Revival, a Creole religion in Jamaica. In G. Saunders (Ed.), *Culture and Christianity: The dialectics of transformation* (pp. 91–116). New York: Greenwood.

Wedenoja, W. (1989). Mothering and the practice of "balm" in Jamaica. In C. S. McClain (Ed.), *Women as healers: Cross-cultural perspectives* (pp. 76–97). New Brunswick, NJ: Rutgers University Press.

Wedenoja, W. (1995). Social and cultural psychiatry of Jamaicans, at home and abroad. In I. Al-Issa (Ed.), *Handbook of culture and mental illness: An international perspective* (pp. 215–230). Madison, CT: International Universities Press.

Wedenoja, W. (2002). Jamaica (I). In S. M. Burgess & E. M. Van Der Mass (Eds.), *The new international dictionary of Pentecostal and charismatic movements*, revised and expanded ed. (pp. 141–145). Grand Rapids, MI: Zondervan.

Wedenoja, W. (2012). The quest for justice in Revival, a Creole religion in Jamaica. In M. D. Palmer and S. M. Burgess (Eds.), *The Wiley-Blackwell companion to religion and social justice* (pp. 224–240). Chichester: Wiley-Blackwell.

11

SPIRITUAL BAPTISTS IN THE CARIBBEAN

Wallace W. Zane

Introduction

Spiritual Baptists are followers of an Afro-Caribbean religion found predominantly on the islands of St. Vincent, Trinidad, Tobago, Grenada, and Barbados, and that, carried with migrants, has a presence in England, Canada, and the United States (Zane, 1999).[1] Like other religions in the West Indies, its practitioners are sought out for healing by adherents and non-adherents alike.

The Spiritual Baptists have been called different names in different islands and at different times in their history: Converted, Penitent, Shakers, Shouters, Wesleyan Baptists, Tie-heads. The name most used today is "Spiritual Baptists," or sometimes just "Baptists." This has caused some concern among North American Baptist denominations as they feel the name should belong to their tradition alone (Hazell, 1994).

Though influenced by Africa, the Spiritual Baptist religion is a form of Christianity that reflects the British colonial reality at the time of the formation of the religion. The basic initiation ritual and most of the practices that make up a typical church service are African in origin, but apart from form, are not African, as they are given Christian meanings. Other practices of the Spiritual Baptists are primarily derived from British Methodism. The religion is not dogmatic, but mystical and revelatory. For example, customs and items found in the church service that Spiritual Baptists claim to come from Africa are often more easily traceable to other sources. However, that fact does not matter to the Spiritual Baptists; any contradiction is perceived only as a surface contradiction, possibly even laid by God to confound those who have worldly as opposed to deep knowledge gained in the spiritual world.

Spiritual Baptists, though a minority in each of the islands, have significance beyond their numbers, in part because it shows an alternative to the lived social reality of limited opportunity for poor people. Hence, an understanding of the Spiritual Baptist tradition is critical in order to understand the social context of Caribbean people as well as their conceptualizations of illnesses and their cures.

This chapter begins with a consideration of the history of Spiritual Baptists and an outline of their beliefs. Then, healing practices are detailed, with an emphasis on the spiritual nature of both healing and of learning the techniques of healing. Finally, the chapter will make recommendations for how this knowledge may be used by health and mental health specialists who encounter Spiritual Baptists in their practice.

History and Development

Spiritual Baptist tradition is a Christian religion that originated in the 1800s in the Caribbean, and has antecedent sources in the Fon and Kongo cultures of Africa (see, for example, Bilby & Bunseki, 1983). It is not an African religion adapted to Christianity, nor a form of Christianity molded out of an African religion; it is its own phenomenon, a syncretic product of the colonial encounter. Various researchers have labeled them as Protestants (Houk, 1995; Simpson, 1966), as an "African-Protestant synthesis" (Herskovits & Herskovits, 1947), as a monastic order (Malm, 1983), as polytheistic (Glazier, 1983; 1988), and as related to shamanism (Gullick, 1998; Zane, 1999). The adherents themselves often call their religion a mystery, and people who want to understand the faith and practice are told, "Come and taste." In other words, the only way to truly understand the religion is to convert and join them in their work.

The Spiritual Baptist religion increased in popularity in the early 20th century, and with its insistence that spiritual power can be conferred by God alone and does not need to be given by a temporal authority (including an ecclesiastical one), the European-dominated legislature on St. Vincent voted to make the religion illegal under the Shaker Prohibition Ordinance of 1912. Other islands followed, with Trinidad in 1917, and Grenada in 1927 (Zane, 1999). In the struggle to make the religion legal, worshippers continued their practices under a variety of names. The name that met with the least resistance was the Trinidadian name "Spiritual Baptist," and although a fairly recent term, is the name most often used by followers in the Caribbean and in the Caribbean diaspora today. The cultural power of Trinidad in the Eastern Caribbean is reflected in the fact that the Trinidadian name has wider recognition than the Vincentian term for the religion, the "Converted." In fact, Vincentian Converted are just as likely to call themselves Spiritual Baptists.

The Spiritual Baptist religion was finally made legal in Trinidad in 1951 and in St. Vincent in 1965. In 1996, the government of Trinidad and Tobago declared Spiritual Baptist (Shouter) Liberation Day would be a national holiday to be celebrated every March 30th. By the early 21st century, the religion had become politically normalized, although its adherents are still often looked down upon by others in the islands.

When speaking with West Indians one may sometimes hear the term "Shango Baptist," a reference to the Trinidadian religion, Orisha.[2] There are Spiritual Baptists who also practice Orisha. In both traditions, the spirits are experienced as realities in the spiritual world, even though the Spiritual Baptist tradition originated in St. Vincent and Orisha developed on Trinidad. The tradition is referred to Spiritual Baptist or to Orisha (or commonly Shango or Shango Baptist), not to both interchangeably. Historically, both traditions are quite separate, Spiritual Baptists originating from a Fon and Kongo base while Orisha is predominantly Yoruban.

Beliefs and Practices in the Spiritual Baptist Tradition

Spiritual Baptist symbolism of items and images in a church setting, and the meaning given to spiritual events and to Bible verses, differs between islands. Rituals that have the same name in different islands may have quite different meanings.[3] Between churches even within the same island, rituals may be performed differently. The religion is mystical, and practitioners believe that God may decide to reveal one item, ritual, or meaning to one individual or congregation or island and a different one to another. Overall, we can consider Spiritual Baptist practice to be a framework for individual and group spiritual exploration and revelation, leading to wide differences between local Spiritual Baptist traditions.

The core of the Spiritual Baptist religion is work. The necessary skills to do the work are obtained on spiritual travels. The work itself, healing non-members or guiding other Spiritual Baptists on their spiritual path, largely requires symbolic travel in spiritual lands. These travels are accomplished in trance sessions, sometimes alone or in groups.

As in many religions, the supernatural world is a reflection of the secular world; in the Spiritual Baptist spiritual world, each city has a port, a school, a hospital, and a watchman at the gate. While the school may resemble an ordinary school, the teacher is a spirit and, like many teachers, the spirit teacher may punish students who are unruly or inattentive. One must study in order to learn one's work or role: captain, nurse, teacher, or other spiritual roles. Although this world may only be experienced while in trance, the spiritual jobs that one learns become titles for church members. In the (physical) church sessions, it is not unusual to hear members referred to as Captain John, or Nurse Susan.

All authority and healing power are received by members as gifts from God during their spiritual world travels and, as previously mentioned, this takes place during trance states. This, like many other features, are common to the religion; however, its revelatory nature leads the tradition to manifest differently in the various places where it is found. Laitinen noted of the Spiritual Baptist religion, "Because of its inherent innovativeness, it evades essentialist notions of religion and culture as pure, bounded, and static" (Laitinen, 2002a, p. 323).

Spiritual Baptist Healers and Healing Practices

Spiritual Baptists are consulted for healing by many in the Caribbean and in its diaspora. Many health problems are often believed to be the result of a "jumbie," an evil spirit that causes physical illness or insanity. If that is the case, individuals may seek out the help of Spiritual Baptists. Spiritual Baptists can also counteract the effects of "Obeah" and are sought if Obeah is suspected. Lum (2000) found that the Spiritual Baptists are used by Caribbean people specifically to cure mental health problems, with enduring success. However, if a person under Baptist care is not spiritually prepared, he or she may be afflicted with a particular kind of insanity. In Trinidad, the condition is referred to as "Baptist-crazy," a mental illness "said to be the result of a bad experience during the ceremony" (Lum, 2000, p. 73).

As Gullick (1998) and Duncan (2008) observed, Spiritual Baptists treat people of the community, even those who do not belong to the religion. For ordinary sickness, a home remedy is likely to be applied, or, if it is a serious illness, medical assistance is advised. If either of those does not work, then a supernatural cure from the Spiritual Baptists may be considered. Spiritual Baptists are a normal part of the traditional mix of health options available to Caribbean people.

The essence of the Spiritual Baptist religion is a call to service that begins with "mourning." During mourning, members of the religion enter days-long trances in which they symbolically travel to a number of spiritual lands, attend schools there, and learn spiritual occupations. The highest status jobs acquired spiritually are similar to those in the "physical world." Furthermore, since the Spiritual Baptists tend to be the poorer people in the islands who would be unlikely to be able to afford higher education, going to school in the spiritual lands is one way of gaining the status and power that are denied to them in the physical world.

The jobs are ranked with the higher levels devoted to healing.[4] The healing ranks such as "pointers," "pointing mothers," "mothers," and sometimes "leaders" or "healers" take a number of years and many spiritual journeys to acquire. Most healers are given ranks of assistant nurse, assistant pointer, or assistant mother before they attain the full rank. This allows for several years of attending alongside the more experienced healers before beginning healing independently. A pointer is the highest in the Spiritual Baptist spiritual hierarchy. A female pointer is called a "pointing mother" or sometimes just "mother." The pointer is the spiritual role that most resembles a shaman in Spiritual Baptist practice, entering the spiritual world at will to retrieve lost souls, initiate others into the healing role, and to heal both physical and spiritual sickness. Spiritual jobs, both healing and non-healing, are ranked in a hierarchy.

Spiritual Baptist churches will often operate under a dual hierarchy. On one side is a government recognized denominational hierarchy of pastors, bishops, and archbishops, who have the ability to marry, bury, and christen. Alongside is a hierarchy derived solely from gifts given in the spiritual world, including the gift of healing. While few in the religion have a position in the secular hierarchy, all have a spiritual title, from water carrier to pointer or pointing mother, and all are eligible, and often required to assist in the spiritual work. The hierarchies are not mutually exclusive; each bishop is also a pointer, as are most of the pastors.

The primary training of a Spiritual Baptist healer is undertaken in the spiritual world. Very experienced pointers or mothers will be able to enter the spiritual world simply by closing their eyes with the intention to travel, a process called "meditation." Others who are experienced may need to make special vigorous ritual motions named "doption" or "adoption," which is a type of kinetic driving used to assist in entering an altered state. Typically, "doption" will appear as rhythmically stomping the feet at a quick pace, while shouting on the stomp and throwing the body forward and downward simultaneously so that the torso bends forcefully at the waist.

Whether the healer is able to enter the spiritual lands by doption or meditation, in each case they must have received the ability to enter first by mourning. This is a period of blindfolded seclusion lasting for 7 to 14 days depending on the local tradition (see, for example, Kremser, 2004). Mourning is also done for baptism. In preparation for baptism, one mourns for three days only. Baptism is not necessarily training to become a healer; baptism itself can be seen as a type of healing (Duncan, 2008).

Healing takes place both privately and publicly and both sets of rituals are conducted by a pointer. In addition to healing, wakes or memorials are services that Spiritual Baptists provide to the larger community on one of the traditional wake nights, usually 9 or 40 days after a death (see also Gullick, 1998). Regardless of the denomination of the deceased, the Spiritual Baptists may be called to conduct the wake. As people privileged by God to do spiritual work, Spiritual Baptists feel that they must provide the service and often do it for nothing more than a nominal gift in kind.

The private work that Spiritual Baptists do for the community is varied; for example, in Tobago, "Exorcising evil spirits is part of a healer's duties" (Laitinen, 2002a, p. 329). The idea of evil spirit possession is not found among Vincentian Spiritual Baptists (Zane, 1999). Further, in Tobago,

> Healing can take place within a church service; for example, a healer can see to an infant as it is being dedicated, or to a sick person who has come to the service. Most times people come to seek help at the home of the healer, though.
>
> *(Laitinen, 2002a, p. 329)*

It is worth noting that, in Tobago, dedicating an infant in the church is equated with healing; on other islands, it is a ritual associated with identity. Otherwise separate categories often overlap for the Spiritual Baptists.

In St. Vincent, "lock up" is the most common condition treated by a Spiritual Baptist healer. The symptoms of "lock up" are: lethargy, sadness, the feeling of a heavy weight on one's chest or shoulders. The method of treating "lock up" appears similar to some types of Western talk therapy. The session begins with a discussion of life history, then proximal events to the "lock up," and finally to the treatment itself which consists of ritualistic actions on the part of the healer, but also active input from the patient. Symbolically, or spiritually, but certainly experientially, the pointer will travel in the spiritual lands to the particular spiritual city where the soul is locked up. The pointer will obtain release of the soul from the spiritual jailor by singing the song of the city, or paying (spiritual) money to the jailor. Many adherents and non-adherents report a great sense of relief at having their soul back after treatment by a pointer.

For natural or spiritual illness other than "lock up," the most common physical action prescribed or performed is a spiritual bath. Some pointers bathe the individual themselves; some give bathing instructions to the person seeking help. A pointer who may give a spiritual bath is also called a doctor or a spiritual doctor, or may be referred to by his specialty as a "bush doctor" or "bark doctor" (use of leaves, bark, and roots), or "chemical doctor" (use of perfumes and oils). The process of giving a spiritual bath is sometimes called "barking" someone. The physical effectiveness of the plants and chemicals used is of little import: the problems the pointers treat are spiritual (see for example, Laitinen, 2002a). Some pointers may perform a ceremony known as "smoking" that uses the smoke of rosemary or other aromatic herbs. In St. Vincent smoking is only used to cleanse a baby from sickness caused by covetousness (that is, someone loving the baby too much) or envy, known locally as "maljo." The baby is held over the smoke and the sickness goes away (Zane, 1999).

Other illnesses are caused by curses, spirits, including a number of local spiritual monsters, and by acts the patient may have committed such as stealing or adultery, resulting in punishment from God or other actors in the spirit world. The treatment in these cases is still spiritual or spiritually-inspired. Illnesses from natural causes are normally treated at home, but may also be treated by a Western-oriented specialist or a Spiritual Baptist.

Spiritual Baptists and Mental Health Practices

Two main issues make Spiritual Baptists worth noting for health professionals, namely, the normalization of the religion within Caribbean communities and migration. Frances Henry (2003) has shown that the Spiritual Baptist religion has come to be an accepted part of the plurality of religions in Trinidad. Where, in the past, affiliation with the religion may have been hidden due to its illegality, it is now openly acknowledged. Caribbean people who are not Spiritual Baptists may sympathize with the Spiritual Baptist religion, seeing it as an authentic Caribbean cultural expression.

Migration between islands has always been a factor in Caribbean history and migration from the Caribbean to North America has increased in the past half-century (McCabe, 2011). Health and mental health professionals who have contact with anyone from the Caribbean may benefit from knowledge of Spiritual Baptists, as it reflects a Caribbean way of viewing the world.

Looking at the adherents themselves, Spiritual Baptist practices have been demonstrated to produce positive psychological benefit. Griffith, Mahy, and Young (1986) and Griffith and Mahy (1984) found that Spiritual Baptist mourning, the long-term blindfolded trance session, is a significant source of improvement in both life satisfaction and physical health. Spiritual Baptists are able to avoid mental health problems by participation in their rituals and involvement with their community:

> Mourners cited six benefits of the practice: relief of depressed mood; attainment of the ability to foresee and avoid danger; improvement in decision-making ability; heightened facility to communicate with God and to meditate; a clearer appreciation of their racial origins; identification with church hierarchy; and physical cures. Mourning appears to be a viable psychotherapeutic practice for these church members.
>
> *(Griffith & Mahy, 1984, p. 769)*

Additionally, much of Spiritual Baptist practice appears similar to Western dream therapies that emphasize intentional dreaming and analysis of one's actions in the dream (La Berge, 1985; Stewart, 1990). Stewart claimed that, with experience, Senoi dream life becomes "more and more like reflective thinking, problem solving, exploration of unknown things or people, emotionally satisfying social intercourse, and the acquiring of knowledge from a dream teacher or spirit guide" (Stewart, 1990, p. 201). The same pattern holds for Spiritual Baptist mourning and other spiritual travel (Zane, 1999).

Given the benefits of mourning as found by Griffith and Mahy, the question may arise as to whether workers in health and mental health should use Spiritual Baptists as a resource for consultation and referral. Some in the Eastern Caribbean and its diaspora will welcome the integration of the two systems. However, Spiritual Baptist religion is still a minority religion that is very different from the mainstream Christianity practiced by most people in the region, and, as such, is not accepted by everyone. For people sympathetic to Spiritual Baptist practice, referral or consultation may be beneficial.

The best outcomes for health and mental health specialists who encounter people in the Caribbean or in North America or England who are Spiritual Baptists would derive from an attitude of understanding. For example, in speaking with Spiritual Baptists, it can be difficult to recognize which parts of their experience are spiritual and which are physical. They recognize this and often use the terms "carnal" or "natural" to refer to their physical experiences and reserve "spiritual" for their spiritual experiences. Yet, they often omit the qualifiers since, to them, all of these are genuine experiences and, in that sense, both are real. Awareness and acceptance that such a distinction may be present can build trust between a health professional and a Spiritual Baptist. Simply asking the question "Is this carnal or spiritual?" can illustrate a willingness to accept their reality as valid. Certainly, their spiritual experiences are valid in the sense that they influence their behavior in the physical world.

Conclusion

Local explanations for medical conditions are sometimes considered by Western-oriented specialists to be superstitions, but these explanations follow local patterns of logic. Spiritual Baptists, in experiencing the spiritual world, are not exhibiting deviant or psychotic traits, but rather behavior derived from the history and culture of the islands. Although the religion is often ridiculed by non-believers because of its close association with African practices, the Spiritual Baptists would say of the outsiders, "They talk bad about us in the day, but seek us out at night."

Notes

1. The author conducted research among Spiritual Baptists in St. Vincent and among Vincentians in New York City (Zane, 1999). Carole Duncan (2008) and Maarit Laitinen (Laitinen, 2002a; 2002b) have provided thoughtful ethnographies on Spiritual Baptists in Toronto and in Tobago, respectively. Stephen D. Glazier has written voluminously on Spiritual Baptists (e.g., Glazier, 1983). There are works that give valuable information about Spiritual Baptists by researchers who primarily focused on other cultural traditions (Goldwasser, 1996; Gullick, 1998; Herskovits & Herskovits, 1947; Littlewood 1993; Lum, 2000). As well, Spiritual Baptist leaders themselves have written on the religion (e.g., De Peza, 2007; Thomas, 1987).
2. These tend to be adherents of the Shango (Orisha) religion who use some Spiritual Baptist practices, or more rarely, Spiritual Baptists who use some elements of the Orisha religion. Actual "Shango Baptists" are fewer in number than either Orisha practitioners or Spiritual Baptist practitioners, but because both have an African focus, non-adherents tend to lump them together in a general non-European African-oriented religious category.
3. For example, in St. Vincent a "pilgrimage" is one church visiting another church in a fun, light-hearted manner; in Trinidad it is a serious religious journey to a spiritual site (Glazier, 1983).
4. Depending on the island or specific tradition within an island, the list of ranks will differ. A typical list of ascending hierarchy is, for males: bell-ringer, cross-bearer, shepherd, messenger, watchman, surveyor, captain, diver, prover, assistant leader, leader, assistant pointer, teacher, pointer, inspector. The list for females will often include: florist, water carrier, flag-waver, bell-ringer, trumpet blower, surveyor, diver, assistant nurse, nurse, nurse matron, African warrior, leadress, shepherdess, assistant mother, pointing mother, inspector. Each of these may have the term "crowned" or "king" or "queen" affixed to them, as in "crowned watchman." Although the "spiritual name" becomes a term of address, as in for instance, "Nurse Smith," the affixes are not normally included in addressing the individual.

References

Bilby, K. M., & Bunseki, F. K. K. (1983). *Kumina: A Kongo-based tradition in the New World*. Bruxelles: Centre d'Etude et de Documentation Africaines.

De Peza, H. A. G. (2007 [1999]). *My faith: Spiritual Baptist Christian*. St. Augustine: Xulon Press.

Duncan, C. B. (2008). *This spot of ground: Spiritual Baptists in Toronto*. Waterloo: Wilfred Laurier Press.

Glazier, S. D. (1983). *Marchin' the pilgrims home: Leadership and decision-making in an Afro-Caribbean faith*. Westport, CT: Greenwood Press.

Glazier, S. D. (1988). Worldwide missions of Trinidad's Spiritual Baptists. *The National Geographical Journal of India, 34*(1), 75–78.

Goldwasser, M. A. (1996). *The rainbow Madonna of Trinidad: A study in the dynamics of belief in Trinidadian religious life* (Ph.D. dissertation). University of California, Los Angeles.

Griffith, E. E. H., & Mahy, G. E. (1984). Psychological benefits of Spiritual Baptist "mourning." *American Journal of Psychiatry, 141*(6), 769–773.

Griffith, E. E. H., Mahy, G. E., & Young, J. L. (1986). Psychological benefits of Spiritual Baptist "mourning," II: An empirical assessment. *American Journal of Psychiatry, 143*(2), 226–229.

Gullick, C. J. M. R. (1998). The Shakers of St. Vincent: A symbolic focus for discourses. In P. B. Clarke (Ed.), *New trends and developments in African religions* (pp. 87–104). Westport, CT: Greenwood Press.

Hazell, B. S. (1994). *The impact of the Caribbean Baptist Fellowship on Christian education ministries in the Windward Islands with implications for its future role* (Doctoral Dissertation [Ed. D.]). New Orleans Baptist Theological Seminary.

Henry, F. (2003). *Reclaiming African religions in Trinidad: The socio-political legitimation of the Orisha and Spiritual Baptist faiths*. Mona, University of West Indies Press.

Herskovits, M. J., & Herskovits, F. S. (1947). *Trinidad village*. New York: Alfred A. Knopf.

Houk, J. T. (1995). *Spirits, blood, and drums*. Philadelphia, PA: Temple University Press.

Kremser, M. (2004). Afro-Caribbean. In F. A. Salamone (Ed.), *Encyclopedia of religious rites, rituals, and festivals* (pp. 22–26). New York: Routledge.

La Berge, S. (1985). *Lucid dreaming*. Los Angeles, CA: Jeremy P. Tarcher, Inc.

Laitinen, M. (2002a). *Marching to Zion. Creolisation in Spiritual Baptist rituals and cosmology*. Helsinki: Research Series in Anthropology, University of Helsinki.

Laitinen, M. (2002b). *Aspects of gender in the Spiritual Baptist religion in Tobago: Notes from the field*. Centre for Gender and Development Studies, University of West Indies, Working Paper Series, St. Augustine Unit. Working Paper, no. 6.

Littlewood, R. (1993). *Pathology and identity: The work of Mother Earth in Trinidad*. Cambridge: Cambridge University Press.

Lum, K. (2000). *Praising His name in the dance. Spirit possession in the Spiritual Baptist faith and Orisha work in Trinidad, West Indies*. Amsterdam: Harwood Academic Publishers.

Malm, K. (1983). An island carnival (CD liner notes). Electra Entertainment. Nonesuch Records 72091.

McCabe, K. (2011). Caribbean immigrants in the United States. *Migration Policy Institute*. Retrieved from http://www.migrationinformation.org/usfocus/display.cfm?ID=834#2

Simpson, G. E. (1966). Baptismal, "mourning," and "building ceremonies of the Shouters of Trinidad. *Journal of American Folklore, 79*, 537–550.

Stewart, K. (1990 [1969]). Dream theory in Malaya. In C. Tart (Ed.), *Altered states of consciousness* (3rd. ed.), (pp. 191–204). San Francisco, CA: Harper.

Thomas, E. (1987). *A history of the Shouter Baptists in Trinidad and Tobago.* Tacarigua, Trinidad: Calaloux Publications.

Zane, W. W. (1999). *Journeys to the spiritual lands: The natural history of a West Indian religion.* New York: Oxford University Press.

PART III

Spirituality, Religion, and Cultural Healing

12

CHRISTIAN SPIRITUALITY, RELIGION, AND HEALING IN THE CARIBBEAN

E. Anthony Allen and Abrahim H. Khan

Introduction

The Caribbean Christian Church traditions of healing and understanding of Biblical teachings implicate the hegemony of Western culture and thought. Rationalism, a hallmark of that culture, has brewed suspicions over claims about miraculous healing (Richardson, 1969). The suspicion is compounded with a culture-bound Cartesian compartmentalizing of spiritual and medical science based healing, and an engendering of a denigration of non-Eurocentric cultural realities (Allen, 1995).[1] Thus, the hegemony has either rejected outright or at the least created a divisive ambivalence around aspects of Biblical interpretation and related healing practices having any resemblance to non-European religious worldview and practice. The ambivalence has hardened to yes/no dichotomy around which has been formed a plurality of spiritual healings within the structure of the Caribbean Church.

Consequently, on account of its own cultural ambivalence, the Caribbean Christian Church has become both victor and victim. As victor, it has a historical role in the total development and resilience of the people in the former British Caribbean region.[2] At the same time, it is an institutional victim of cultural and philosophical contradictions born of imperial and neo-imperial designs. That duality is undermining the availability of the full benefits of Christian healing and contributing to dysfunctional distortions of the reality of the situation. For example, there is interdenominational prejudice with respect to aisle crossing by Mainline and Evangelical Church members seeking healing to Pentecostal denominations (Cole, 2007) and the secretive use of folk healers (Allen, 2003) or even those from other faith traditions. Further, there is denial of the benefits of integrating medicine and health promotion with spiritual teachings and practices in a primary health care system, especially in Jamaica, the first country in the region to become free of British colonialism. However, within the past 40 years, a new integrative or "Whole Person Healing Ministry" movement has developed, embracing most denominations across the Caribbean. The challenge now is for health care providers and trainees to help Caribbean clients engage meaningfully with Christian healing and to utilize its health promoting advantages in working through any dysfunctional ties related to cultural contradictions.

Recognition and social acceptance of healing practices outside medical treatment were not without trauma for the Caribbean Christian Community. By the second half of the 20th century social and political movements were gaining a momentum that would throw into sharp relief the ambivalence and cultural conflict created by resistance of an Afrocentric worldview to a Eurocentric one, with implications for the interpretation of scripture and the understanding of life. The latter worldview was undermining the very presupposition of healing practices, namely, the non-rational notion of God's revelation beyond nature and His supernatural involvement in healing (Richardson, 1969). But by the mid-20th century, resistance to it was increasing as a result of a sociopolitical and cultural synergy in connection with at least four factors: a) the rising tide of national independence across British Caribbean territories, 2) a sense of racial pride and belonging associated with Garveyism in the 1930s and later heightened by the impulses of African nationalism, 3) the ripples of Black Power movement spreading among the younger generation wanting to define their identity for themselves, and 4) the emergence and spread of Rastafarianism in Jamaica[3] and across the Afro-Caribbean region.

Aligned with a Eurocentric view, Mainline Protestant and Catholic Churches were stressing social outreach, along with Evangelical Churches that opted to preach the scriptural "Word." These denominations appealed more to the cultured, Westernized educated classes whose members are mostly of white or lighter complexion, as opposed to black, and belong to upper and middle income level people (Lowenthal, 1972). Their critique of belief in healing rituals is that it is due largely to lack of education and a simplistic interpretation of the Bible (Cole, 2007).

By contrast, aligned with an Afrocentric view, is the Pentecostal Church along with Revivalist and Spiritual Baptist movements[4] that have healing rituals as a main characteristic. They attract largely the lower income, rural, and inner city poor, mainly of African ancestry. The latter movements tend to merge recollections of African realities with Christian ideas. That is, the healing methods combine Christian beliefs (Trinity, angels, and anointing) with beliefs that rely also on the assistance of ancestral spirits, and that include the engagement of strong musical and dance rituals and the use of herbal baths. However, though the Pentecostal denominations unambiguously promote miraculous healings, the supernatural gifts of the spirit, and the ministry of deliverances, they are not to be confused with spiritualism or Afro-Caribbean movements that employ a mix of Christian beliefs and folk healing ritual practices. For the Afrocentric Christian beliefs movements the issue was not to prove the divinity of Christ on earth or to establish certitudes, but to live life before a spiritual presence with the conviction that the creator God has provided all that is needed to be a healthy person. That is, there is a continuous interaction between the physical and spiritual realm, an interaction that can be disrupted by the reality of evil forces from which one must be protected. These beliefs are common to both an Afrocentric worldview and a Biblical cosmology.

The resistance to a Western worldview increased following World War II to the point that healing practices gained not only sociopolitical recognition but also came to characterize Afrocentric Christianity in the Caribbean. This latter form of Christianity gained the upper hand in the ambivalence, largely as a result of 1) declining viability and growth of European originated Mainline and Evangelical churches (Cole, 2007), some of it brought on by members seeking healing choosing to cross over to the Pentecostal churches or to middle class Protestant, charismatic, independent churches having similar beliefs and practices to the Pentecostals, 2) members openly consulting local/native healers without having later any internal conflict and guilt from doing so, 3) the educating of misguided thinking that belief in the miraculous means that treatment by modern medicine is unnecessary, and 4) the absence of promotion of a healthy lifestyle, psychological counseling, and medical screening in churches, and that may mean the members unnecessarily suffer emotionally and die prematurely. All these factors helped in the emergence and receptivity of a new integrative approach to or model of church ministry that would accommodate also healing practices and practitioners.

This chapter identifies traditional principles and practices of Christian healing, correlating practices with prayers and discussing the intercessors along with their training and formation. It is then followed by a postcolonial critique of Christian healing. Next, it presents the new integrative healing paradigm, including how the staff is trained and supervised and the possibility for research. The model of the healing ministry discussed opens up possibilities for a close working relation with medicine, in healing and restoration of health to the infirmed. However, the health care professional needs to understand any client's core beliefs about health, disease, and healing. This is even more relevant when working with Caribbean clients holding a Christian belief system in a population comprising a plurality of ethnicity and culture.

Principles of Christian Healing

Central to the healing practises and theology of the Christian religion is an understanding that the Bible is, according to its adherent, God-inspired. As a literary source, it has two main parts: the Old and the New Testament. The former, narrating the creation story and the prophetic tradition, is a salvation history of God's relationship to a people whom he/she has chosen. The relation is marked by disobedience or sin and evil as the cause of sickness and suffering. Healing and health are possible only through repentance and divine forgiveness.

God's promise is to care and to heal of disease.[5] The New Testament, situating Jesus as part of the prophetic tradition of Judean culture, depicts his activities as being healer and exorcist: enabling the lame to walk, the blind to see, and casting out demons.[6] His saving and healing activity is not just from physical infirmities and afflictions, but primarily from spiritual sickness and death. He advocates for the marginalized and those oppressed by the religious–political establishment of the day. More interesting is that health and healing are linked not just to sin, evil, and repentance but also to his compassion for the afflicted. His followers and Christianity carried his combat spirit against sin and evil along with a show of compassion to new and different cultural situations (Porterfield, 2005). The apostle Paul, for example, tells the Corinthians that healing was infrequent among them because of their intolerant divisiveness.[7]

Further, the history of Christianity is marked by transformative healing experiences: St. Ignatius describing the Eucharist as medicine of immortality and the healing powers of St. Cyprian and St. Agatha (Porterfield, 2005). Other examples include anointing with oil, belief that the relics of saints have curative powers, healing in monastic hospitals in the Middle Ages (Wilhelmi, n.d), and, in the modern period, the healing water of the shrine at Lourdes. These are indicative also of the idea that the vision of healing is unquestionably central to the history of Christianity and specifically connected to crucial concepts in Christian theology: sin, evil, repentance, forgiveness, and redemption. As part of that history, the Caribbean Christian Church with its healing activity shares the vision that can be set out in terms of principles.

Four principles, at the least, encompass divine healing according to scripture. One that is cosmological in scope, affirms briefly that God is the source of all creation, created out of love, or goodness.[8] Dialectically related to the good, evil is understood as that which lacks the good, is manifested as sickness and death, and personified by Satan, a fallen angel in cosmic struggle with the good (Buttrick et al., 1963, pp. 226–227). As the source of creation, God is not limited in his ability to heal and to overcome evil.

Another principle relates to health or wholeness. That is, God has created humans in his/her own image.[9] Thus, the human is more than a material or mind–body being, but also one that is infused with spirit. The theological implication is that each individual is a whole or complete being, having capacity to be to be rational, creative, and relational. As part of their wholeness, individuals are able to sustain a spiritual relation with God and fellow creatures. An I–thou relation, it empowers humans to transcend all sufferings connected with being finite, and survive even physical death. By God holding together our wholeness, health then is not just the absence of disease or infirmity but is also a harmony of mind, body, and spirit. Hence, health is a positive quality of life, the creature sustaining the right relation to the Creator and to the other creatures, including the natural order of life. The New Testament injunction to love God and neighbour[10] is a summary of healthy living that encompasses various lifestyles.

A third principle relates to disease and the healing process. A core Christian belief is that the human potential for wholeness is subject to disruption and hence dis-ease on account of ego-centric rebellion or defiance against the relationship with God and hence neighbour and environment (Buttrick et al., 1963). The term for this defiance or misuse of the freewill is sin, understood as a state in which we are rendered vulnerable to human, natural, and demonic evil. In that state, humans become perpetrators of affliction on others and the environment. They inflict on themselves negative lifestyles, ignore the moral order by which human existence is meaningful, assault the natural order that sustains human existence, and thus bring on themselves illness and affliction. But through acceptance of God's forgiveness, their restoration of wholeness and hence healing of dis-ease is possible. According to Buttrick et al. (1963) salvation is the saving power by which that restoration is effected.

A final and fourth principle relates to the modality of divine therapeutic intervention. Accordingly, divine healing may occur through different pathways: miracles, having faith, or having knowledge in the medical arts and human sciences such as counseling, psychotherapy, and social intervention. Miracles, of which the Bible gives many examples, are signs of God's providential intentions for humanity.[11] Faith as a healing mode implies an attitude of faithfulness that accepts the forgiveness of sins understood as a means of grace that correlates with a spiritual transformation of our being. The human sciences pathway correlates with the tradition of the Biblical prophets in their advocacy for the marginalized and oppressed. In the modern context it may include making accessible to the poor and oppressed medical and health resources: medical knowledge relating to prevention and available cures, improvement of personal hygiene, and seeking treatment for afflictions. This kind of advocacy may have psychological and spiritual implications for the healing of individuals, families, and communities.

Altogether, the four principles presuppose that human self is more than a physical body. It is spiritual as well and susceptible to afflictions that are not always occasioned by sin. Afflictions may result from chance circumstances that include one's ignorance or negligence with respect to the laws of nature, old age, or from God testing and strengthening us to reach an even greater level of wholeness (Buttrick et al., 1963). Further, it does not follow that divine healing removes all infirmities, to recall Biblical narratives: the healing of Sarah's womb was not until old age, Isaac was blind for many years, and Jacob in his old age was both blind and sick. Still further, the greatest of all healings is God's calling home the faithful, through death, to acquire an immortal body and thus to end the pain and sorrow that mark our mortality.

Christian Healing Practices

Healing practices among English speaking Caribbean Christians have central to them prayers that are Biblically based and are in keeping with the tradition of the

Christian Church. Prayers vary, but fall in one of three broad categories and may be integrated as needed, rather than used separately. Further, they are relatively simple, with minimum use of personal charisma, ritual, or sacred objects. Still further, they incorporate Biblical passages appropriate for healing from the Gospels in the New Testament, or the Psalms in the Old Testament, but are by no means limited to those parts of the Bible.

The first category, prayers for miraculous healing or formal healing prayers, are an integral part of congregational or special worship services. They may be said at evangelistic prayer crusades, in private homes, and at health care or other residential institutions. They are comprised roughly of three steps, involving the intercessor, or prayer leader, and the afflicted person. The intercessor is either a priest, church member with special gifts, or lay reader. The first step is for the intercessor to prepare the afflicted for healing by providing encouragement through Biblical exhortations to recognize God's desire and ability to heal. Next, the afflicted individuals state their ailment or health concerns. Or, sometimes through the gift of "a word of knowledge," God may give the intercessor a revelation of the complaint and a confirmation of the healing to come. This leads finally to the third step: the healing prayer or activity itself that may be just a simple word of revelation that indicates restoration is occurring. The steps apply also to prayer for the healing of memories, for past hurts or trauma followed by counseling, and for the casting out of demons or spirits. The latter prayers belong to the ministry of deliverance in the work of Pentecostal or Charismatic non-denominational churches. In the healing activity of this deliverance, someone on the prayer team whom God has given the gift of discernment of spirits invokes the authority and name of Christ as the power that enables the casting out of the demons.[12] Altogether, in healing prayers the intercessor and the afflicted recognize that God in Christ is the healer who operates through humans as agents. Thus, in standard church practice, the Christian seeks healing by calling direct upon the authority, or name of Christ, rather than invoking perceived power, resident in any person, object, or ritual.

Second, prayers with touching of the afflicted, consists of two healings that involve the act of touching the afflicted accompanied by Biblical exhortations. Hands of the intercessor are laid on the forehead of the afflicted, or the thumb of the priest–intercessor is dipped in oil and then used in making the sign of the cross on the forehead of the afflicted.[13] Each activity is done with words spoken in the name of God, for both activities symbolize the touch of God and the bestowing of His spiritual power. In conjunction with either one, the Eucharist or Holy Communion may be administered, or Confession made. Both are sacramental means of God's grace and hence channels of healing. The act of Confession involving the acceptance of the assurance of God's forgiveness is itself a powerful therapeutic aid to healing. Though not a sacrament, fasting by the intercessor may be a potent facilitator in preparation to become a tool of God's power. These rituals, accompanied by prayers, may require repeated performance.

The third category consists of prayers that are supplemental to knowledge of medical and human sciences. Christ expressly stated that it is not the healthy but the sick who need a doctor.[14] By the 4th century the Church had started infirmaries and hospitals—monastery hospitals to care for the sick (Horden, 2005). Today, medical missionary movements of the Church build hospitals, provide doctors, and staff medical schools (Koenig, McCollough, & Larson, 2001). Catholics, Anglicans, and Seventh Day Adventists all run Caribbean hospitals. The healing prayers, considered part of pastoral care during visitation in an institutional setting, are an adjunctive to medical treatment or therapy. They consist of reading Biblical passages, laying on of hands, and anointing, as the occasion might accommodate. More specifically, the healing act in certain cases may require follow-up with psychological counseling, and social work with the family to encourage patience with the afflicted and give interpersonal, emotional, and concrete support to the timid and weak.[15] In an institutional setting a chaplain, church priest, or trained lay reader may serve as intercessor.

Spiritual Healing Practitioners, Their Training and Formation

The Caribbean Christian Church accommodates intercessors who pray for healing of the infirm. Intercessors belong to one of three levels. The Clergy is one level whose members, as part of their pastoral care and spiritual counseling, may include healing for specific concerns. They are pastors or priests, trained at a seminary or theological school and ordained by a Church. Another level consists of lay leaders in the Church or congregation. They pray for others as part of their various responsibilities. A third level are ones with the gift of healing, whether pastors, lay leaders, or other members, to particular ministries of healing. Some gifted persons have become healing evangelists, often operating through para-church organizations. In addition, the Bible exhorts all members of the Church congregation to pray for one another, and for those outside the congregation, as part of the healing community of Christ. Each individual is also encouraged to take personal responsibility for his or her healing prayer. Training and commissioning individuals to a ministry of spiritual healing is in keeping with Biblical as well as Church traditions. The Apostle James encouraged the New Testament Church to send forth elders to pray for the sick and anoint them with olive oil to restore their health and have their sins forgiven.[16] The Gospel Mark reports that Jesus called together his 12 disciples and gave them power and authority to drive out evil spirits and cure diseases, and commissioned them to preach and heal the sick.[17]

All who pray formally for the sick are usually required to be Christians of exemplary character, making no claims to personal or intrinsic ritual power, operating ethically within congregational structures and not for personal gain. There is always the danger of factionalism, of cultic mind control, and of forbidding medical and psychological interventions due to over-enthusiasm or inadequate experience and training. Usually there is the corrective ideal of appropriate training and practical supervision for each of the three levels of intercessors, including areas relating to Scripture, personal growth, moral life, and approaches to ministry.

Collaboration and an Integrative Healing Model

The task, if the church is to play a significant role in the lives of the Caribbean people, is to bring together and integrate different healing approaches and strategies so as to relieve afflictions and promote health and well-being. Already, training in understanding and assessing spirituality has been introduced to medical, theological, and psychology students at the University of the West Indies, Mona campus with good initial reception (Allen & Paul, 2003). It is a first step for Caribbean students and clergy, for more training, and supervision of professional development, which overworked clergy in a congregation can hardly provide, are areas requiring attention. Further, ethnographic research, along the lines of the recent work by Griffith (2010) on the Spiritual Baptists, is needed as is research on clinical expressions of issues, phenomena, and inner conflicts surrounding the Western/African indigenous interface. Still further, the measurable health assets of churches, best practices, and public health impact in the Caribbean and its diaspora are also areas requiring research. Training, research, and professional development go hand in glove with an approach that seems to be addressing the task, and thus becoming an adopted model.

The Whole Person Ministry is offered as a model that incorporates different healing approaches and strategies. Integrative, it is congregationally based, takes into consideration the whole person, and is guided in its understanding by Biblical paradigms. This model adopted by the Bethel Baptist Church in Jamaica, comprises medical services, counseling, prayer and spiritual care, social care, and outreach activities (Allen, 2005). Medical services are community based and comprehensive, meaning that they are promotive, preventative, curative, and rehabilitative. Curative services are integrated with the aid of a Wholistic Assessment Questionnaire. On the basis of the questionnaire, patients/clients are then assigned to the appropriate medical doctors, psychological counselors, prayer counselors, conflict resolution counselors, or the church's social worker. Preventative and divine healing services include the spontaneous laying on of hands, special healing services, invitations for healing in regular services, and a prayer "hot line."

The healing and spiritual assessment approach is open-ended to assisting both counselors and clients. It enables counselors to become culturally competent in understanding the relationship of the client's possible ethnic and social class-influenced culture and the culture conflicts (if any) with their healing worldviews and expectations. The assessment elicits the client's self-understanding of faith and lived experiences: practices, crises, ego strengths and weaknesses, and desire for change. It provides an opportunity for clients to share their spiritual worldview/cosmology and their understanding of health, illness, cure, and living, and to relate them to their own situation or dis-ease for which they seek remedy. Further, clients may gain clarity as to whether the healing modality is to be one that is mental, physical, social, spiritual, or other. Still further, the approach is instrumental for clients with problems concerning any cultural conflict that may exist (Allen, 2005).

Counselors and volunteer assistants of the Whole Person Healing Ministry try to discover the available relevant "functional" and ethical healing resources within the Christian belief system. They try to understand the terms of reference, and denominational and cultural nuances of the client's situations as disclosed in the assessment. They network to learn of available culturally sensitive religious clergy who might assist specific clients. They encourage the client to reflect on self-help approaches that are auxiliary to prayer for healing, and to take advantage of wholistic peer support in their home congregation. Counselors do not seek to influence the client's beliefs through coercion or use of a spiritual healer. Rather, they understand their approach as co-participatory and ethically responsible. As a healing congregation, Bethel church provides over 15 non-professional volunteers who work with 17 paid staffers to render multidisciplinary services.

The integrative model allowing for spiritual healing, or some other aspect of Whole Person Healing Ministry, has been adopted elsewhere in Jamaica and in other Caribbean countries. Among the island's capital of over 500,000 persons, Copeland (1992) listed at least 46 such ministries run by 13 denominations, most being in poverty-stricken areas. A healing ecumenism encompassing Mainline, Evangelical, and Pentecostal churches is forming around the wholistic needs of Caribbean people and out-shadowing culture-conditioned doctrinal debates. In Jamaica, for example, there have been many joint workshops sponsored by ecumenical faith and health coordinating and capacity building agencies and the Ministry of Health. Trinidad, Barbados, and the Leeward Islands and Haiti are also involved.[18] The Caribbean Conference of Churches (2008) has been facilitating initiatives in churches related to HIV/AIDS, substance abuse and violence. In a transnational and metropolitan world, Caribbean immigrants have taken with them culture conflicts and solutions about healing. Apart from a continuance of Pentecostal healing, some evangelical and mainline leaders have set up aspects of new integrative healing programs for Caribbean diasporas in England and America.

The Whole Person Healing Ministry is not without challenges. One is the need for more members' presence and participation in low income communities, and for integrating healing practices and wholistic evaluations (Allen, 2003). Another is that the Mainline churches, having opted for the integrative model, have been content to practice a health ministry that combines insights gained from psychology, medicine, and sociology, and to abandon for the most part the practice of miraculous healings to Pentecostal and Charismatic churches (Henlin, 2006).

Conclusion

The Whole Person Healing Ministry, as an integrative model, offers Caribbean Christian clients the opportunity to engage meaningfully with biblical healing, while taking into consideration a traditional and Afrocentric cultural matrix, and utilizing the insights from medicine and the human sciences. Tried and tested for almost 40 years, it is being embraced by different Christian denominations in the Caribbean region. However, there are challenges to it as mentioned above. Still, there remains one challenge that as an integrative healing model it can least afford to overlook. For to present oneself before God for healing, in the cultural context of Caribbean Christians, it would make no sense to embrace all aspects of African culture, to reject all of Western thought, or to dismiss the insights about wholeness of life from cultural neighbours in the population: Chinese, East Indians, Amerindians, and other ethnicities. They too are Caribbean, and make up its Christian community.

Notes

1. Traditionally the village or urban church has been one of the central influences of formal aspects of Caribbean mores and community life (Austin-Broos, 1997).
2. The Pentecostal movement originated during a 1906 revival in a black church in the USA. A black preacher, W. J. Seymour, was their main pioneer (Hollenwager, 1974, pp. 18–19).
3. Rastafarianism holds that the Messiah is the Emperor of Ethiopia, Haile Selassie, that the Promised Land is Ethiopia, and that modern Babylon is Western culture. It takes as biblical authority Psalm 87: 4–6, and has its roots also in the Back to Africa movement of Marcus Garvey in 1920s and 30s.
4. The history of the Baptists in Jamaica illustrates a culture clash in Caribbean spirituality. The Baptist movement, begun by freed US slaves, experienced in the 1860s a revival and spiritual fervor that initiated an outbreak of Pentecostal manifestations that included the spiritual gift of healing (Bisnauth, 1996, pp. 175–176; Gayle, 1982). Partly due to the strong opposition of the relatively new British missionaries, several thousand members left the Baptist Church to form their own indigenous African-Jamaican syncretistic religious movements (Austin-Broos, 1997, p. 62). Today these movements and their offspring which thrive among the West Indian underclass include Revivalists and Pocomania in Jamaica and the Spiritual Baptists in Barbados and Trinidad. The first two mix Christian beliefs, veneration of the Trinity and angels with employing the services of ancestral and other spirits. Healing methods are a main feature of these movements. Typically, they combine prayer with strong musical and dance rituals, herbal baths, and medicines. Most of these groups are described by Bisnauth (1996, pp. 165–184).
5. For example, see Exodus 23:25–26; Deuteronomy 7:11–12, 15; Genesis 20:17–18.
6. For example see Matthew 4:23–24; Matthew 9:20–22, 27–30al; Acts 3:16.
7. Corinthians 11:29–30.
8. For the creation myth see Genesis, Chapter 1, in the Bible.
9. Genesis 1:26–31; 1 Corinthians 26; and 1 Timothy 4:4.
10. Luke 10:27.
11. See John 9:3, Jesus' response when queried about healing the congenitally blind man.
12. Mark 1:34 and 6:13.
13. Mark 6:5 and 6:13; Acts 5:16; and James 5:14.
14. Matthew 9:12 and Luke 5:31.

15. Thessalonians 5:14.
16. James 5, pp. 14–16.
17. Mark 9, pp. 1–2.
18. These are based on person communication by Rachel Vernon (2000); and Oral Thomas (2010).

References

Allen, E. A. (1995). *Caring for the whole person*. Monrovia, CA: MARC Publications.
Allen, E. A. (2003). Capacity building for healing, faith and reconciliation in mission through biblical wholism: A Caribbean case study. *World Council of Churches' Consultation on Faith, Healing and Missions*. Santiago de Chile.
Allen, E. A. (2005). The congregation as a healing community: The story of Bethel Baptist Church, Jamaica. *Indian Journal of Pallative Care, 11*(1), 37–43. (adapted)
Allen, E. A., & Paul, T. J. (2003) *Spiritual health assessment in the undergraduate medical curriculum at UWI, Mona*. Presented at the UWI Medical Alumni Association Conference, Nassau, Bahamas.
Austin-Broos, D. J. (1997). *Jamaica genesis – Religion and the politics of moral orders*. Kingston, Jamaica: Ian Randle Publishers.
Bisnauth, D. (1996). *History of religions in the Caribbean*. Kingston, Jamaica: Kingston Publishers Ltd.
Buttrick, G. A., Kelper, T. S., Knox, J., May, H. G., Terrien, S., & Bucke, E. S. (Eds.) (1963). *The interpreter's dictionary of the Bible*. Nashville, TN: Abingdon Press.
Caribbean Conference of Churches. (2008) *About CCC: Introduction*. Retrieved from Caribbean Conference of Churches at http://www.ccc-caribe.org/eng/intro.htm.
Cole, R. J. (2007). What can the Euro-Christian churches in the Caribbean learn from indigenous Caribbean religion? *Caribbean Journal of Religious Studies, 21*(1), 16–27.
Copeland, S. (1992). *An analysis of churches related clinics in Kingston and St. Andrew and their contribution to healthcare delivery* (Dissertation). University of the West Indies, Kingston.
Gayle, C. (1982). *George Liele: Pioneer missionary to Jamaica*. Kingston, Jamaica: Jamaica Baptist Union.
Griffith, E. H. (2010). *Ye shall dream a dream*. Mona, Jamaica: University of the West Indies Press.
Henlin, K. E. (2006). *Healing in the ministry of Jesus – An examination of the ministry and practices of Jesus as recorded in the Synoptic Gospels* (Dissertation). The University of the West Indies, Kingston, Jamaica.
Hollenwager, W. (1974). *Pentecost between black and white*. Belfast: Christ Journals Ltd.
Horden, P. (2005). The early hospitals in Byzantium, Western Europe, and Islam. *Journal of Interdisciplinary History, xxxv*(3) (Winter), 361–389. Retrieved from jacklaughlin.ca/readings/spiritual life/horden_hospitals.pdf
Koenig, H. G., McCullough, M. E., & Larson, D. B. (2001). *Handbook of religion and healing*. New York: Oxford University Press
Lowenthal, D. (1972). *West Indian societies*. London: Oxford University Press.
Porterfield, A. (2005). *Healing in the history of Christianity*. New York: Oxford University Press.
Richardson, A. (1969). *Dictionary of Christian theology*. Philadelphia, PA: The Westminster Press.
Wilhelmi, B. (n.d.) Differentiations: Christian Healing Tradition. Retrieved April 8, 2012, from http://www.ihp.sinica.edu.tw/~medicine/ashm/lectures/paper/paper8.pdf

13

RASTAFARI

Cultural Healing in the Caribbean

Kai A. D. Morgan

Introduction

RastafarI[1] was born out of a need to challenge the ever-prevailing Eurocentric ideology and restore the Caribbean's African history and identity in order to restore us to our traditional greatness (Afari, 2007). Africans, from the beginning of time, have always respected nature and its elements (i.e., fire, water, air, and earth), and the plants thereof, and have always utilized nature in its ritualistic processes of maintaining health and healing sickness (Somé, 1998). With Eurocentric ideology came the stripping of these practices as primitive and worthless. RastafarI has evolved from these beginnings, endorsing the spirit of peaceful revolution, attempting to build institutions, and respecting rituals which honor our Africanness, and today the movement has expanded from Jamaica to the wider Caribbean and the world, speaking to its globalization (Boxill, 2008).

With the Rastafarian culture comes the absorption and the glorification of the African heritage of black people, and with it the many practices that are aligned with nature and an intuitive spirit. This belief system encompasses the Rastafarians alternative approach to general health (i.e., Africentric and natural/herbal medicines) and represents a perspective that has broadened into mainstream practice today.

In the area of mental health in particular, the oppressive history of the Rastafarians in Jamaica and the ensuing personality patterns detected also calls into question the existence of a "healthy paranoia," against Babylon[2] system, much like the "healthy paranoia" that has been identified and described amongst African Americans, against white supremacy. Therefore the issues of psychosis, delusions, and paranoia, in the area of mental health, become salient topics of discussion. Rastafarian ideology equally applies to healing; however, like any other culture, RastafarI continues to evolve.

After almost 500 years of colonialism, erasing the blueprint of Eurocentrism is almost impossible. However, very often, the answer lies within our awareness of our African ancestry, the establishment of our personal and collective identity from which an acceptable, possibly integrative model can be generated. Rastafarl currently struggles with this issue as some isolate themselves from Western influence as much as is possible, while others live amongst the Caribbean community trying to combine the two with the strengths of each. The debate about whether this is a weakening of Rastafarl philosophy or a strengthening of a combined and new cultural identity continues. In this postcolonial reality, we must understand, as Chevannes (2006) articulates, that we stand "betwixt and between" these two worlds, therefore, finding our path is dependent upon this very truth.

In this chapter, the original tenets regarding health and mental health, and the process of evolution and how this has altered these tenets will be explored. I begin with looking briefly at the origins and development of Rastafarl, outlining some of the major tenets. This is followed by an account of Rastafarl beliefs regarding health and ill health, then more specifically addresses practitioners and their approaches to Rastafarl. Finally this chapter concludes with a discussion of the integration between Rastafarl beliefs and contemporary medicine and the recommendations of how to approach this group from a health care perspective.

Rastafarl: Origins and Development

Rastafarl began in Kingston, Jamaica, in the 1930s with Leonard Howell, Archibald Dunkley, Claudius Henry, Joseph Hibbert, and much later Vernon Carrington (Hickling, Matthies, Morgan & Gibson, 2008) who with their contributions shaped Rastafarl into what it is today. Borne out of political strife, racial and classicist oppression, the movement espoused black consciousness and identity, the strength and sacred nature of Mother Africa and her children, a reverence and respect for Marcus Garvey and the divinity and/or greatness of His Imperial Majesty, Emperor Haile Selassie I of Ethiopia (Barrett, 1997). Several mansions (much like religious denominations) of Rastafarl exist which advocate varying principles and these include the Nyabingi House, The Bobo Shanti or Ethiopian National Congress, and The Twelve Tribes (Barrett, 1997). However, some basic principles abound: Haile Selassie as Jah (God), Zion (Ethiopia) as heaven on earth, an orientation towards African culture, spiritual use of cannabis, dietary restrictions, and the wearing of dreadlocks (Zips, 2006).

In the years that followed the origins of Rastafarl, the culture has developed from one in the 1930s of passive/peaceful resistance, with alienating dogma, fear-inducing responses and ostracism, to the late 1960s when there became a greater acceptance of Rastafarl by the wider society, until 2012 where attitudes, ideals, and even practices (e.g., language, dress, eating habits) are being embraced. This is a time and place where Rastafarl commands respect.

The Rastafarian culture has evolved and though some of the core principles have shifted, the Rastafarians have indefatigably shaped the rhetoric on African identity through their convictions. This concept has guided many youth in a positive way toward an understanding of their Africanness. The ideology and practices have been on the rise in Jamaica, the Caribbean, and its diaspora with the population of Rastafarians globally estimated at 1 million, with about 200,000 in Jamaica alone (Barnett, 2008). This major global impact is due to several figureheads such as Marcus Garvey and Bob Marley, as well as the social and political consciousness, love, and unity which have appealed to the masses (C. Campbell, personal communication, February 2, 2010).

Principles and Practices of RastafarI

The principles and practices of Rastafari including those regarding illness and health are based in the philosophy of His Imperial Majesty, Haile Selassie I born Tafari Makonnen, a figure of central importance to RastafarI, and his Empress Menen Asfaw (see Selassie & Ullendorff, 1976 for a discussion). In addition, the teachings of Marcus Garvey (Lewis & Bryan, 1991), the emotional and spiritual richness of Kemet (now Ethiopia), and the beauty that Africa brings forth for its people has been an abounding concept in RastafarI. Furthermore, Africa, the Motherland, and its value and respect for the power of nature and alignment with creation and healing into its reasonings, is also critical to the RastafarI rhetoric. The mind and the promotion of a good "livity" (natural way of life or totality of one's being in the world) form the unique rituals that have become associated with RastafarI and are also closely derived from African practices. These include such things as meetings, ceremonies, and reasonings. The "Nyabingi" or "Bingi" is the most important and recognized of such functions, of which music, drumming, prayers, smoking, and singing are integral activities (Barrett, 1997).

There are also various guidelines for what one consumes. Food must be as "ital" (derived from vital; meaning natural, pure, and clean) as possible. Some Rastafarians endorse a purely vegan (no meat, fish, dairy, nor poultry) or vegetarian (no meat, or poultry, some fish) diet, while others endorse or include the eating of poultry (K. K'nife, personal communication, 2010). What is standard across all mansions of RastafarI is that the ingestion of pork is forbidden. Salt is avoided, no chemicals, no alcohol, no cigarettes, and no drugs (herbs are not considered drugs) is endorsed (Barrett, 1997). Cooking in a clay pot is popular among Rastafarians due to the metals that can sometimes be disposed from aluminum pots (C. Campbell, personal communication, February 2, 2010). In general, Rastafarians perceive food as a way to be one with nature and also as medicine for the body.

The herb known scientifically as *Cannabis sativa*, and affectionately as ganja (cultivated Indian hemp from the female plant), marijuana (of Mexican-Spanish roots) and many other terms, all representing different forms of the herb, has been a source of great debate amongst scientists, naturalists, herbalists, Rastafarians, and non-Rastafarians. While it is a herb and therefore one of the healthy food sources, it has been the source of much controversy due to its illegality in Jamaica, yet it is an important facet of Rastafarl cultural practices. It becomes integral to this discussion relating to health and mental health.

Rastafarl Illness and Health Beliefs

Rastafarians, like our African ancestors and compatriots, believe in the monistic concept of mind and body and have rejected the idea of Cartesian dualism, which has sought to divide the elements of the human mind from the body and therefore juxtaposing us against ourselves, providing an imbalance which at its extremities causes pain and suffering. Therefore, from the Rastafarian perspective of universal oneness, one's diet (vegetarian or vegan) and livity become critical in maintaining a totally healthy system (mental, physical, and spiritual) (Boxill, 2008; Chevannes, 2006).

In Rastafarian culture, the body is regarded as a temple and must be treated with care. The rules which govern how the body is attended to somewhat depends on the mansion to which one belongs. However, the sacredness of the body goes beyond mansions. Both the outer and the inner bodily systems are revered. Therefore one usually applies natural products (e.g., shea butter, black soap, essential oils etc.) to the outer skin and nourishes the inner organs with essential foods (e.g., nuts, vegetables, fruits, legumes etc.).[3] The body has a direct connection to the mind. If the body is pure, then it is a perfect conduit for the energy that will intertwine with the mind, also aiding its purity.

The mind is a source of great energy. All Nyabingi reasonings are exercises for the mind, assisting the process of energizing the mind–body connection to its ultimate for the good of the Rastafarian community and for the good of the entire nation. Preservation of the mind is achieved through utilizing herbs, including marijuana, which allows one to reach the "heights of meditation," reading certain books, praying, and by being disciplined with observed rituals (A. Amen, personal communication, February 3, 2010). The principle and strength of mental exercise is duly recognized and appreciated by Rastafarians.

A Rastafarian who is in the best of optimal health is physically and mentally sound. There is no separation between the mental and the physical. "Firmness" (physical strength) is a must and one must be sure about what one's position is in the global scheme of things, one's position and understanding of Rastafarl, and one's environs; these are all symbols of mental soundness (A. Amen, personal communication, February 3, 2010). Likewise, symbols of an unhealthy "livity" include over-involvement in the dancehall, alcohol drinking, sexual promiscuity or casual sex (A. Amen, personal communication, February 3, 2010).

The etiology of ill health can be explained in a number of ways. Kadamawe K'nife explains that Rastafarl began as an intuitive system of knowledge, especially because of the low level of literacy—the original elders started a largely oral tradition with the Bible as a guiding principle. The "ones" (Rastafarian people) knew intuitively what to eat and what not to eat. The "irations" (logic or reasonings) surrounding such ideology were very simple. For example, one may not eat food from *under* the ground as one is seeking spiritual *upliftment*; or one may not eat anything that grows on a vine because it causes sexual energy to rise (as the vine rises) and sexual energy is not a focal point of one's purpose on Earth[4] (K. K'nife, personal communication, 2010). Nevertheless, what ensued was certain deficiencies in one's diet, especially B12, which could cause a multitude of illnesses. Over the years, RastafarI has learned about these deficiencies and are relying more on scientific findings to counteract them. RastafarI firmly believe that one can maintain a healthy lifestyle through one's nutritional habits, which is the beginning of one's spiritual cleanliness.

In the Caribbean, illness is often believed to be caused by spiritual forces or violation of cultural taboos. This is no different for the beliefs of the Rastafarian populations; however, the addition of unhealthy nutritional practices (consumption of table salt, red meat, animal-based products, processed products, white flour, and white sugar) can also lead to some of the common chronic illnesses such as diabetes and hypertension. Livity also refers not only to spiritual cleanliness, but to personal cleanliness/hygiene, good moral standards/highly ethical behavior, good nutrition, and a reverence for nature and truth (C. Campbell, personal communication, February 2, 2010). All these factors intertwine—"cleanliness is next to Godliness"—to ensure total spiritual cleanliness and therefore strong immunity against the disease process. Clearly, these belief systems affect health-seeking behaviours; if one believes that illness is caused by spiritual forces, then one will seek remedies that connect with the spiritual realm.

The rhetoric on the etiology of mental illness has not been clearly defined or established by the Rastafarian community, thus this is classified based on one's personal/individual belief system (C. Campbell, personal communication, February 2, 2010). Therefore, one may become ill due to demon possession (e.g., Obeah), due to predisposition to mental illness brought on by stressors and exacerbated by smoking marijuana or taking hard drugs (e.g., cocaine) or due to an unnatural livity. According to Kadamawe K'nife (K. K'nife, personal communication, 2010), mental illness is derived from possessing a "superactive brain" and there must be certain genetic predispositions to same. By the same token, the curative agents for mental illness are as varied as their etiological factors and may consist of medicinal herbs, traditional medicine, psychotherapy and the reduction or cessation of marijuana and hard drugs, and finally calming techniques (yoga, relaxation, and exercise) to soothe the "superactive brain." It is thus apparent how with the evolution of RastafarI, members of the community have begun to merge their ideology and will utilize the traditional approaches to healing. Rastafarians are not so separate and apart from the population that they do not recognize the dictates of mental illness, and what it may take for healing to occur.

The typical profile of the Rastafarian youth who enters the psychiatric ward for treatment is a male in his early 20s who smokes marijuana and is inevitably diagnosed with either schizophrenia or other psychotic disorder, including cannabis-induced psychosis (i.e., ganja-induced). The initiation into RastafarI is often wrongly interpreted by many youths as the smoking of marijuana (J. Niah, personal communication, February 3, 2010; L. Moyston, personal communication, February 3, 2010). Many Rastafarian youth, ignorant of the totality and the foundation principles of RastafarI, begin their "trod" (journey) into RastafarI with the heavy smoking of marijuana. This sometimes lands them into problems with their reality testing and they end up on the psychiatric ward. On the contrary, marijuana is not a mandatory practice of all Rastafarians. In fact, Mutabaruka, dub poet and renowned Rastafarian, has always espoused that he has never smoked marijuana. Nevertheless, many immerse themselves into the practice of smoking marijuana, a practice that is, as most Rastafarians will indicate, not for everyone and has varying effects for each individual, sometimes based on dosage. Most Rastafarians understand that the relationship between ganja and self is an individualistic one.

Healing Practitioners and Practices

Caribbean people use a mix of traditional and biomedical healing practices. The degree of use of traditional means, including spiritual healing, is inversely related to class status. Consequently, most illnesses are treated holistically. When traditional means fail, modern medicine is tried (C. Campbell, personal communication, February 2, 2010). This is no different from RastafarI who sometimes utilize a quasi-folk healing approach. There is a well-known physician and Rastafarian, Dr. Carlton "Pee Wee" Fraser, who is trusted and frequently accessed by the RastafarI community including infamous Mortimo Planno, the late Bob Marley, and many others in their times of ill health. This individual is favoured by the community because he espouses a natural healing tradition and a holistic concept of livity, combined with his Western medical training (L. Moyston, personal communication, February 3, 2010). There are other practitioners, who despite their Western training, have adapted a more holistic approach, some with naturopathic/homeopathic training also, which are more suited to any treatment regime that a Rastafarian would employ and be compliant with. These practitioners in the Caribbean setting are few and far between, and are typically general practitioners. Most RastafarI who utilize mental health services (particularly inpatient services) do so involuntarily, though this is not very different from the motivation ascribed to other members of the population. This is also dependent on the type of mental health service. From the institutionally-based facilities to the psychiatric wards on a general hospital to the general wards at a hospital and private psychiatric and psychological care to the attendance of social worker, the perception and stigma is different. At one extreme, the Rastafarian who wants nothing to do with the

Babylon system, will fight against the usage of not only the mental health services, but also any medical or health service. Some will utilize a combination of medications, prescribed by the medical doctor as well as additional herbs and supplements to treat any disease process he or she may observe.

In a preliminary assessment of a number of mental health professionals, very few had in-depth knowledge of the needs of Rastafarian individuals as they had not been exposed to them as outpatients, neither psychiatrically nor psychologically. Inpatients on the other hand fit the profile previously mentioned and these youths are brought in by family members and loved ones who are concerned about the drastic shift in their behavioral and cognitive patterns (S. Longmore, personal communication, 2010).

Compliance is a difficult challenge for mental health professionals who manage patients with chronic illnesses such as schizophrenia and bipolar disorders (S. Longmore, personal communication, 2010). With the complexity and livity of the Rastafarian, that challenge is multiplied. With the reality that there are no Rastafarian or, at the very least, holistic psychiatric practitioners, that challenge is magnified further, as the first line of treatment for such chronic mental illnesses is indeed conventional medicine, such as antipsychotics (e.g., Seroquel or Risperdol) and mood stabilizers (e.g., Epilim or Depakote).

In the Rastafarian community, the importance and healing properties of herbs and nature in general is espoused in a folk herbalist tradition. "Ganja" is a plant that is termed the "healing of the nation." For some Rastafarians, ganja is essential to bring the heights of reasoning and is an important herb for medicinal purposes and mental development. For these Rastafarians, there is no place for psychotropic medication, which allows one to further lose control of one's faculties, diminish one's personality, while becoming dependent on the prescribed drug and ignoring the causative factors (C. Campbell, personal communication, February 2, 2010). While for other Rastafarians, mental or psychological development is more suited to the therapeutic realm, where the etiology of the symptoms are explored and real healing can begin and maybe there can sometimes be a place for psychotropic medication (C. Campbell, personal communication, February 2, 2010). In addition to this, exercise, nutrition, and meditation become critical to the healthy sustenance of the whole person.

Some approaches to mental health wellness espouse the eradication of the smoking habit, while others espouse a reductionist perspective. In other words, an attempt to compromise is utilized with the reduction in the amount of the herb ingested being encouraged and focus on the clear relationship (usually how the herb exacerbates the illness) that may have been established between the herb and the psychosis. When that rapport between practitioner and patient is established, this methodology appears to work best.

Healing through music is an important factor in the Rastafarian tradition. From Count Ossie (a Rastafarian musician) to the drumming at a Bingi to the reggae tunes of Peter Tosh and Bob Marley, to the genre of roots reggae (Rastafarian reggae music), music has been integral to the foundation of RastafarI. Reggae was the avenue that promoted RastafarI across the world. Drumming utilizes the natural power of rhythm and music and applies it to an individual or group for the purpose of healing. Group drumming breaks down social barriers, promotes freedom of expression, nonverbal communication, unity, and cooperation. It decreases depression, anxiety, and stress, boosts the immune system functioning, and benefits physical health.

Collaboration and an Integrative Healing Model

Mental health professionals generally utilize Western approaches to medicine when confronted with RastafarI in their midst; however, there are a few practitioners who very skillfully cross the barrier and successfully interweave the traditions and cultures of RastafarI into the healing process. These professionals not only understand the Rastafarian tradition and the current struggles and issues related to its formation and development, but they also understand the terrain that they must maneuver in order for compliance and healing to take place. What the average mental health professional may term grandiosity (delusions of grandeur) can sometimes be explained as the reasonings of the "normal" Rastafarian. In order to best deal with Rastafarians, one must have a general understanding of the traditions; some find it easier to reason and talk with Rastafarians, and to formulate compromises such as those discussed earlier with the herb.

Another consideration in clinical practice is the concept of "healthy paranoia." Rastafarians are well-reputed for their lack of trust in anything that belongs to Babylon's system. It is therefore not unusual for a sense of mistrust to prevail for outsiders and typically one has to liaise with a member of the Rastafarian community in order to enter the community. This sense of mistrust must not be mistaken amongst mental health professionals as a clinical, pathological paranoia as it serves an adaptive function and is based on reality of experience (Anderson & Morgan, n.d.).

The use of psychology, as an important part of the mental health profession, also becomes a salient point of discussion. Psychological approaches become important in how one orients to the cultural needs of such individuals. Psychotherapy is more about "reasoning" and it is here that perhaps the Rastafarian would be more willing to engage in rhetoric about his or her healing, given that, again, the understanding of his or her traditions can be carefully considered and interwoven into the fabric of treatment.

Mental health professionals must also recognize the evolutionary process that RastafarI has undergone with a shift in the economic, racial, technological, and social environments; the challenge always exists to explore and understand culture as a stable yet dynamic entity, paying special attention to issues such as gender roles, sexuality, and age to name a few. A holistic approach incorporating psychiatry, psychotherapy, nutrition, exercise, meditation, and other possible facets of healing can be critical to the "buy-in" of any RastafarI to the healing process.

The use of cognitive–behavioral therapy, music therapy, and psychological processes to the end point of strengthening the mind is more amenable to Rastafarl than are the practices of psychiatry. The psychologist can be perceived as part of the community, an elder, the replacement for that person in the community who would usually listen to one's woes and burdens and assist one with solving them (A. Payne, personal communication, February 5, 2010; K. Banton, personal communication, February 5, 2010). The techniques of the health psychologist, developmental psychologists, clinical and counseling psychologists are in line with strengthening the mind and are therefore more in line with Rastafarl (C. Campbell, personal communication, February 2, 2010; A. Amen, personal communication, February 3, 2010). It is abundantly clear that a Rastafarian client/patient would feel more comfortable with a Rastafarian practitioner. This is not unusual in the literature on multicultural competencies and preferences of clients in multicultural settings. They feel more open and trusting with ones who they believe understand them more keenly. However, the reality is that the existence of such practitioners is not sufficient (I know only of two in Jamaica), and so the emphasis is on cross-cultural understanding and how best our practitioners can bridge this gap that so evidently exists.

The Rastafarian community in its evolutionary process currently has a few of its believers who are mental health professionals. This is no doubt an important gap in bridging the divide between the Western and traditional approaches. The evolution of Rastafarl is an important concept in the rhetoric on the mental healing of the nation. There are glaring differences between the elders and the youth developing the culture, the way of life, the entire livity, with the youth being more integrative into the Babylon system which allows them to be more open to accessing mental health services, but serves as double-edged sword as it is this same integrative, evolutionary factor that allows the youth to wear more "Western" garb, eat salt, misconstrue the boundaries of sexuality, and in general to stray from strict adherence to the doctrine of Rastafarl.

Future hopes lie in having Rastafarian hospitals and more Rastafarian-based schools (e.g., Bunny Wailer's Solomonic school) as an integral part of the nation's healing. The further exploration of marijuana, which has so many healing properties, is crucial. It is one of the most powerful seeds that this earth produces and one of the most environmentally- friendly plants in the world. We know very little about the cannabis plant, only knowing about three to four properties of the 450 plus that exist (A. Amen, personal communication, February 3, 2010). Why are we not investigating these properties more carefully instead of trying to focus on its role in mental illness and as a gateway drug?

Indeed, the prevalent use of marijuana in the Rastafarian community brings about a conundrum of concerns regarding the interplay between marijuana and psychosis and the differential diagnoses of cannabis-induced psychosis and any other psychotic process (e.g., schizophrenia). The literature is replete with warnings about the linkage between ganja smoking in adolescence and psychosis in adulthood (Andreasson, Allebeck, Engstrom, & Rydberg, 1987; Arseneault et al., 2002; McGrath et. al., (2010). However, there has been much debate about the conclusiveness of such studies (NORML, 2010); about the cross-cultural relevance of such studies (Dreher, Nugent, & Hudgins, 1994); the lack of comparative data when one reviews the rising trends in marijuana usage which do not concur with the rates of schizophrenia; the lack of clarity in determining which actually comes first, mental illness or cannabis use, and the ensuing ambiguous relationship between cannabis and psychosis. These individuals and groups (e.g., Coalition for Ganja Law Reform, National Organization for the Reform of Marijuana Laws (NORML)) recognize the possible health risks and therefore call for legal regulation, much in the same way that ibuprofen and other drugs that have particular and potentially damaging side effects are regulated (NORML, 2010).

Research is necessary to further explore the issues of Rastafarl within this postcolonial reality. Most authors of books and articles about Rasta are not Rasta and are not even Jamaican. Although this can have its advantages, for example encouraging objectivity, it also has its drawbacks due to a lack of cultural understanding. The Afro-Caribbean has mainly espoused an oral tradition, so we have failed to articulate and document our own Caribbean history. The issues of Rastafarl and health, Rastafarl and mental health, Rastafarl and personality, identity, and politics all need to be researched and incorporated into the training of our practitioners.

Currently, cross-cultural studies of minority groups (i.e., African Americans, Native Americans, Asian Americans, and Latin Americans) are a mandatory part of American Psychological Association (APA)-approved doctoral psychology programmes, as mandated by the APA in its role in curriculum development. Likewise, Rastafarian practices and belief systems should be made mandatory for our Caribbean people to understand. This is a critical training issue.

Conclusion

A present challenge for mental health professionals is to deal with this conundrum of Rastafarl. This is critical because of the growing number of people, especially youth, that are being drawn into such a livity at varying levels, and are being affected by ganja smoking; because of the high rates of non-compliance with current treatment regimes; and, finally, because of the resonance of Rastafarl as something fundamentally Jamaican/Caribbean. We must therefore speak to all its aspects appropriately from our own Caribbean story, as articulated by us. The ideology that surrounds mental illness is not clearly defined from a Rastafarian perspective and so one must be flexible in one's approach, release stereotypes, and listen to the voice of the individual.

Notes

1. RastafarI is spelt throughout this chapter with a capital I at the end of the word to emphasize the central concept of empowerment through words, especially with "I."
2. Babylon is a name given to the establishment, represented by the police, governmental organizations and so on and hails from the experiences of Rastafarians with these systems, which indeed did oppress them, and attempted to destroy the foundations of the Rastafarian uprising back in the 1960s.
3. As part of the evolution of RastafarI over the past 70 years, the originally endorsed livity is not always strictly adhered to. For example, consumption of substitute meats made from wheat gluten (e.g., veggie chunks, veggie steak) and soy products (e.g., tofu) are an acceptable part of a Rastafarian diet. While still others include live foods, as the consumption of cooked food destroys the enzymes that promote healing and nourishment for the body.
4. This ideology mainly belongs to some Boboshanti peoples, the most orthodox of the RastafarI mansions.

References

Afari, Y. (2007). *Overstanding Rastafari: 'Jamaica's gift to the world.'* Kingston, Jamaica: Senya Cum Publishers.

Anderson, C., & Morgan, K. A. D. (n.d.). Looking at RastafarI: The impact of culture & religion on personality (unpublished).

Andreasson, S., Allebeck, P., Engstrom, A, & Rydberg, U. (1987). Cannabis and schizophrenia: A longitudinal study of Swedish conscripts. *Lancet, ii*, 1483–1485.

Arseneault, L., Cannon, M., Poulton, R., Murray, R., Caspi, A., & Moffitt, T. E. (2002). Cannabis use in adolescence and risk for adult psychosis: Longitudinal prospective study. *British Medical Journal, 325*, 1212–1213.

Barnett, M. (2008). The globalization of the Rastafari movement from a Jamaican diasporic perspective. *Ideaz, 7*, 98–114.

Barrett, L. E. (1997). *The rastafarians.* Boston, MA: Beacon Press

Boxill, I. (2008). The globalization of Rastafari. *Ideaz, 7.* Kingston, Jamaica: Arawak Publications.

Chevannes, B. (2006). *Betwixt and between.* Kingston, Jamaica: Ian Randle Publishers.

Dreher, M., Nugent, K., & Hudgins, R. (1994). Prenatal marijuana exposure and neonatal outcomes in Jamaica: An ethnographic study. *Pediatrics, 93*(2), 254–260.

Hickling, F. W., Matthies, B., Morgan, K., & Gibson, R. C. (Eds). (2008). *Perspectives in Caribbean psychology.* Kingston, Jamaica: CARIMENSA Publishing

Lewis, R., & Bryan, P. (1991). *Garvey: His work and impact.* New Jersey: Africa World Press.

McGrath, L., Welham, J., Scott, J., Varghese, D., Degenhardt, L., Hayatbakhsh, M., Alati, R., Williams, G., Bor, W., & Najman, J. (2010). Association between cannabis use and psychosis-related outcomes using sibling pair analysis in a cohort of young adults. *Archives of General Psychiatry, 67*(5), 440–447.

NORML (2010). NORML responds to latest warnings regarding marijuana use and schizophrenia. Retrieved on February 13, 2011 from http://norml.org/news/2010/03/05/norml-responds-to-latest-warnings-regarding-marijuana-use-and-schizophrenia

Selassie I, H., & Ullendorff, E. (translator). (1976). *The autobiography of the Emperor Haile Selassie I: "My life and Ethiopia's progress" 1891–1937.* Harare, Ethiopia: School of Oriental & African Studies.

Somé, M. P. (1998). *The healing wisdom of Africa: Finding life purpose through nature, ritual, and community*. New York: Tarcher/Putnam.

Zips, W. (Ed.) (2006). *A universal philosophy: Rastafari in the third millennium*. Kingston, Jamaica: Ian Randle Publishers.

14

HINDU HEALING TRADITIONS IN THE SOUTHERN CARIBBEAN

History and Praxis

Keith E. McNeal, Kumar Mahabir, and Paul Younger

Introduction

Hinduism found its way to the Caribbean in the hearts and minds of South Asian migrants under a new system of "indentureship" devised by the British—and soon followed by the French and other colonial powers—to supply West Indian planters with alternative sources of labor in the aftermath of slavery. Indenture was characterized by a five-year contract, often renewed one or more times, and maintained by criminal legal sanctions. Recruits were unfree while indentured, and—by the late 19th century—return passage to India had to be self-paid should one decide to quit the West Indies upon completion of servitude. Halted in 1917 due to political agitation in India, over two and a half million Indians emigrated from the subcontinent under this transoceanic system of labor migration, though less than a quarter of them returned to the subcontinent after serving their indenture (see Brereton & Dookeran 1982; Clarke, Peach, & Vertovec, 1990; Jayawardena, 1968; La Guerre, 1985; Look Lai, 1993; Mangru, 1987; Vertovec, 1992; Younger, 2002: 2010). Colonial discipline saturated the lives of indentured laborers, with frequent prosecution by employers and wretched living conditions presenting serious challenges to stable family life in addition to the maintenance of health and psychological well-being. Enslaved Africans had faced these problems as well, thus indentureship has been described as a "new system of slavery" (Tinker, 1974).

What happened from the mid-19th century onward was the gradual reorganization and consolidation of diverse beliefs and practices brought from various parts of South Asia into a more standardized type of Hindu sociocultural system: "from village and caste beliefs and practices to wider, more universalistic definitions of Hinduism that cut across local and caste differences" (Jayawardena 1968, p. 444).

This chapter therefore outlines the development of Hinduism in the southern Caribbean and considers the ways varied healing traditions stemming from South Asia have adapted to and been reconfigured by their experience in the West Indies. We focus on Guyana and Trinidad since they are home to some of the most dynamic Indo-Caribbean healing traditions, which have also had the greatest impact throughout the region as well as abroad in North America. Our discussion situates practices of religious and popular healing within changing political and theological contexts in order to analyze the most prominent contemporary forms of Indo-Caribbean therapeutic praxis: a psychosomatic healing prototype known as *jharay*, as well as practices of cathartic, trance-based psychotherapeutic treatment and devotional exorcism offered by heterodox *Shakti* temples. The colonial legacy and postcolonial transformations are examined with regard to their implications for health and mental health.

Hinduism in the Southern Caribbean

The first indentured Indians arrived in British Guiana in 1838, and almost 239,000 Indians were brought to this tiny coastal strip of northeast South America by the time the system was abolished (Younger, 2010). They likewise arrived in Trinidad, which Britain had taken from Spain at the turn of the 19th century, except the process began later there, in 1845, and involved approximately 144,000 people. The majority hailed from the Gangetic plains of northeast India, having sailed through the Bengali port of Kolkata (Calcutta) en route to the Americas. A mix of people from varied caste backgrounds arrived, though Brahmins were few and lower castes likely represented a larger percentage than in the regions from which they came. The experience of radically novel economic routines and power relations spawned a range of modified, as well as new, sociocultural forms. Though the majority was Hindu—with a small, but significant number of Muslims in the mix—an important early distinction concerned whether one was a northerner who had sailed through Kolkata or a southerner via the port of Madras (Chennai) on the coast of Tamil Nadu, i.e., a *Kolkatiya* versus *Madrassi* (La Guerre, 1985).

Indians were seen as hailing from an inferior Oriental civilization, thus condescension animated the official colonial position on Hinduism and Islam, a legacy that translated into a stubborn local tendency to refer to people of South Asian descent as *East*—rather than West—Indians, thereby framing them as "outsiders" and complicating their political claims on the state in both colonial and postcolonial incarnations (Khan, 2004; Munasinghe, 2001; Segal, 1989; 1993; 1994; Sheller, 2003; Williams, 1991). Given conventional assumptions about the "essential" relationship between caste and Hinduism in South Asia, it is ironic that growth of mainstream Hinduism was in fact facilitated by attenuation of the caste system in the West Indies, where caste could not be transplanted as an integrated system of social structure, economic relations, and ritual hierarchy (Van der Veer & Vertovec, 1991).

The result was a "leavening" process (Haraksingh, 1986; 1988) in which beliefs and practices from varied localities and communities in India were submerged and reformulated in relation to one another. Hinduism and caste ideology were simplified under the oppositional principles of high/low, pure/impure, Brahmin/Chamar, and North/South Indian: protean categories mediated by the contingencies of local power relations.[1] Structural transformations reflected by these categorical modifications enabled aspiring Indians to take advantage of the overseas experience by shedding connections with previous status and elevating themselves as New World higher "castes" of a sort. To the extent that the discourse of caste persisted at all, it became a cipher deployed in the negotiation of new class relations within the changing political economy of capitalism (see Jayawardena, 1968; Schwartz, 1967; Younger, 2010).

The process of social leveling fostered by indentureship meant that the expansive number of those claiming Brahmin status were able to establish themselves as leaders of the "North Indian" community. Their leadership was as much sociological as it was religious, and a thriving new temple tradition evolved in the wake of indentureship to meet the emergent needs—including health and psychological—of the Hindu community. These *mandir* (temple) traditions became the locus for congregational communities that met on Sundays for worship typified by devotional singing and listening to the Brahmin give a "sermon," or *katha*. Pandits (priestly Hindu specialists who oversee and direct ritual observances and life cycle rites) also provided pastoral care to families throughout the week. This form of Hinduism is strongly Vaishnavite—i.e., oriented to Vishnu—in theological orientation and characterized by an emphasis on *bhakti* devotionalism (Vertovec, 1992). Drawing support from conservative Hindus, the development of standardized West Indian Hindu accelerated in the 1920s under the canopy of Sanatanism in response to the provocation of *Arya Samaj* reformism emanating from India. A "Sanatanist" is a follower of *Sanatan Dharma*—known as "Eternal Order" or "Traditional Religion"—and Sanatanism had already begun to consolidate in the subcontinent in response to the Samajjist challenge (Younger, 2010).

The overall point here is that a dominant form of Hinduism emerged in the 20th century West Indies under the neo-traditionalist sign of Sanatan Dharma. The waxing and waning of an internal Samajjist–Sanatanist dialectic was overdetermined by the fact that Christianity retained hegemony as the dominating cultural barometer of social status and moral legitimacy throughout the colonies, putting Hindus on the defensive. Thus the Indo-Caribbean community internalized values espoused by colonial elites and adopted them as their own terms of reference in an effort to forge a "respectable" Hinduism. This orthodoxy is predominantly devotional and Vaishnavite in orientation, identified with "North Indian" tradition, proctored by a transculturated Brahmin ceremonial elite, has become standardized as well as centered upon a limited set of "high" Sanskritic deities, and is as much sociological as it is religious in practice. Though the apical position of Brahmins is hardly watertight—especially in the postcolonial era—Hinduism may be understood as having become progressively ethnicized under their stewardship in the Caribbean. Van der Veer and Vertovec (1991, p. 158) observe that West Indian Brahmins have, in important ways, achieved an even more central social position than in India itself.

Yet the other side of this homogenizing Brahmanical coin has been the marginalization of ostensibly "low" or "impure" folk practices falling outside of the alleged "orthodox" orbit. Most Brahmins relaxed their attitude toward lower "castes" and took on a role comparable to that of a parish priest, multiplying their functionality in diaspora while closely guarding the sanctity of the office through secrecy and some degree of endogamy. Caribbean Brahmins widened their purview as proletarian Hindus progressively embraced their vision, thereby consolidating the hegemony of Sanatanism. In negative terms, mainstream West Indian Hinduism has distanced itself from "heterodox" healing practices, as well as actively marginalized ostensibly "primitive" ritual modalities such as animal sacrifice, ritual fire-walking, trance performance, and spirit mediumship signifying abject aspects of the Indian past (McNeal, 2011).

Jharay and *Shakti*: Hindu Caribbean Healing Practices

This process of orthodoxification is reflected in curricula for the training of pandits developed late in the 20th century, which are not especially focused upon healing, per se. They do focus on astrology; however, this is only indirectly relevant to therapeutic praxis in that identifying auspicious times for doing important things or fulfilling various ritual obligations is pertinent for the general pursuit of well-being. Pandits may treat sufferers by offering to *jharay* them, discussed further below, which they often learn to perform by observing their gurus or growing up in a family of pandits, rather than formal didactic training. *Mantras* (mystical chants) and *yantras* (talismans)—of which there are two local types: *tabij* (amulets) and *totka* (apotropaic magic)—are also commonly used among Hindus for spiritual protection, yet they are increasingly looked down upon as "superstitious" by educated or higher-class Hindus.

Anthropologist Steven Vertovec (1992) observed that the system of folk Hindu magic known as *ojha* overlaps and intermingles extensively with the Afro-Creole tradition of *Obeah*, and that *ojha-men*—or "seer-men"—serve clients of all ethnic and religious backgrounds. Indeed, anthropologists Arthur and Juanita Niehoff (1960) earlier concluded that Indo-Caribbean incorporation of black ritual and religious forms was historically much greater than usually imagined. Ojha specialists traditionally offered a number of services—sometimes for significant prices—such as casting spells or protecting people from them, counteracting cases of the evil eye (known as *najar* in patois Hindi, or *maljo* in the more predominant Creole tongue), soothsaying, concocting love potions, and locating lost items. Ojha was used to deal with various culture-bound syndromes that have become progressively recessive among Indo-Caribbeans of the late 20th and early 21st centuries, such as affliction by *rakas* (dastardly infant demons), *patnas* (which attack only unmarried girls), *jumbies* (wayward ghosts), and other folk spirits (Mahabir, 2010). It is clear that ojha had already begun to be seen as a "lower" status activity by the 1950s, if not before (Klass, 1961; Niehoff & Niehoff, 1960).

Jharay

One of the most prominent types of healing within the local Hindu repertoire is known as *jharay*, the only component of the folk healer's therapeutic armamentarium that continues to be used while the rest of the ojha tradition has dissipated. The term "jharay" is used in the West Indies as both verb and noun, e.g., "the pujari jharays" and "I got a jharay." It refers to purification administered through ritualized "brushing" or "sweeping" of the seeker by a mystical specialist. Healers use various implements in order to jharay supplicants—commonly *cocoyea* broom (palm frond) straws, but also sometimes peacock feathers, *doob* grass, or vibhuti pinched within one's fingers or held in hand—and utter mantras that empower their work. One may be jharayed for conditions as varied as insect stings or snake bites, head and stomach aches, jaundice, or cases of maljo, as well as anxiety or depression, or for good fortune during trying times.

The efficacy of jharay as a therapeutic ritual technology varies depending upon the circumstances at hand. We see psychosomatic illnesses as more amenable to religious cure than organic diseases. There is no one singular form of jharay, but the underlying model recurs across a range of popular modalities. Thus a masseuse may jharay at times, but only if they are sufficiently adept. Jharaying is widespread among Hindu Obeah men or ojha men and women, yet it is unclear how much pandits employ this technique—some do, but many do not, as a result of dominant trends in both orthodox religion and biomedicine outlined above.

Shakti

Jharaying is itself embedded at the heart of the other main form of Hindu healing in the contemporary southern Caribbean—known as *Shakti Puja*, or Kali Worship—which takes place in temples dedicated to therapeutically-oriented trance performance and spirit mediumship. This practice of healing is widely considered a "Madrassi" tradition; yet, such a characterization is more apt for Guyana, than Trinidad (McNeal, 2011; Younger, 2002; 2010). Shakti refers to the cosmic energy activating the universe in its polymorphous complexity, and is associated with the *devis*—or goddesses—in Hindu cosmology. Puja refers to ritual worship directed towards a deity. West Indian Shakti Worship revolves around devotion to—and healing received from—deities conjured through spectacular trance performances by spirit mediums, all of which now takes place within temples under the overarching aegis of Mother Kali (in Trinidad) or Mariyamman (in Guyana), even though it also traffics in masculine deities. The tradition is deemed "heterodox" from the Sanatanist perspective since it is predicated upon practices of popular mysticism considered "primitive" and less than "respectable," although this bias may be relatively lesser in Guyana than Trinidad.

A reconstituted Madrassi ritual tradition coalesced early in the 20th century in British Guiana due to the substantial number of south Indians living in the compacted coastal colonial society. In contrast to the north Indian-inflected "Hindu" tradition, Madrassi ritual praxis was less political and more mystical, centered on devotions to the goddess Mariyamman and other flanking deities. Guyanese Madrassi religion became temple-based and premised upon regular offerings to the gods—including live animal sacrifice in addition to fruits, flowers, coconuts, lit flame, and so forth—in order to cultivate devotional relationships with them and seek their healing interventions through the trance performances of ecstatic mediums.

In Trinidad a much smaller percentage of Madrassis in colonial society became more encompassed by the evolving tradition of Sanatanism. Their lively wedding and funerary traditions—as well as devotions to Mariyamman and a spectacular tradition of firewalking—were practiced throughout the period of indentureship, but more or less eclipsed by the mid-20th century. There were also north Indian traditions of Kali Puja involving animal sacrifice and trance performance as part of community devotions to Mother Kali in colonial Trinidad, as well as *Di* Puja (pronounced "Dee"), in which the spiritual "Master of the Land" is entreated for agricultural fertility or protection of the household. All of these practices— Madrassi and otherwise—were deemed "heterodox" by the muscular Sanatanism that gained such traction after World War II. Yet links were made by several aspiring Indo-Trinidadians with Pujari Naidoo in Guyana, who helped establish the first postcolonial mandir dedicated solely to shakti healing in Trinidad. This first temple community was followed by a series of extensions and schisms, producing a set of temples that continues to proliferate to this day.

Shakti Puja is often observed on a weekly basis in temples that range in size from makeshift shacks to compounds capable of holding hundreds of people. Most are oriented around a central *murti* (sacred statue) of Mariyamman or Kali, around which—in turn—are positioned her accompanying gods and goddesses at concentric levels of remove. Divinities of "orthodox" north Indian provenance are also present in these temples, but they are secondary to the "heterodox" deities that operate as the most central sacred personae within these ritual precincts. Devotees arrive early before the puja armed with flowers, milk, fruit, and other items offered to any or all of the *deotas* before the formal service begins. The general structure of the temple puja consists of *pujaris* (ritual leaders and their assistants) and an attending group of devotee–observers moving to each and every deota "stand" (location of the *murti*) in order to make offerings of fruit, flowers, green and dry coconuts, incense, lit flame, and possibly install a *jhandi* (spiritual flag representative of each divinity). Ritual performance is accompanied by devotional songs and musically driven by the rhythmic percussion of typically three or five or more *tappu* (special goat-skin) drums. The round of puja offerings to the deities culminates climactically in collective devotion to the great central goddess herself, via her *murti* as well as her performing spirit medium. If the temple makes blood offerings via live sacrifice, it is at this point that the animals are beheaded for whomever they are being offered.

People bring all sorts of issues and problems to be dealt with by deotas. These "consultations" are conducted openly within the space of the mandir; however, everyone except those directly involved stands back in order to create a buffered space of semi-privacy for the divine interchange. The entranced "manifestation" of the deities through experienced adepts is the highpoint of Shakti Puja and many people visit such temples on puja days with the specific purpose of consulting with the deotas via their ecstatic oracles about a wide range of existential problems such as illness, domestic or work conflicts, infertility, sexual dysfunction, or *tabanka* (love depression). As one devotee put it: "Yuh go to Kali when you have to, not when you want to!" The end of the puja is also a time when especially severe cases of illness or spiritual affliction may be dealt with more privately by the primary healers of the temple. Leaders of some temples may also be available during other days of the week in order to "see about people" with special concerns or urgent thera-peutic needs. There are also cases of practitioners who run private healing centers out of their home without holding public puja. The more involved or complicated the case, the more the pujari's pastoral care expands, often leading to long-term social relations with the primary healers and temple community more generally.

One senior pujari observed that his temple "come like a clinic," continuing:

> We can heal the sick with shakti. But it is not we that is doing it, it is God. So the divine Mother Kali and all the deities – they are using the bodies of these people, of these pujaris, to cure and heal the sick.

Trance performance within these temples is conceived as the activation of shakti energy within the human body.

This temporary "elevation" of shakti in a spirit medium makes the practice of jharaying with *neem* leaves—a sacred Indian plant closely associated with devi worship—especially powerful during ecstatic consultations in temple puja. Jharaying in shakti praxis is conducted with a bundle of ritually prepared neem fronds, which are brushed all over the head and body of the supplicant or devotee. This is a potent gesture transmitting the healing power of the god's shakti to those who seek it. Jharaying in shakti temple puja is usually accompanied by an interchange with the deity through its ecstatic votary, such as making a confession or seeking advice, receiving instructions about how to focus one's devotions in order to "get through" difficult times. Ecstatic mediums take flaming cubes of camphor into their mouths, or hold them in their hands, as a performative sign of authentic mystical activity taking place, the logic being that only superhuman power can withstand the heat and avoid getting burned.

Lay members as well as visitors to shakti temples also commonly become entranced by shakti "vibrations," but this form of "catching power" is a lower-level, more generic type of mystical energy not identifiable as any specific divinity. This baseline form of ecstasy experienced by lay devotees or spiritual seekers may be intensely cathartic, as it offers the opportunity to phenomenologically transcend oneself within a supportive, ritualized context. In retrospect, such experiences may come to be seen as the beginning of one's career as a medium, if one ends up graduating to the higher level of performance and much more complex register of experience. These experiences feed reciprocally into prayer and personal devotion outside the ritual arena, creating a ramifying chain of experience that may gain transformative momentum over time—what psychotherapy refers to as the "expanding circle of mental health."

William Guinee's (1990) survey data demonstrate that people involved in Kali Worship in contemporary Trinidad are often poor and suffering, with nowhere else to turn. They have attempted to relieve their distress through more conventional routes without success. Thus they become open to an alternative community that welcomes them and their problems. Once meeting with success through ecstatic temple puja—accessing the healing power of the Mother and her associates via trance performance—their motivation shifts and they may become more deeply affiliated with the temple community. They may even themselves become involved in care-giving for others over time. The clientele of temple-based Shakti Puja is also considerably more ethnically and religiously hetero-geneous than that of orthodox Hindu mandirs.

Guinee's (1992) extraordinary study of suffering and healing in one of the largest Kali Temples in Trinidad shows how the practice of ecstatic Shakti Puja operates as an embodied theodicy, forging new attitudes and transformative relations over time when successful. Spiritual diagnoses of problems made at the mandir offer hope and an explanation for misfortune or suffering, as well as provide a devotional recipe for bringing about relief and change. The supplicant participates in a series of exchange relations with deotas (deities) mediated by both mediums and the temple community, fostering cathartic devotional praxis that alleviates one's sense of helplessness—and thereby fosters a more buoyant, grounded, proactive sense of self—through participating in procedures that do something concrete and compelling about it. There is much more nuanced research to be done on the psychospiritual complexities and self-transformative "magic" of such healing practices.

One important difference between the practice of shakti healing in Trinidad and Guyana is that Guyanese practitioners are much more committed to appeasing and soliciting the gods through live sacrificial animal offerings, as compared with Trinidad, where the dominance of Sanatanism has been amplified by greater socioeconomic mobility. More than in Guyana, this sphere of religious practice has progressively abandoned live animal sacrifice as part of orthopraxy in Trinidad, although several "holdout" temples continue to resist the switch to the wholly vegetarian approach to puja known as *sada*.

Ecstatic Shakti Puja is important not only because this complex practice is one of the most prominent forms of healing in the contemporary West Indian Hinduism, but also because it is the therapeutic practice that has traveled most extensively among Indo-Caribbeans throughout the north Atlantic world. Extensions of Trinidadian-style Kali Worship have also spread further afield in several major metropolitan centers of the United States.

Yet, it may be Trinidad that has recently taken the lead in spreading the gospel of Shakti Worship within the Caribbean region itself. Ritual linkages have recently been forged between a prominent Trinidadian temple and a small, but symbolically significant community of Hindu-identified Martiniquans of African and mixed-African descent. Mahabir (2011) observes that people of Indian descent in Belize and Guadeloupe also look towards Trinidad for inspiration and support in recent attempts at reclaiming their history and culture. Trinidad and Tobago has substantial oil and natural gas resources that make it the industrial and financial powerhouse of the West Indies, thereby able to project national cultural power throughout the region.

In addition, the proliferation of new digital media as well as the continued circulation of Caribbean people throughout the Atlantic world foster dynamic patterns of cross-fertilization and reciprocal influence among varied healing modalities and nationally inflected temple traditions that have yet to be adequately documented and analyzed.

Collaboration and an Integrative Healing Model

It is important to note that the forms of therapeutic engagement and spiritual healing discussed here—especially jharaying and Shakti Puja—may involve conclusions reached on the part of the healer that a supplicant, or "patient," would be better served by a biomedical doctor, and thereby make such a "referral." We (especially McNeal) have encountered such assessments in collecting the life histories of various devotees, and witnessed these referrals made on the part of shakti mediums dealing with people in search of healing power. Hindu hospital patients are sometimes jharayed by ritual healers while their doctors turn a blind eye.

Kumar Mahabir (2012) considers all of the therapeutic forms discussed above along with other folk healing practices such as herbalism, midwifery, massage, and chiropractics in his typology of ethnomedicine in Trinidad, seeing them as sorely under-appreciated within the local infrastructure of health care. Indeed, Mahabir argues these ethnomedical traditions represent "untapped development potential" in the late modern era of neoliberal globalization and structural adjustment programs, which downsize the public health sector and scale back formal health care. Indo-Trinidadian massage especially stands out in this regard, since its benefits span a wide range of conditions and there were as many practitioners on the island in the mid-1990s as there were doctors and nurses. While biomedicine is dominant, largely militating against whatever legitimacy ethnomedicine might otherwise garner, the relationship between bio- and ethnomedicine is complex, including the persisting relevance of some traditional therapeutic traditions at the proletarian level, as well as aspects of biomedicine filtering down into ethno-medicine in less overt, yet nonetheless significant ways.

It must be emphasized that practitioners of vernacular Caribbean Hindu healing do not view their traditions as inherently or necessarily in competition with biomedicine despite the fact that most biomedical practitioners see popular healing practices as "primitive" holdovers destined to eventually die out. Yet such thera-peutic practices are successful in certain ways, at certain times, and under certain conditions. They are especially efficacious when used to deal with psychological illnesses and psychosomatic conditions. Healers recognize this with distinctions such as differentiating between "Mother Work" and "Doctor Work," for example. However, the line between ethno- and biomedical therapy is neither static nor distinct in personal experience or ritual practice. Indeed, according to Singer, Araneta, and Naidoo (1976) it was Pujari Naidoo's years of observing psychiatric intake assessment and clinical interviews conducted between doctors and patients in Guyana's colonial-era mental hospital that inspired his dispensing with liturgical pidgin Tamil speech by ecstatic mediums in his mandir in the 1960s, effecting a change that would better approximate psychotherapy, as well as exert ramifying effects throughout the region.

Conclusion

The understanding and experience of spiritual illness—as well as its treatment and various therapeutic outcomes—change over time in dynamic interrelations with healers, family members, and other factors. The idiom of "spirit" affliction is a protean one that may obliquely express a multifarious range of conflicts and problems in one's life, making it an elusive object, yet also meaningful precisely because of this ineffability. The operation of spirits in oneself may reflect intrapsychic pain or interpersonal conflict, yet also provide a fulcrum for spiritual intervention and vehicle for self-transformation. Indo-Caribbean Hindu healers understand this. Their therapeutic engagements are geared toward cultivating and harnessing the sacred power of trance praxis in order to care for others and ameliorate their suffering or alienation.

Their interventions are not always successful, but in this regard they are akin with biomedicine and psychotherapy, neither of which is infallible, but contingent upon person, problem, and circumstance as well. Indeed, Indo-Caribbean Hindu healing traditions are resilient and respond to the times. Biomedicine may be ascendant, but it coexists with these practices that express the soul as much as the body—and for this reason, they are unlikely ever to be wholly superseded. The question is what sorts of new complex configurations the future holds. Much research remains to be done.

Note

1. *Chamar* refers to a demographically large, low-caste group in India who worked traditionally as cobblers in leather-working trades and therefore considered ritually unclean. However, the term has been broadened throughout much of the diaspora as a derogatory gloss more generally.

References

Brereton, B., & Dookeran, W. (Eds.). (1982). *East Indians in the Caribbean: Colonialism and the struggle for identity*. Millwood, NY: Kraus.

Clarke, C., Peach, C., & Vertovec, S. (Eds.). (1990). *South Asians overseas: Migration and ethnicity*. Cambridge: Cambridge University Press.

Guinee, W. (1990). Ritual and devotion in a Trinidadian Kali Temple (master's thesis). Indiana University.

Guinee, W. (1992). Suffering and healing in a Trinidadian Kali Temple (Doctoral Dissertation). Indiana University.

Haraksingh, K. (1986). Culture, religion and resistance among Indians in the Caribbean. In U. Bissoondoyal and S. B. C. Servansing (Eds.), *Indian labour immigration* (pp. 223–237). Mauritius: Mahatma Gandhi Institute.

Haraksingh, K. (1988). Structure, process and Indian culture in Trinidad. *Immigrants and Minorities, 7*(1), 113–122.

Jayawardena, C. (1968). Migration and social change: A survey of Indian communities overseas. *Geographical Review, 58*, 426–449.

Khan, A. (2004). *Callaloo nation: Metaphors of race and religious identity among South Asians in Trinidad*. Durham, NC: Duke University Press.

Klass, M. (1961). *East Indians in Trinidad: A study of cultural persistence*. Prospect Heights, IL: Waveland Press.

La Guerre, J. (Ed.). (1985). *Calcutta to Caroni: The East Indians of Trinidad*. St. Augustine, Trinidad: University of the West Indies Press.

Look Lai, W. (1993). *Indentured labor, Caribbean sugar: Chinese and Indian migrants to the British West Indies, 1838–1918*. Baltimore, MD: Johns Hopkins University Press.

Mahabir, K. (2010). *Indian Caribbean folklore spirits*. San Juan, Trinidad: Chakra.

Mahabir, K. (2011). Editorial. *Indian Arrival Day Magazine*, Trinidad.

Mahabir, K. (2012). *Traditional medicine and women healers in Trinidad*. San Juan, Trinidad: Chakra.

Mangru, B. (1987). *Benevolent neutrality: Indian Government policy and labour migration to British Guiana, 1854–1884*. London: Hansib.

McNeal, K. (2011). *Trance and modernity in the Southern Caribbean: African and Hindu popular religions in Trinidad and Tobago*. Gainesville, FL: University of Florida Press.

Munasinghe, V. (2001). *Callaloo or tossed salad? East Indians and the cultural politics of identity in Trinidad*. Ithaca, NY: Cornell University Press.

Niehoff, A., & Niehoff, J. (1960). *East Indians in the West Indies*. Milwaukee Public Museum Publications in Anthropology, *6*.

Schwartz, B. M. (Ed.). (1967). *Caste in overseas Indian communities*. San Francisco, CA: Chandler.

Segal, D. A. (1989). *Nationalism in a colonial state: A study of Trinidad and Tobago* (Doctoral dissertation). University of Chicago.

Segal, D. (1993). Race and "color" in pre-independence Trinidad and Tobago. In K. Yelvington (Ed.), *Trinidad ethnicity* (pp. 81–115). Knoxville, TN: University of Tennessee Press.

Segal, D. (1994). Living ancestors: Nationalism and the past in postcolonial Trinidad and Tobago. In J. Boyarin (Ed.), *Remapping memory: The politics of timespace* (pp. 221–239). Minneapolis, MN: University of Minnesota Press.

Sheller, M. (2003). *Consuming the Caribbean*. London: Routledge.

Singer, P., Araneta, E., & Naidoo, J. (1976). Learning of psychodynamics, history, and diagnosis management therapy by a Kali cult indigenous healer in Guiana. In A. Bharati (Ed.), *The realm of the extra-human: Agents and audiences* (pp. 345–370). The Hague: Mouton de Gruyter.

Tinker, H. (1974). *A new system of slavery: The export of Indian labour overseas, 1830–1920*. London: Oxford University Press.

van der Veer, P., & Vertovec, S. (1991). Brahmanism abroad: On Caribbean Hinduism as an ethnic religion. *Ethnology, 30*(2), 149–166.

Vertovec, S. (1992). *Hindu Trinidad: Religion, ethnicity and socio-economic change*. London: Macmillan.

Williams, B. (1991). *Stains on my name, war in my veins: Guyana and the politics of cultural struggle*. Durham, NC: Duke University Press.

Younger, P. (2002). *Playing host to deity: Festival religion in the South Indian tradition*. New York: Oxford University Press.

Younger, P. (2010). *New homelands: Hindu communities in Mauritius, Guyana, Trinidad, South Africa, Fiji, and East Africa*. New York: Oxford University Press.

15

ISLAMIC INFLUENCE IN THE CARIBBEAN

Traditional and Cultural Healing Practice

Abrahim H. Khan

Introduction

Islam came to acquire a recognizable presence in the Caribbean from 1837 with waves of Indians arriving to supply the labor force for British sugar plantations. Its influence on the traditional and cultural lore of the region is reflected in at least one healing practice known by *dam karna*, an Urdu expression that means roughly, "blowing breath." Still occurring, the practice is part of religion "as it is lived," or of vernacular religion that American folklorist Primiano (1995) distinguishes from "official" or elite religion understood primarily with respect to philosophic-theological doctrines or group rituals. It belongs also to the genre in the history of understanding oneself with respect to human survival and well-being, in countries that once were part of the British colonial Caribbean sugar plantation and political economy and relied on indentured Indians for its labor force.

Health care provision in the harsh indentureship conditions was a bare minimum, planters defaulting in the contractual obligations, according to Mangru (1987); reliance for remedying ailments was on local practices informed by the cultural lore shaped by religion. Despite the comparative ready access of modern medicine in Guyana and Trinidad, the persistence of *dam karna* is an indication of continued belief in its efficacy, and thus is a reason to consider it as an adjunctive therapy and treatment in existing or primary health services in the Caribbean.

In scholarship the medical literature shows signs of a correlation between religion and health, especially in the area of mental health and well-being (Bhut, King, Dein, & O'Connor 2008; Koenig, 2001; Cinnirella & Loewenthal, 1999). At a primary health care level, religious beliefs and practices are increasingly accorded recognition in North American medical practice as a resource for coping with trauma from life's adversity and suffering (Newberg & Lee, 2006). But this recognition has yet to be extended to the role of religion in Caribbean traditional and cultural healing. A discussion of *dam karna* would assist at the least in better formulation of ideas and research projects appropriate to health care in the region.

This chapter has for its underlying argument that *dam karna* belongs originally to a form of life, aspects of which have to be recovered for the practice to become an adjunct to existing health care services. It explains how the expression *dam karna* gained currency in the vernacular of the English Caribbean colonies and hence remained in use even among the Indo-Caribbean diaspora in North America. This is then followed by an exposition or recovering of the healing practice relative to Islamic principles, practitioners, and remedies. Finally, considerations are offered for its acceptance as an adjunctive therapy in a primary health care system.

Methodologically, the study proceeds along ethnological and humanistic lines in the academic study of religion. Its explanation and analysis presuppose that *dam karna* is intelligible in the context of vernacular religion. According to Primianio, the concept of vernacular religion allows for recognizing religious beliefs as involving a complex of conscious and unconscious negotiations of and between religious believers in unequal power relations, and as having a bidirectionality influence in relation to the environment, each affecting and being affected by the other.

Though official Islam and Hinduism eschew recognizing the interactional phenomenon, a widening (see, for example, Bowman, 2003; Khan, 2004: Smith, 1967) in the academic study of religion makes it possible to consider the phenomenon "vernacular religion." The exposition on *dam karna* is based on first hand acquaintance with the associated form of life while growing up in Guyana and augmented by conversations with Caribbean Muslim diaspora members in Toronto and Orlando. Archival materials are employed as further checks and balances—travelogues, diaries, and historical, literary, cultural studies (socio-political) and newspaper reports from Guyana, Trinidad, and Jamaica, with respect to factors coming into play to form a unified and organic system of belief for religious individuals.

Presence of Islam in the Caribbean

From 1838 to 1917, India under British rule dispatched to the Caribbean 619,988 immigrants as indentured workers to the sugar plantations that faced a sudden shortage of labor force due to the abolition of slavery. The plantation workers went primarily to four countries: Guyana received the largest number 238,909; followed by Trinidad 143,939; Guadeloupe, 43,326; and Jamaica, 36,420. Roughly 13% of the total immigrants were Muslims and Urdu speaking. The remainder was considered to be largely Hindus, and mainly Hindi speaking. Today, however, the majority of Muslims are in two countries. Guyana has approximately 13% of its estimated 800,000 population, and Trinidad 8% of its 1,400,000 population. With their arrival, Islam gained its foothold in the

Caribbean region, and *dam karna* became transplanted (Birbalsingh, 1989; Lal, 1983; Seecharan, 1997).

Not unexpected, a fluidity in customs, religious practices, and beliefs at the quotidian level in that indentured situation existed between Islam and Hinduism as forms of life. That is, conscious and unconscious negotiations between the two religious traditions were occurring to form a unified and organic system at the vernacular level that helped to deal with the harsh living conditions. The fluidity helped at a communal or neighborly level to deal with harsh living conditions associated with indentureship and plantation life. With respect to relief from ailments that seemed mental/psychical, *dam karna* is a case in point about the fluidity. This was not peculiar to the diaspora, for it has its antecedents in areas from where more than 90% of the immigrants had come, and what is today the State of Utter Pradesh (Flueckiger, 2006; Sengupta, 2009). The search for health and well-being clearly seems to trump religious strictures associated with orthodoxy in Islam or Hinduism and that define the identity of many of the adherents of each religion, especially in Guyana and Trinidad (Khan, 1998; 2004). In those two countries today Islamic culture thrives alongside that of Hinduism and Christianity to the point that it is recognized in the form of national holidays by each county.

Before the Indian indentureship, Islamic influence had reached the Caribbean through the slave trade that brought African Muslims. Even prior to British slave trade, Islam may have had a presence in Jamaica through Moorish mariners, and later through free Muslim Moors or Maroons, according to Afroz (2008). Religious gatherings and practices were done secretly by Maroons working as slaves, but under supervision of kinfolks considered as spiritual guides, or friends of Allah (*Awliya' Allah*) (Solaiman, n.d.).[1] The *awliya'* are pious one, making intersession to God on behalf of those requesting divine assistance. The dominance of Christian conversion and influence in the plantocracy led to erosion and erasure of Islamic gatherings and practices.

However, recent archival and anthropological work in Trinidad (Khan, 2004) is showing Islamic influences and suggesting cultural fluidity or blending with Hinduism. Remnants of Islamic practice are being identified by the academic research of Afroz (1999; 2001). In Jamaica, one example of a remnant is the use of the term *bucra* by Maroons and slaves to characterize the animal attitude of a fellow human. According to Afroz (2008), the term is a corrupt form of the Arabic *baqarah* meaning cow, and the name for a chapter of the Qur'an—Surah al Baqarah. Verses 67–71 about self-sufficiency and obstinacy reference a type of individual, notes Afroz, whose human development is arrested and with loss of the ability to recognize that he or she is no longer spiritually alive. When used by Maroons and slaves, the term *bucra* was meant as amusing, in mockery of the oppressors or sugar planters that they were that type of individual–spiritually dead.

Muslims account for 0.15% of Jamaica's estimated 2.4 million people. Reports on Friday prayers puts the attendance at 100, though festival celebration days may see as many as 10,000 according to Dawes (2005). Given the comparatively small size of the community, it is not surprising that for Muslims in Jamaica there is a similar cultural fluidity to Guyana and Trinidad. That fluidity extends to treating the sick or to traditional healing practices correlating with beliefs that define a Muslim or Islamic view of life.

Islamic Principles and Belief System

The interplay between religion and health is by no means exclusively associated with an Islamic context. According to its over 2,000 year history, Mesopotamian, Persian, and Egyptian civilizations linked disease or illness befalling a person to the actions of a demon or evil deity (Reynolds & Tanner, 1983; Tempkin, 1973). Greek and Hebraic–Christian religious traditions, for example, evidence the intermeshing. Religions seek not only to relieve suffering, or to heal, but offer as well an explanation for the human condition. They explain the prevalence of disease, sickness, and evil as human failings to live in truth—be it through disobedience, defiance, or forgetfulness as in monotheistic religions; or by ignorance and unmindfulness as in non-theistic religious traditions. In this respect, Islam is no different. Its sacred text, the Qur'an, especially the last Surah, Chapter 115, known as An-Naas,[2] is a call to trust in Allah as protection from evil or the practice of witchcraft. In the healing practice known as *dam karna*, sometimes confused or identified with *jharay* (and hence evidencing cultural fluidity), Qur'anic verses come to play an important role, as do the pious ones or *awliya'* mentioned earlier.

Islam has central to its life view the notion of faith (*iman*) that is adumbrated by six basic articles. They are expressed here briefly as belief in 1) the unity or oneness of Allah/God, 2) angles of God, 3) the Qur'an as a revealed book or God's guidance as is the Torah, Psalms, and Gospels comprising the Christian Bible, 4) prophecy—Muhammad is another prophet in the tradition of the Hebrew or Old Testament prophets, 5) the day of judgment in the afterlife, and 6) divine decree— God having decreed for human kind free choice remains the creator and knower of all. They, in one way or another, are presupposed by *dam karna.*

At the very heart of human life according to Islam is the idea that guidance is from God alone through the Qur'an. Practicing and especially God-fearing (*taqwah*) Muslims know by heart the Qur'an as a holy book (Khan, 2004). Those who know and practice its commands, and live a devout life are perceived as potent in healing. They are the intercessors (*awliya'*), having become friends of God by purifying their hearts through *dhikr* or remembrance of God. They in fact impart to healing its Islamic influence.

Healers and Healing Remedies

The traditional and cultural folk healing practice we are discussing is sometimes referred to colloquially by different names: *dam karna, maangna du`ā`*, and *jharay*.[3]

Etymologically, each alludes to performance or action. The first, *dam karna*, an Urdu expression, is derived from the Persian *damiidan* which is to blow or breathe, and associated with the Arabic "*dam*/blood." This associative meaning, in connection with healing, is intensified by the meaning of the noun *dam* = breathe, air, life, scent, and stewing over a slow fire (Alavi, 2008; Steingass, 1892). These meaning ranges are suggestive of spreading over the whole that which is essential or life giving. The Urdu verb, *karnaa*, derived from Persian, means "to do"; hence *karna* is the act of doing, and *dam karna* is to do the blowing after making the supplication that includes reciting a passage of the Qur'an, which for adherents is a life-giving or affirming book. In this connection, it is important to note that the Qur'an is received by Muslims as a miracle, the only miracle associated with Muhammad when asked by his detractors to show one, as proof that he is a messenger of God.

The expression, *maangna du'ā'* is an Urdu one meaning "supplication," but often rendered as prayer, and used here as such. It is clearly different from the liturgical *salāt* or prayer done five times daily. The word *maangna* written also as *māngnā*, is to ask or beg as in knocking from door to door for alms;[4] the Arabic *du'ā'* is a humble supplication/prayer of which there is a different one for each occasion or circumstance (Platts, 1884). Hence, the expression works out to "asking humbly with hands held out to receive a blessing/healing by God." The hands, at the end of the petition may then be wiped over the face as token of having received blessings, according to Padwick (1969). In Toronto, Jamaican Muslims at rehabilitation institutions with an imam as chaplain use the term *du'ā'* in requesting the imam to say on their behalf a fitting Qur'anic prayer and to do the blowing of breath. However, used colloquially by Guyanese and Trinidadians, the expression refers to a performative act—that of praying as in pleading with God for health, to dispel dis-ease or infirmity

Central to the performative act are Qur'anic recitations as prayers. They include verses from *al-Fatihah*, the open surah of the Qur'an (seven verses), followed by other verses. Qur'anic verses used as prayers are from the surah al-Fatihah, quite likely surahs al-Falaq and al-Nas, Chapters 113 and 114, respectively; and the verse/*ayat* al-Kursi or 2:225 as may be fitting. Other verses appropriate to the request may be in order. Though not part of the performative act, the treatment may include the ill person wearing a *tabeej*/amulet (in Arabic *ta'wiz*), or a yellow dress for a number of days, or facing the sun and saying a mantra or prayer, as the healer may consider appropriate. For the sick or seeker of remedy, knowledge of the source or content of the recitation matters not at all. Rather, it is belief in the efficacy of the performance or healing act that counts.

As a healing act, *dam karma* has at least two components. One is the supplication or prayer/*du'ā'* that involves the reciting of the appropriate verses for the Qur'an. The other is the blowing of breath over the affected area of the person. It is not the breath itself that has the efficacy, but the spoken words of God, given by the Qur'an. Those words are spread over the body or infirmed part by reciting the verses and immediately blowing on the body or infirmed area. Sometimes, instead of blowing on the body, the blowing is done over a cup of water and given to be drunk by the sick. The term for requesting the performative act is *maangna du'ā'* as if it references the two components, but in fact it literally means "asking for supplication." Sometimes too, the Qur'anic verses are written in digits on a piece of paper, folded and given to be kept in the pocket or carried in a *tabeej*/amulet worn on the body, either arm, shoulder, or waist, using a string. Digits are used to represent the syllables of the verses of the Qur'an, whose words are considered sacred, life-giving, and requiring reverence and ablution before opening the book itself. The digitalized form mediates the reverence for the text and the reality that one is inescapably exposed to pollution in daily living but must nonetheless have the self become permeated with the word of God. It may even be the case that the paper with Qur'anic verses written by the maker of the *du'ā'* is put in water to dissolve as much as possible and drunk.

Remedies sought are, for example, those for a continually crying child, presumed to be suffering from an evil eye or gaze (Urdu-Hindi: *nazar*) cast on the child or from a seemingly unexplainable pain or dis-ease. Sometimes the gaze or stare is cast innocently, that is, the person may not be aware of having the gaze, and casts it through an innocent comment or praise about a child's good looks. Sometimes it occurs when there is envy or jealousy. Ailments in individuals would include pains that are abdominal, limbic, or elsewhere on the body, and might be accompanied by diarrhea, or refusal to take food and drink. Sometimes the cure sought is for a mental health condition, or one associated with an evil spell and spirit possession. Sometimes the condition is connected with dreadful dreams. Conditions are often ones that medical prescriptions have failed to remedy, or have not been medically diagnosed correctly. Thus they turn to alternative medicine or forms of healing.

To be sure, in connection with *dam karna* there is no healer but only a person performing or doing it—reciting the texts and blowing the breath. Such persons are regarded as living a morally exemplary and religiously devout life, reputed to be learned about matters of healing, or known to be the head of a brotherhood, and may be perceived as having *karamaat*/charisma (blessed) by being a friend of Allah, close to God. Whether male or female, that person is often in the community or village and presumed to have the knowledge of what to say and do. Sometimes a family member, considered spiritually and morally upright and who has seen it done frequently in his/her own family may be called upon, in urgency, to do *dam karna*. Generally an older person, he or she is addressed respectfully in the vernacular by names such as *sadhu, babu, maiya ji, shaykh, didi, mamu,* that are customarily used in the village or life situation. Further, persons doing the recitation and blowing are knowledgeable about the Qur'an, can read and know what verses to recite and are often imams (Khan, 2004). Some imams in conversation with me were reluctant to acknowledge that they are approached for healing purposes. But one indicated that as many as 90% of the imams known to him would read and do the blowing. In short, the infirmed seeks out assistance from one who is knowledgeable about the Qur'an, and knows how to read or recite by heart this Arabic text, especially the verses appropriate for the situation for which healing is being sought. In all of this, the reciter is not a healer nor pretends to be one, for the presumption is that it is Allah through the Qur'an by which healing is effected.

Sacred–secular intersections or religious observances are often considered auspicious for healing and making petitionary prayers. It might be expected that the 10th of Muharram or the first month in the Islamic calendar is one such point. For Shi'ite Muslims in Trinidad and Jamaica that day is observed as the Hosay festival, and in Guyana is identified as *tadjha* day,[5] commemorating the martyrdom at Karbala. For Sunni Muslims it is a joyous day, commemorating the day Adam and Eve were created, Noah's ark landed, and Solomon received his kingdom. During the indentureship period the Hosay festival became widely popular, with all ethnicities participating to the point that it ceased to be a heartening and life-affirming occasion (Khan, 2004). By the mid-20th century, it had fizzled out in Guyana, but continues to be observed in Trinidad in a carnival-like style or spectacle, and to a very lesser extent in Jamaica. Neither archival research[6] nor conversations with knowledgeable members of the community give any indication that the Hosay festival functions in the Caribbean as it does in Africa and elsewhere, as a sacred–secular intersection for divine healing to occur.

Collaboration and an Integrative Healing Model

Contextualized and described, *dam karma* as a healing practice is not unique to the Caribbean. It has cultural variations and is fairly widespread in the Muslim world. Case studies of healing practice among some Bangladeshis in England, and Muslims in Pakistan, South Africa, Palestine, and the US offer evidence and are comparatively more detailed in their social science methodology. Further, in a study of Bangladeshis in England, Rozario (2008) distinguishes between two kinds of illness: one that is medical, and another that is caused by evil spirits or *bhuts*, and requiring remedy by a spiritual practitioner.

In Palestine, the majority of folks find no contradiction, according to anthropologist and folklorist Sharif Kanaana (2004), between folkloric daily practices and the practice of official Islam. Though official religion condemns their folkloric practices, they seem unaware of each practice belonging to a different (sub) system, or where one ends and the other begins. Sharif Kanaana's description of one subsystem is that of holy men, engaged in prayer, fasting, reading the Qur'an, and able to do *karamaat*/miracles. They are the vehicle through which remedies are effected. Altogether, from those studies mentioned, the pattern of healing practice bears striking family resemblance to that of *dam karna* in the Caribbean. Based on my conversations with Caribbean Muslims in Toronto and Orlando, that practice continues among diaspora members today. What is important to note is all the variant healing modes associated with Islam, whether in the Caribbean, Asia, the Middle East, or Africa, clearly rely on the centrality of the word of Allah or Qur'an (see, for example, Abdulla, 1992; Mason, 2002; Naidoo, 1985).

The persistence of *dam karna* in the Caribbean region has also to be understood relative to the accessibility and quality of medical care in the region, especially among former British colonies. Reasons for its persistence are fairly intuitive. Use of prescription medication would sometimes fail to take into consideration sociocultural conditions that hinder properly following medicinal instruction. Another is the lack of urgency in updating the medical practitioner's training, a consequence of which is incorrect diagnosis, prescription, or techniques in caring. Other contributing factors to the lack of urgency include inadequacy in methodology of the science and the availability of refined techniques and/or state of the art equipment. These factors, not all empirical knowledge related, are connected with socioeconomic and political priorities. They are determinants of accessibility to medical treatment for rural area people, and especially those having to eke out a bare daily existence. In times of crisis or when health is at risk, the individual sufferer turns to what is available and known to bring relief, regardless of whether it is folk or modern medicine. In short, there is an alternative to interpreting or understanding the reality of suffering or impediments to health and well-being, not readily accommodated always by the practice or paradigm of modern medicine.

Unlike rural folks, urban people are less constrained from gaining access to health care services. Yet, they also tend to rely on traditional and cultural healing practices such as *dam karna* and consider that one kind of practice complements the other. In fact, one professional in Trinidad from the Muslim community indicated that there was no need to rely on such healing practices when everyone in his country could have access to medical services. Further along the conversation he began relenting when asked why *dam karna* still seems to linger.

A likely and important insight about *dam karna* may have been overlooked by the community member in his zeal for modern medicine (Y. Asgarali, personal communication, 2010). It is that *dam karna* may at one level have therapeutic value or significance, namely that physiological processes are influenced by emotions and stresses that are reducible through religious beliefs and rituals. This mind–body connection is one that modern medicine, psychiatry, and psychotherapy are beginning to more readily acknowledge and, where appropriate, to integrate or modify the medical paradigm regarding the nature of the reality that is called suffering, health, and well-being (Abruzzi & McGandy, 2003). In other words, there is more awareness of drawing a distinction between disease and illness, and for that matter curing and healing, and of acknowledging that traditional healing practices may correlate with etiology that is related to a humoral pathology, or bodily energy disequilibrium (see, for example, Foster, 1976; Hisham & Kabbani, 1997). Efforts to explore alternative conceptions of reality with respect to illness and in fact just what is meant by objectivity with respect to medicine is relatively recent, beginning just after World War II (Hisham & Kabbani, 1997; Kleinman, 1995; Koenig, 2001).

A strong warrant, in short, exists for considering *dam karna* as adjunctive therapy in a health care delivery system. That is, while some health disorders are culture bound, it is equally clear that some others have a non-naturalistic etiology. Their causes are personalistic, traced or imputed to the intrusion of a spiritual entity and thus the disorders or ailments do not fit neatly the disease patterns normally correlating with the diagnostic categories of Western medicine. Such are some of the cases that have received, for an intervention, *dam karna*, where Allah/God is understood as the healer. Included in that genre are the well documented cases of miracles, one of the criteria in the Christian tradition, for canonization by the Vatican (Duff, 2008).

Conclusion

To continue withholding recognition of *dam karna* when it is clearly efficacious for certain disorders makes little sense in light of emerging interests in the connection between healing religion and medicine. There are antecedents, if not good reasons, for considering how it and similar healing practices might contribute to health and well-being in the cultural and political economy of the Caribbean. Such consideration does not mean an abandonment of the quest for intelligibility in becoming an adjunctive therapy to existing health care services. For without that quest no human science is possible nor, for that matter, the academic study of the interplay between religion and medicine.

Clearly, *dam karna* provides another investigative area in medicine and mental health. In particular, it opens up opportunities for exploring further connections between areas such as counseling psychology and spirituality, or Islamic hospital chaplaincy. It is at this level that its practitioners can be annexed by a mainstream health care system to be in dialogue with health care workers and thereby begin a process towards regularizing the healing practice.

Notes

1. Solaiman (n.d.). Chapter 2 discusses the spiritual influence of this brotherhood or *Tariqah* from West Africa. Chapter 3 discusses the coming of Indian Awlyia to Guyana.
2. Especially verse 4, referring to the mischief of those practicing secret arts or witchcraft. In fact the last three chapters are quite important for warding off evil and becoming healed. *Surah* 114 is also with respect to protect from evil and witchcraft.
3. Derived from the Hindi *jhāṛā* to sweep away, remove, clean off, or drive away, either with fire, bush brush, or a bramble broom. Jhadu is to cast off evil spirit (Shakespear, 1834), and is phonetically similar to Arabic *jharrah*, used in 19th century north India to refer to the local doctor/hakim or barber.
4. Platts (1884), for *dar-dar māṅgnā* is knocking/beating door to door asking. See also *bhīkh-maṅgā* in Platts (1884).

5. An etymological deviant of the Arabic *ta'ziya* that means mourning or consolation, *tadjha* refers in general to the gathering for commemorating the martyrdom of the grandsons of the Prophet Muhammad at Karbala, and is marked by a day of Atonement called '*Aashura*, that is the 10th day of Muharram.
6. No evidence is found in studies by scholars familiar with and who have published on the community: Bisnauth (1993); Ferguson (2006); Khan (1998); Korom (2003); Mangru (1993); and Thaiss (1994; 1999).

References

Abdulla, I. H. (1992). Diffusion of Islamic medicine into Hausaland. In S. Feierman & J. M. Janzen (Eds.), *Health and healing* (pp. 177–196). Berkeley, CA: University of California Press.

Abruzzi, R., & McGandy, M. J. (Ed.) (2003). *Medicine: Encyclopedia of science and religion.* Macmillan-Thomson Gale (pp. 552–556). Retrieved March 20, 2010, from http://www.bandung2.co.uk/Books/Files/Religion/Encyclopedia%20of%20Science%20and%20Religion.pdf

Afroz, S. (1999). From Moors to Marronage: The Islamic heritage of the Maroons in Jamaica. *Journal of Muslim Minority Affairs, 19*(2), 161–179.

Afroz, S. (2001). The Jihad of 1831–1832: The misunderstood Baptist Rebellion in Jamaica. *Journal of Muslim Minority Affairs, 21*(2), 227–243.

Afroz, S. (2008). As-Salaamu-Alailum: The Muslim Marroons and the Bucra Massa in Jamaica. *Slavery and Abolition, 29*(4), 543–713.

Alavi, S. (2008). *Islam and healing: Loss and recovery of an Indo-Muslim medical tradition.* Basingstoke: Palgrave Macmillian.

Bhut, K., King, M., Dein, S., & O'Connor, W. (2008). Ethnicity and religious coping with mental distress. *Journal of Mental Health, 17*(2), 141–151.

Birbalsingh, F. (1989). *Indenture & exile,* Toronto: TSAR

Bisnauth, D. (1993). *History of religions in the Caribbean,* Kingston: Kingston Publishers.

Bowman, M. C. (2003). Vernacular religion and nature: The "Bible of the Folk" tradition in New Foundland. *Folklore, 114*(3), 285–295.

Cinnirella, M., & Loewenthal, K. M. (1999). Religious and ethnic group influences on beliefs about mental illness: A qualitative interview study. *British Journal of Medical Psychology, 72*, 503–524.

Dawes, M. (2005, April 23). The Muslim way in Jamaica. *Jamaica Gleaner.* Retrieved March 20, 2010, from http://www.jamaica-gleaner.com/gleaner/20050423/%28spirit%29/%28spirit%291.html

Duff, J. (2008). *Medical miracles: Doctors, saints, and healing in the modern world.* Oxford: Oxford University Press.

Ferguson, J. (2006). The Muslim minority in Jamaica. *Jambeat, 1*(2). Retrieved March 1, 2010, from http://jamfash.tripod.com/muslim.html

Flueckiger, J. B. (2006). *In Amma's healing room.* Bloomington, IN: University Press, 171–175.

Foster, G. M. (1976). Disease etiologies in non-Western medical systems. *American Anthropologist, 78*(4), 773–782.

Hisham, S., & Kabbani, M. (1997). Spiritual healing in the Islamic tradition. Presented at Harvard Medical School. Retrieved June 25, 2009, from http://naqshbandi.org/events/benson/paper.htm

Kanaana, S. (2004). Folk religion among Palestinians, Inash Al-Usra Society. Retrieved February 20, 2010, from http://www.zajel.org/article_view.asp?newsID=3460&cat=20

Khan, A. H. (1998). Indian identity and religion in Caribbean literature: *Shikwa*/Complaint. *'Ilu Revista de Ciencas de las Religiones, 3*, 133–145.

Khan, A. (2004). *Callaloo nation: Metaphors of race and religious identity among South Asians in Trinidad*. Durham, NC: Duke University Press.

Kleinman, A. (1995). *Writing at the margin*, Berkeley, CA: University of California

Koenig, H. G. (2001). Religion and medicine III: Developing a theoretical model. *The International Journal of Psychiatry in Medicine, 31*(2), 199–216.

Korom, F. J. (2003). *Hosay Trinidad: Muharram performance in an Indo-Caribbean diaspora*, Philadelphia, PA: University of Pennsylvania.

Lal, B. V. (1983) *Girmitiyas: The origins of the Fiji Indians*. Canberra: Journal of Pacific History.

Mangru, B. (1987). *Benevolent neutrality*. London: Hansib Publication

Mangru, B. (1993). *Indenture and abolition: Sacrifice and survival on the Guyanese sugar plantations* (pp. 18–43). Toronto: TSAR Publications.

Mason, J. E. (2002). "A faith for ourselves": Slavery, Sufism, and conversion to Islam at the Cape. *South African Historical Journal, 46*, 3–24.

Naidoo, L. R. (1985). *Indigenous healing among Indian South Africans*. Paper presented at a cross-cultural symposium by the Department of Psychiatry, Medical School, University of Natal. Retrieved March 2, 2010, from http://www.docstoc.com/docs/19823497/1-Indigenous-Healing-Among-Indian-South-Africans-LR-Naidoo-1

Newberg, A. B., & Lee, B. Y. (2006). The relationship between religion and health. In P. McNamara (Ed.), *Where god and science meets religion*, vol. 3 (pp. 35–66). Westport, CT: Praeger.

Padwick, C. E. (1969). *Muslim devotions*, London: SPCK.

Platts, J. T. (1884). A *dictionary of Urdu, classical Hindi, and English*, London: W. H. Allen & Co.

Primano, L. N. (1995). Reflexivity and the study of belief. *Western Folklore, 54*(1), 44–46.

Reynolds, V., & Tanner, R. (1983). *The biology of religion*. New York: Longman.

Rozario, S. (2008). Allah is the scientist of the scientists: Modern medicine and religious healing among British Bangladeshis. Asia Research Institute, *Working Paper Series No. 101*, 11–13.

Seecharan, C. (1997). *"Tiger in the stars": The anatomy of Indian achievement in British Guiana 1919–29*. London: Macmillan.

Sengupta, S. (2009, March 17). Braids of faith at Baba's Temple: A Hindu-Muslim idyll. *New York Times, International*. Retrieved February 19, 2010, from http://www.ny times.com/2006/03/17/international/asia/17varanasi.html

Shakespear, J. (1834). *A dictionary, Hindustani and English*, 3rd ed. London: Parbury, Allen, & Co. Retrieved February 19, 2010, from http://dsal.uchicago.edu/dictionaries/shakespear/

Smith, W. C. (1967). *Questions of religious truth*. New York: Charles Scribner.

Solaiman, M. A. (n.d.). *A short history of the Awliya' Allah in Guyana*. Retrieved March 19, 2010, from http://www.wimnet.org/t&t/Guyana%20Awliya.PDF

Steingass, F. J. (1892). *A comprehensive Persian-English dictionary, including the Arabic words and phrases to be met with in Persian literature*. London: Routledge & K. Paul. Retrieved March 17, 2010, from http://dsal.uchicago.edu/dictionaries/steingass/

Tempkin, O. (1973). *Dictionary of the History of Ideas* (Vol. II) (pp. 395–407). New York: Charles Scribner and Son.

Thaiss, G. (1994). Contested meanings and the politics of authenticity: The *Hosay* in Trinidad. In A.S. Ahmad & H. Donnan (Eds.), *Islam, globalization, and postmodernity.* London: Routledge.

Thaiss, G. (1999). Muharram rituals and the Carnivalesque in Trinidad. *ISIM Newsletter, 3*(99), 38.

PART IV

Traditional Healing and Conventional Health and Mental Health

16

COMMUNITY MENTAL HEALTH IN THE ENGLISH SPEAKING CARIBBEAN

Gerard Hutchinson

Introduction

The development of mental health services in the English speaking Caribbean has occurred in parallel with the training of mental health professionals in the region. The philosophy of this process has always been community service driven and has been influenced by the growth of the training opportunities in mental health offered by the University of the West Indies. The vision of the university to train professionals to serve the region (Sherlock & Nettleford, 1990) has been integral to the community mental health treatment services that are currently being provided. However, these services have struggled to fully meet the needs of the communities they serve because they have been thus far unable to fully reconcile the complex health related traditions and belief systems of Caribbean people with the imported models of science based illness models that have been imported though adapted from the dominant Euro-American cultural axis.

As the poet Martin Carter (1977) wrote, "I walk slowly in the wind, watching myself in things I did not make" (p. 58).

The Caribbean constitutes one of the world's most mobile societies exporting the largest percentage of its constituent population in the world. Internal rural to urban migration, and continued migration to the USA, England, and Canada has also tampered with the social and family fabric, already challenged by the sense of poverty and dissatisfaction with the possibilities of life in perceived backward and underdeveloped islands. This has created among other phenomena the concept of barrel children, referring to children who are nurtured through the contents of barrels sent to them by their parent/s who live abroad. The reparation of money to the region by relatives living abroad is also a great source of income in some island economies (Bakker, Engils-Pels, & Reis, 2009). This loss of direct nurturing by parents and the dependence on the financial and material support from abroad alongside the decline in community support has been partly blamed for the rise in delinquent and criminal behaviour among adolescents in the region. The pervasive cultural influence from the metropolitan centres in the United States and Britain has also been thought to contribute to an increase in maladaptive behaviour such as self-harm, drug use, and a range of developmental disorders including Attention Deficit Hyperactivity Disorder (ADHD) (Crawford-Brown, 1999).

Additionally, the geographic location of the West Indian islands have facilitated their use as transshipment points for cocaine, moving between its production base in South and Central America to its main demand bases in North America and Europe. This has led to major mental health and social problems including cocaine addiction, escalating gun crime, and the psychosocial problems associated with drug dependence, in some instances permanently scarring communities and families and eroding the effects of material progress within Caribbean society (Pan American Health Organization, 1986; Reid, 2005). In this way, mental health in the region has developed primarily along a socially conscious needs based trajectory. However, there is still a pervasive perception that mental health problems are caused by supernatural or spiritual factors rather than by changes in brain or central nervous system functioning. As much as 30% of medical students in Trinidad for example believe that mental health problems are caused by supernatural practices or influences. This reflects a dominating cultural view as many people continue to believe that mental health problems are caused by supernatural if not spiritual forces (Hutchinson, Neehall, Simeon & Littlewood, 1999). This has inexorably led to a conflict between traditional religio-magic thinking and the more recently embraced Western empirical tradition from which the training of the mental health professionals has been drawn.

The shifts in Western philosophy about psychiatry and mental health paradoxically still provide the intellectual guidance for the training of our psychiatric practitioners in the region in the absence of a clear philosophical ethos to guide the practice of Caribbean mental health treatment (Hutchinson, 2005). The Diagnostic and Statistical Manual (DSM) system of the American Psychiatric Association has become the diagnostic standard in the region although there is ongoing debate about the cultural applicability of some of its categories (Thakker &Ward, 1998). These issues have implications for the expectations that are placed on mental health service delivery and the ways in which services have developed to meet these expectations.

This chapter discusses the evolution of training as a means of community mental health provision and assesses the particular mental health concerns that affect the region. Issues such as religion and the role of traditional healers in the context of adapting the services to the needs of the people are also discussed. Finally, it addresses the need for adjunctive mental health service providers from the private sector as well as non-governmental organizations.

History of Mental Health Provision

Community mental health treatment in the English speaking Caribbean has been evolving in theory and practice over the past 45 years and has grown in parallel with training in psychiatry and psychology at the University of the West Indies (UWI); however the embrace of formal community mental health care has not been comprehensive (Beaubrun, 1992). An appreciation of the need for educating medical professionals more extensively in psychiatry was first articulated by Michael Beaubrun in a paper entitled "Psychiatric education in the Caribbean" (Beaubrun, 1966). At that time (the mid-1960s), Beaubrun noted that mental health treatment was concentrated in asylum type mental hospitals in the larger islands of the Caribbean, Jamaica, Trinidad, Barbados, and Guyana, and in some of the smaller ones as well. He advocated for an expansion and extension of mental health services that would provide better community care and for increased public education about mental illness. He wrote that the existing situation did not adequately meet the needs of the West Indian population and directed the establishment of a 25 bed psychiatric unit at the University Hospital in Mona, Jamaica, and eventually began training psychiatrists by the end of that decade to serve the needs of the West Indian community. This was a landmark initiative because it was the first public attempt to bring mental health care into the mainstream health domain and by extension out of the mental hospital. He also identified the need to train mental health nurses, psychiatric social workers, and psychologists. The psychiatric unit in a general hospital was seen by Beaubrun as a prototype and the first step toward the development of community mental health services. It led to the eventual establishment of Psychiatry Units in most of the major general hospitals in the larger islands of the West Indies and served to predict the expansion of mental health services into the community. Beaubrun (1977) also pioneered the training of community mental health nurses who provide the backbone of the community mental health care by traveling into the communities and providing mental health support.

This of course paralleled and reflected an increasing awareness in the metropolitan world that patients with mental health disorders could function effectively in the community and that a mental health diagnosis was not synonymous with a lifelong stay in a mental hospital. It provided a model for the development of mental health services within general hospitals and to locate psychiatry in this context. It also encouraged the process of moving the diagnosis and treatment of mental health disorders closer to the community in both literal and figurative senses, demystifying the closed door sensibility of a mental hospital/asylum. However, this is a pendulum that has swung back and forth over the course of the history of mental health treatment (Sumathipala & Hanwella, 1996).

Mental Health Training in the Caribbean Context

Beaubrun (1966; 1992) implied that the cultural focus on training in psychiatry should be in the environmental setting in which practice was to take place (as compared to the previous practice of travelling to Britain or the USA). This was consistent with the philosophy of the independence era in the West Indies at that time (Trinidad and Tobago and Jamaica were granted independence from Britain in 1962, and Barbados in 1965). This also inadvertently nourished the notion that the most effective mental health care in particular should be sensitive to the sociocultural context of the people it was designed to serve. This anticipated the ideas of multiculturalism and cultural sensitivity in mental health practice.

The growth of community mental health services has therefore been facilitated by a supply of psychiatrists and more recently psychologists in the region through the development of training programs at the three regional campuses in Jamaica, Trinidad, and Barbados which serve the English speaking Caribbean. Postgraduate training in psychiatry now occurs at each of these sites. Training in psychiatry in the region has to be reconciled with the principles of training as espoused by the Royal College of Psychiatrists and the American Psychiatric Association (Horwitz, 2002; Moller, 2001). These principles while rooted in the biopsychosocial model emphasize the biology of the brain as the main focus of psychiatric interest. This has situated the individual as the site of pathology and the focus of intervention, thereby diminishing the community context in which he or she functions (Novas & Rose, 2000). This has in turn led to an emphasis on biological interventions as being the preferred options for clients of mental health.

Definitions regarding the nature of mental health have therefore mostly focused on mental illness, and mental health perceived as the absence of this demonstrable illness. This has probably occurred because the focus of treatment in mental health has been predominantly psychiatry driven in the region until this new decade. In some islands, however, there are no psychiatrists and care must be delivered by psychologists with referral to general physicians and surgeons when necessary. Psychology has become the undergraduate degree with the highest demand at the University of the West Indies (Hickling, Mathies, Morgan, & Gibson, 2008) and there are now postgraduate training programmes in each of the campuses for clinical and counselling psychology. This is suggestive of a greater sensitivity to the need to understand the behaviour of Caribbean people in the context of greater access to information and the exposure to the globalized world. The impact of eroding community supports that had hitherto been taken for granted, such as supervision of children, community sport, and cultural activities, has resulted in a renewed attempt to establish a sense of psychological well-being in the context of overall wellness (Williams & Griffith, 2005). A study in Jamaica suggested that the mediators of psychological well-being and life satisfaction in the community were related to perceptions of physical health and social status in terms of religion and marriage (Hutchinson et al., 2004).

The Mental Health Clinic and the Community

The public perception of mental health care remains almost entirely derived from the pattern of mental health service development that focuses on a major mental hospital, perhaps small psychiatry units in general hospitals, and satellite clinics geographically dispersed throughout each island. These clinics are located usually in health centres that devote specific days to mental health treatment. In islands where there are no psychiatrists, a situation now that is rare, psychiatric nurses and /or psychologists provide the mental health input, and the medical management would come from general physicians and surgeons This pattern is the standard for mental health care in the English speaking Caribbean.

Community clinics have been instrumental in bring a greater awareness of local needs to the attention of the wider mental health services while also making the delivery of mental health care more personal. Since these clinics are conducted in the primary care health facilities, they reinforce the medical model as the basis for treating with mental health problems from a purely biological medication based perspective. While there is a place and need for this, there is sorely lacking a more whole person approach and interventions that focus more specifically on psychological and social issues rather than medical and psychiatric ones. Since the base for these services remains the hospital, genuine community outreach is often a result of the instinctual cultural orientation of the practitioners rather than an institutionalized service development paradigm (Hickling & Maharajh, 2005; Maharajh & Parasram, 1999). In this way, the philosophy of training has created the existing awareness of the value of mental health care and has largely followed the trends that have taken place in the metropolitan world.

The concept of sectorisation, which refers to the use of geographically defined units to locate mental health teams, appeared early in the 1970s and attempted to establish services in as close a proximity to where people lived as possible (Hickling & Gibson, 2005). However, the axis around which care turned remained the inpatient treatment facility. These facilities have continued to be large asylum type mental hospitals which have persisted in the larger islands of Jamaica, Trinidad, and Barbados as well as some of the smaller islands such as Grenada and St Vincent for example.

This has led to the maintenance of the pervasive belief system that mental health problems only require significant intervention when the afflicted are demonstrably a risk to themselves or others as evidenced by aggressive or violent behaviour or consistently inappropriate socially disruptive behaviour. Roland Littlewood (1996) described this as a kind of benign stigma which posits a general tolerance of aberrant behaviour until it becomes threatening and/or embarrassing. The problem is that because it has been psychiatry led, it has remained rooted in a medical model.

In addition, the use of substances both licit and illicit remains the most frequently utilized response by people experiencing stress in the population, particularly those in rural areas who are not well served by the community health system (Valtonen, Sogren, & Cameron-Padmore, 2006). This then leads to a treatment gap which is partially addressed by services being provided by churches and other religious organizations, non-governmental organizations providing services to families and victims of various kinds of trauma, and the healers of the religio-magic variety. Interestingly there has been a resurgence of interest in this type of approach paralleling the rise in the West of interest in alternative treatment strategies such as acupuncture, yoga, meditation, and a range of other interventions including those directed specifically at the spirit (Aarons, 1999). There is, however, growing suspicion about the use of medication for these kinds of problems as perpetrated by the medical and pharmaceutical industry which champions the medical model of psychiatry. This has been partly due to a lack of balance because of a relative shortage of other mental health professionals such as psychologists, psychiatric social workers, and occupational therapists. As these services have become more accessible, there has been a growing demand for counseling type services not just from mental health practitioners but also from churches and other community groups (Allen, 2001).

Nevertheless, the inability to further the community mental health agenda has been partly due to a lack of resources, and to the stigma and perception that those deemed to be mad are permanently afflicted and likely to be eventually violent. However, many non-governmental organizations provide community mental health initiatives, although these are usually for specific populations, for example rape victims, trauma affected families, alcohol and drug abusers, and activity within non-governmental organizations varies across the islands. There are also, in some islands, Employee Assistance Programmes (EAPs) which are funded by the employer in order to provide psychological and social services to their workers who may be experiencing these kinds of problem (World Health Organization, 2011).

Community Mental Health and Traditional Healing

The initial aims have therefore not entirely been met and the evolution of the provision of mental health treatment has continued to be primarily housed in the mental hospital in a firmly grounded medical perspective. This perspective has not fully or successfully endeared it to the communities it seeks to serve in the way it was perhaps first envisaged. In other words, it remains apart from the community and has not become an integral component of community psychosocial health (Maharajh & Parasram, 1999).

Self-harm behaviour is increasing and in some countries suicide rates are high, while homicidal behaviour is a cause of concern throughout the region, with particular issues related to gang formation in deprived communities and the ever popular but sinister drug trade (Blum et al., 2003). Interest in the effects of alcohol dependence and more recently cocaine has been necessary because both are the consequences of geography and history. The West Indies were the major producers of sugar in the New World (Williams, 1970) and one of the by-products of this industry was the rum industry. Drinking alcohol excessively has long been one of the major community health problems, contributing to poor physical health as well as a number of psychosocial problems which directly or indirectly impact on mental health. The use of cannabis and cocaine are also problematic in the context of transshipment issues described in the Introduction and the widespread availability of cannabis which continues to attract young urban users.

Although there is increasing secondary and tertiary education, many children with learning disorders go undiagnosed until their teenage years and some for their lifetime, because of the absence of trained mental health professionals who can conduct these assessments. This too has affected the psychosocial fabric of the West Indies, hindering societal development and affecting the behavioural norms that are consistent with community development. Individuals who are not able to fulfill their potential because of these minor cognitive deficits become targets for the drug trade and other non-progressive activities. Another recent hypothesis is that some of the behavioural problems in the Caribbean population are a consequence of personality issues which are negatively impacting interpersonal and intimate relationships, parenting, family nurturing, and responses to authority (Hickling et al., 2008). Among young West Indians, there seems to be a disconnect with both authority and history, leading to a sense of disenfranchisement and consequent antisocial behaviour at worse and at best a lack of commitment to personal development in the context of regional development. This nihilism may be contributing to the escalating problems of criminal behaviour, drug use, and self-harm (United Nations Office of Drugs and Crime, 2007).

There has also been a shift in the psychosocial organization of communities in the West Indies, where there has been a rise in individualism and a consequent loss of collectivism. This focus on personal benefit has seen a decline in many community activities beneficial to mental health such as community based sport and cultural endeavours. Community supervision of children, insistence of standards of social conduct, and nurturing of socially positive values have all given way to a pervasive by any means necessary philosophy to acquire material and/or social prestige even in the midst of profound deprivation (Girvan, 1997). It has also fostered the transformation of gangsters into community leaders who have acquired their status by providing material community support through the dispensation of largesse principally obtained from their drug and gang related criminal activities (Mathies, Meeks-Gardner, Daley, & Crawford-Brown, 2008). They also act as role models perpetuating the romanticized notions of violence and social intimidation as the vehicle of leadership and material success (Chevannes, 2001).

Gender relation is the other area which is impacting significantly on community mental health and is in a state of flux. Greater empowerment of females has led to a declining tolerance for domestic abuse and an increased presence of women in the traditional male dominated areas of education and employment. A difficulty with adjustment among males is creating increasing relationship and gender related conflicts. The Jamaican educationist Errol Miller (1991) wrote several years ago that men were at risk and the evidence supporting this assertion is growing significantly and spreading throughout the region where girls are outperforming boys at every turn while boys continue to be overrepresented in violence, drug use, and criminal activity. Interestingly women are greater utilizers of mental health services and indeed all health facilities and it may be this willingness to seek help that has cemented their ongoing drive for improvements in their psychosocial environment.

A greater understanding and sensitivity of the processes that inform help-seeking behaviour in postcolonial multiethnic developing societies is necessary given the distrust of institutions and a suspicion about the benefits and side effects of psychotropic medication. There must be a direct investment in the further development and expansion of the skill base in mental health to ensure that adequate and relevant training informs best practice. Wider public education to facilitate a better and faster recognition of mental health problems throughout the lifespan, and active and constructive partnerships between the various elements of community treatment must be established. There have been some attempts to realize this through training in psychology for ministers of religion and perhaps there should also be exposure to the practices of the dominant religious and faith based communities for mental health practitioners (Allen, 2001).

Religion is a powerful force in the negotiation of community mental health. There has been an increasingly collaborative relationship between religious and mental health practitioners, though the borders of this collaboration remain blurred both for clients and for practitioners themselves. In Jamaica, there is one psychiatrist/psychotherapist who is also a trained pastor and marries the two ideologies in his practice (Hickling & Gibson, 2005). Psychology education has also become an integral part of training for those undertaking theological training and the first postgraduate programme in counselling psychology was in fact established by the School of Theology in Mona, Jamaica.

Still, these two have not always been merged successfully or satisfactorily and remain independently functional with some tension. There is still widespread use of an assortment of healers, pundits, priests, and Obeah men as the population seeks to deal with the problems of their existence and their relationships with others. However, research among the African American and Caribbean community in the USA has demonstrated the psychological value of the Baptist church in the ongoing negotiation of psychological distress among its membership and there is also emerging vindication of the social support role of membership and participation in church related activities as a protector against the conversion of psychological distress to mental illness (Griffith, 1995).

Religion therefore has a pivotal role to play in the process of preventative mental health and treatment. The Caribbean remains a place where religious belief and behaviour play significant roles in community perceptions of itself. I have already alluded to the belief in the supernatural and the spiritual and these are fuelled by the growing evangelism and even in the growth of Islam in the region. Bridges must be constructed to create working alliances between mental health practitioners and the religious establishment to ensure the creation of common agendas and mutual support in the management of psychological distress in the communities which they serve. Many religious organizations host health clinics for the treatment of physical illness in their congregations and the next step would be to incorporate mental health clinics into this process. It has been shown that up to 25% of those patients utilizing primary health care facilities have either primary or concomitant mental health problems (Maharaj, Reid, & Misir, 2010) and it is conceivable that avid participation in religious activities may also be a sign of underlying physical distress.

Many people seeking help from the mental health clinics also engage in a parallel system of help-seeking with herbalists, alternative health practitioners, religion, and spiritual and supernatural supports. There is clearly a need to work together with traditional healers and religion to mount an effective response to the mental health needs of the region.

Indeed, holistic healing should be the goal; however, the way in which this can be achieved must be explored more fully. This should be informed by a better understanding of our unique history which demands a true multidisciplinary and muti-sectoral approach to engage and incorporate indigenous knowledge and instinct. There is some evidence that in the pre-colonial Caribbean community mental health care was informed by communalism and the community did in fact care for their mentally ill using a community perspective (Hickling & Gibson, 2005). The more recent indigenous support systems such as community activism, sport, and cultural activity have been undermined by globalization and access to images from the dominant North American culture. Consonant with this, there has been an exponential growth in evangelical Christian churches, all preaching a gospel of prosperity and well-being as being a direct result of Christian faith and participation. This has reinforced the idea that psychological phenomena such as depression are really a result of a lack of faith rather than inherent disorders of brain function, and further retarded the desire to seek treatment except through reinforcement of the religious paradigm.

It has been estimated that mental health problems and substance use are fast becoming the number one health problem in the region of the Americas (Periago, 2005). There is also a pressing need to articulate and catalyze a research agenda in mental health, an issue acknowledged in the documentation of a health research agenda in the Caribbean. The priorities identified include reviews of mental health legislation and policies, the epidemiology of mental illness, and the relationship between mental health and chronic disease (Caribbean Health Research Council, 2011). It is suspected that more than 50% of those needing community mental health services are not accessing them, therefore amplifying the negative effects and care giving burden in the communities where they live. Therefore, the treatment gap remains wide and it is likely that the number of untreated individuals exceeds the number that is being treated (Periago, 2005).

Conclusion

The people of the Caribbean are becoming an increasingly savvy and well informed population and therefore require responsive and proactive mental health service delivery. This population is also more aware that they are affected by the stress and psychological challenges of daily life and will demand support for this. It is to Beaubrun's (1966) credit that he introduced mental health training to the region in anticipation of this development. This was done also with a view to catering specifically to the needs of the Caribbean population in terms of having homegrown culturally sensitized psychiatrists able to respond to the needs of the populations they served. However, more work needs to be done to create a training environment that better reflects the reality of Caribbean life. This will certainly require an incorporation of the models of care currently practiced by the more indigenous traditional and spiritual healing methods so that uptake of services will be improved. This will undoubtedly improve the mental health of the region and establish a more supportive platform for human development.

References

Aarons, D. E. (1999). Medicine and its alternatives. Health care priorities in the Caribbean. *The Hastings Center Report, 29*(4), 23–27.

Allen, E. A. (2001). Whole person healing, spiritual realism and social disintegration. A Caribbean case study in faith, health and healing. *International Review of Missions, 90*(356/357), 118–133.

Bakker, C., Engils-Pels M., & Reis, M. (2009). *The impact of migration on children in the Caribbean.* UNICEF Office of Barbados and the Eastern Caribbean, paper #9.

Beaubrun, M. H. (1966) Psychiatric education in the Caribbean. *West Indian Medical Journal, 15*(1), 52–62.

Beaubrun, M. H. (1977). *A mosaic of cultures.* Geneva: World Health Organization.

Beaubrun, M. H. (1992). Caribbean psychiatry, yesterday, today and tomorrow. *History of Psychiatry, 3*(11), 371–382.

Blum, R. W., Halcon. L., Beuhring, T., Pate, E., Campbell-Forrester, S., & Venema, A. (2003). Adolescent health in the Caribbean – Risk and protective factors. *American Journal of Public Health, 93*(3), 456–460.

Caribbean Health Research Council (2011). *Health research agenda for the Caribbean.* St Augustine: Caribbean Health Research Council.

Carter, M. (1977). *Poems of succession.* London: New Beacon Books.

Chevannes, B. (2001). *Learning to be a man. Culture, socialization and gender identity in five Caribbean communities.* Kingston: University of the West Indies Press.

Crawford-Brown, C. (1999). *Who will save our children. The plight of the Jamaican child in the nineties.* Kingston: University of the West Indies Canoe Press.

Girvan, N. (1997). *Societies at risk? The Caribbean and global change.* Management of Social Transformation (MOST) Discussion Paper No. 17.

Griffith, E. E. H. (1995). Personal storytelling and the metaphor of belonging. *Cultural Diversity and Mental Health, 1*(1), 29–37.

Hickling, F. W., & Gibson, R. C. (2005). The history of Caribbean psychiatry. In F. W. Hickling & E. Sorel (Eds.), *Images of psychiatry: The Caribbean.* Mona: Department of Community Health and Psychiatry.

Hickling, F. W., & Maharajh, H. D. (2005). Mental health legislation. In F. W. Hickling & E. Sorel (Eds.), *Images of psychiatry: The Caribbean.* Mona: Department of Community Health and Psychiatry.

Hickling, F. W., Mathies, B. K., Morgan, K., & Gibson, R. C. (2008). Introduction. In F. W. Hickling, B. K. Mathies, K. Morgan , & R. C. Gibson (Eds.), *Perspectives in Caribbean psychology.* Mona: CARIMENSA, University of the West Indies.

Horwitz, A. (2002). *Creating mental illness.* Chicago, IL: University of Chicago Press.

Hutchinson, G. (2005) Sociology and mental health. In F. W. Hickling & E. Sorel (Eds.), *Images of psychiatry: The Caribbean.* Mona: Department of Community Health and Psychiatry.

Hutchinson, G., Simeon, D. T., Bain, B. C., Wyatt, G. E., Tucker, M. B., & LeFranc, E. (2004). Health and social determinants of well-being and life satisfaction in Jamaica. *International Journal of Social Psychiatry, 50*(1), 43–53.

Hutchinson, G., Neehall, J. E., Simeon, D. T., & Littlewood, R. (1999). Perceptions about mental illness among medical students in Trinidad and Tobago. *West Indian Medical Journal, 48*(2), 81–84.

Littlewood, R. (1996). *Pathology and identity. The work of Mother Earth in Trinidad.* Cambridge: Cambridge University Press.

Maharaj, R., Reid, S., & Misir, A. (2010). Validation of the interviewer administered modified Zung scale for detecting depression in a West Indian population. *Caribbean Medical Journal, 72*(1), 6–8.

Maharajh, H. D., & Parasram, R. (1999) The practice of psychiatry in Trinidad and Tobago. *International Review of Psychiatry, 11*(2/3), 173–183.

Mathies, B. K., Meeks-Gardner, J., Daley, A., & Crawford-Brown, C. (2008). Issues of violence in the Caribbean. In F. W. Hickling, B. K. Mathies, K. Morgan, & R. C. Gibson (Eds.), *Perspectives in Caribbean psychology.* Mona: CARIMENSA, University of the West Indies.

Miller, E. (1991). *Men at risk.* Kingston: Jamaica Publishing House.

Moller, H. J. (2001). Viewpoint. Biological psychiatry, past, present and future. *World Journal of Biological Psychiatry, 2*(3), 156–158.

Novas, C., & Rose, N. (2000). Genetic risks and the birth of the somatic individual. *Economy and Society, 29,* 485–513.

Pan American Health Organization (1986) Drug use in Latin America and the Caribbean. *Epidemiological Bulletin, 7*(2), 1–7.

Periago, M. R. (2005). Mental health. A public health priority for the Americas. *Pan American Journal of Public Health, 18*(4/5), 226–228.

Reid, S. D. (2005) Substance abuse. In F. W. Hickling & E. Sorel (Eds.), *Images of psychiatry: The Caribbean* (pp. 197–232). Mona: Department of Community Health and Psychiatry.

Sherlock, P., & Nettleford, R. (1990) *The University of the West Indies. A Caribbean response to the challenge of change.* London and Basingstoke: MacMillan Caribbean.

Sumathipala, A., & Hanwella, R. (1996). The evolution of psychiatric care – a spiral model. *Psychiatric Bulletin, 20*, 561–563.

Thakker, J., & Ward, T. (1998) Culture and classification: The cross-cultural applicability of the DSM-IV. *Clinical Psychology Review, 18*(5), 501–529.

United Nations Office of Drugs and Crime (2007) *Crime, Violence and development: Trends, costs and policy options in the Caribbean. A joint report of the United Nations Office of Drugs and Crime and the Latin American and Caribbean Region of the World Bank.* March, Report # 37820. New York: United Nations.

Valtonen, K., Sogren, M., & Cameron-Padmore, J. (2006). Coping styles in persons recovering from substance abuse. *British Journal of Social Work, 36*(1), 57–73.

Williams, E. (1970) *From Columbus to Castro. A history of the Caribbean.* New York: Harper Row.

Williams, I. C., & Griffith, E. E. H. (2005). Exploring new policy horizons in Caribbean mental health. In F. W. Hickling & E. Sorel (Eds.), *Images of psychiatry: The Caribbean* (pp. 315–360). Mona: Department of Community Health and Psychiatry.

World Health Organization (2011) *WHO-AIMS report on mental health systems in the Caribbean.* Geneva: WHO.

17

PSYCHOLOGY, SPIRITUALITY, AND WELL-BEING IN THE CARIBBEAN

Omowale Amuleru-Marshall, Angela Gomez, and Kristyn O'Rita Neckles

Introduction

Recently, two important publications (Hospedales, Samuels, Cummings, Gallop, & Greene, 2011; Samuels & Fraser, 2010) documented that the Anglophone Caribbean, with a population of mainly African-origin people, is the worst affected by chronic non-communicable diseases—the so-called lifestyle diseases—in the region of Latin America and the Caribbean. These authors make the following observations which should be arresting to anyone who is involved in the practice of counseling or healing in the Caribbean. In Barbados, the prevalence and mortality rates of diabetes-related lower extremity amputations are reported to be among the highest in the world. Diabetes mortality in Trinidad and Tobago and in St. Vincent and the Grenadines is 600% higher than in North America, and the cardiovascular disease mortality rates in Trinidad and Tobago, Guyana, and Suriname are 84%, 62% and 56% higher, respectively, than in North America. In Trinidad and Tobago, obesity and overweight among females are 50–60% higher than most countries and cervical cancer rates are 3–12 times higher. It should be noted that these are highly preventable diseases, the prevention of which require changes in personal, familial, communal, and societal behavior. Behavioral changes are the domain of counselors and other psychologists presumed to have the science and practice to intervene to effect cultural, social, and personal behavior change. Yet their interventions will not be effective unless they are informed by the historical and social circumstances out of which Caribbean cultures are formed.

The countries in this region were established by violence, with epic dehumanizing campaigns of colonialism, genocide, slavery, and indentureship conditioning the psychology of the people. Any analysis of Caribbean behavioral health, therefore, must take this history into account (Sutherland, 2011; Ward & Hickling,

2004). This is not intended to distract attention from more contemporary psychological stressors and oppressors. Indeed, an increasingly widening condition of poverty, unemployment, and socioeconomic decline endangers the psychological and overall well-being of large segments of these populations (Lewis, Joseph, & Roach, 2009; Girvan, 2001).

Nonetheless, very little has happened to individuals, or to their collective formations, in these Caribbean places that can be disconnected from the enslavement and traumatization of African persons. Despite the attainment of political independence, the postcolonial experience provided neither the time nor the policies and programs to repair its psychocultural damage to the region's African-origin majority. Byrd and Clayton's (2000) analysis of the African American "Slave Health Deficit," illustrates that even if corrective interventions were attempted, the available time would have been grossly inadequate.

Placing the earliest arrival of enslaved Africans in the Caribbean between 1630 and 1640 (although their arrival has been dated as early as 1517 (Murdoch, 2009)), the entire period of African life in the Caribbean would be at least 372 years by 2012. Fifty-three percent of that time was spent in a horrific and unrelenting assault on the Africans' physical and psychosocial health (Murdoch, 2009; Sheridan, 1985). Given different dates of independence, another 33 to 39% of the total time was spent, following emancipation, in colonized arrangements which delivered a protracted series of booster shots to reinforce the psychocultural damage and distortions installed during slavery (Bulhan, 1985). While political independence was formally attained at different points, no country's population enjoyed the relative self-determination of independence for more than 13% of the total historical experience. Even if concerted efforts to repair the psychocultural malformations or deformities were being consciously attempted, 13% of the total exposure is patently insufficient to repair the psychocultural pathology engineered over 87% of the total period of cultural deracination and human degradation imposed with multiple forms of violence, often quite horrific in nature and consequence (Sheridan, 1985).

In this chapter, we review some of the complex range of psychosocial maladies engulfing the region's people, consequent to the dehumanizing circumstances out of which these societies emerged. This is followed by a consideration of professional groups who might potentially engineer the repair of Caribbean individuals, and their communities, with some attention paid to their availability and accessibility. A brief discussion of selected elements of counseling or psychotherapy which appear to be appropriate to Caribbean cultural conditions is provided before, finally, the incorporation of spiritual systems and healers of different Caribbean stripes and popularity is discussed as a necessary enhancement of whatever is created or refined to heal Caribbean psyches.

Sun, Rum, Fun, and the Coexisting Psychic Trauma

The Caribbean has a cultural brand as being a space for fun-loving, pleasantly inebriated, easy-going people who see and have "no problem, man." Yet an analysis of mental health needs in the region reveals, in addition to the prevalence of conventional psychopathological states, a rather broad range of behavioral problems which demand attention (Kohn et al., 2005, cited in Maass, Mella, & Risco, 2010; Morgan & O'Garo, 2008). While the rates of psychosis, depression, anxiety disorders, and dementia appear to be within the range that is reported in other countries, the incidence rates of affective disorders appear to be sketchier (Hutchinson & Hickling, 2005; Maharajh & Rampersad, 1999).

Some ethnic and gender differentiation has been noted. For example, the prevalence of suicide, especially among women in the Caribbean, presents certain unavoidable ethnic patterns, disfavoring Indian-origin women, while homicide is distributed in patterns that suggest increased risks for African-origin men (Hutchinson & Hickling, 2005; Maharajh & Rampersad, 1999). There appear to be increases in suicides, as well as substance abuse, child abuse, gender violence, and veiled personality disorders in some Caribbean countries and emerging rates of anxiety-based and stress-related problems have also been noted (Maharajh & Rampersad, 1999). Sutherland (2011) identified a range of psychocultural pathologies developing among African Caribbean people which included excessive materialism, wanton individualism, disrespect for elders, women and children, violence, hopelessness, and the devaluing of blackness. Moreover, the increasing patterns of unhealthy behaviors and lifestyles, which predispose chronic diseases, complicate the array of psychobehavioral problems, associated with ". . . slavery [and] . . . the degradation of the soul . . . that we are still dealing with . . . [as] very real issues today" (Morgan & O'Garo, 2008, p. 11). These are gravely unmet needs and the relative unavailability of professional helpers makes matters worse (Maass, Mella, & Risco, 2010).

Current Mental Health Resources in the Caribbean

There is a variety of professionals who are trained to intervene in the development and progression of psychobehavioral problems and all employ talk therapy or counseling exclusively or with medication. Psychologists, psychiatrists, different types of counselors, and social workers are among the professional groups that are normally expected to be engaged in therapeutic activities to remediate psycho-behavioral conditions. In the case of psychologists, their comparative unavailability presents challenges as countries seek to monitor and respond to the needs of vulnerable groups, locked in pockets of poverty (Maass, Mella, & Risco, 2010). The presence of professional psychologists varies widely across the Caribbean (Lefley, 1981). Some countries, such as Puerto Rico and Martinique, have relatively large proportions of them while in other places, especially in the Eastern

Caribbean, professionally trained psychologists are virtually invisible (Ward & Hickling, 2004; World Health Organization, 2011). In the larger Caribbean states particularly, there have historically been more psychiatrists than psychologists (Lefley, 1981; Maharajh & Parasram, 1999), but social workers are often as scarce as psychologists in many Caribbean places.

Even when helping professionals are available, their deployment can often present financial and geographical inaccessibility. They tend to be more typically located in cities and towns and offer services to individuals or families in fee-for-service, private practice arrangements which betray their class allegiances. The bourgeois aspirations of the available psychologists, psychiatrists, counselors, and social workers would seem to exacerbate problems caused by their inadequate numbers. Efforts to launch wider-reaching and effective models of health care have been seen to threaten the "proletarization of professionals" (Maass, Mella, & Risco, 2010, p. 397). Counselors must come to recognize how their privileged position in society often blinds them to many of the injustices that underlie clients' psychological distress (Duran, Firehammer, & Gonzalez, 2008). Indeed, the ways in which professional helpers understand the problems which they are seeking to confront do not only inform how and where they offer their services but ultimately what these services, themselves, are conceptualized and planned to accomplish.

Effective Psychological Counseling and Healing

Counselors' ability to work effectively with Caribbean persons raises questions about the types of psychological or counseling interventions that are appropriate in this historicultural context. A culturally-appropriate healing experience would require that the impact of the people's history and social circumstances is brought into the clinical narrative (Duran, Firehammer, & Gonzalez, 2008; Sutherland, 2011). This is precisely why the importation of a "culture-bound" diagnostic nosology that focuses on the examination of the person, rather than the situation, is viewed as an alienating approach to psychology in the Caribbean (Hickling & Paisley, 2011).

Hickling (2007) proposes that a Caribbean approach to psychotherapy must focus on the "psychohistoriography" of the region and not on ahistorical, culturally-dislodged ideas of individual pathology. Building on a protracted experience of teaching, research, and service in community psychiatry in Jamaica, he distilled, with interdisciplinary influences, culturally-based, indigenized therapeutic strategies. Adequate training of psychological counselors for the Caribbean must include making them aware of, and prepared to confront, various forms of cultural oppression and social injustice that impact the mental health of historically disenfranchised groups. The master's degree in cultural therapy, proposed by the Caribbean Institute of Mental Health and Substance Abuse at the University of the West Indies, Mona, is a vanguard step in this direction (Gibson, Matthies, & Hickling, 2007).

The work of Hickling and his associates, drawing heavily on cultural therapy, is somewhat similar to the classic efforts of Paulo Freire (1972) and his notion of conscientization, or a change in consciousness, constructed on clients' deconstruction of their historical and cultural experience to inseminate a psychology of liberation (Duran, Firehammer, & Gonzalez, 2008). What is needed are more sociogenic approaches which would cultivate a professional willingness to examine sociohistorical factors that contribute to the psychological oppression of individuals, their families, and communities in the Caribbean (Duran, Firehammer, & Gonzalez, 2008; Sutherland, 2011). The focus must shift from intrapsychic dynamics to the ". . . bloodthirsty and pitiless atmosphere, the generalization of inhuman practices, and the firm impression that people have of being caught up in a veritable Apocalypse" (Fanon, 1968, p. 251).

Serious attempts to construct an appropriate psychology for the Caribbean cultural experience must revisit the work of this iconic Martinican psychiatrist. Several decades ago, he posited that Caribbean societies—colonial societies—damage psyches and leave them devoid of the requisite psychocultural framework to even understand, much less to dismantle, the violent forces and systems that shape and condition their humanity. According to Fanon (1967a), "Psychologists, who tend to explain everything by movements of the psyche, claim to discover this behavior on the level of contacts between individuals . . . Such attempts deliberately leave out of account the special character of the colonial situation" (p. 33). Clearly, etiological primacy must be placed in the sociocultural situation in which individuals are involuntarily sequestered as ". . . every neurosis, every abnormal manifestation, every affective erethism in the Antillean is the product of his cultural situation" (Fanon, 1967b, p. 152).

Fanon asserted that the goal of psychotherapy must be to rebuild the identity, culture, and a progressive sociopolitical trajectory of people in these former colonies through a liberating praxis (Fanon, 1967b). His legacy is the quest for a psychology that de-emphasizes individualism and seeks, instead, to nurture sociality and collective liberty (Bulhan, 1985). It is noteworthy that this perspective is finally finding a place in the discourse of effective clinical skill sets for psychologists working with historically-marginalized groups. Ecological, sociopolitical, and historical forces delivering differential effects on individuals and groups must not be minimized any longer (Fouad & Arredondo, 2007).

An example of drawing on the historicity of Caribbean populations is offered by Dudley-Grant (2001). Recognizing the preponderance of African heritage in the Caribbean, she offers family therapy as an important ". . . means of intervening in the social decay that is rapidly taking hold in the Virgin Islands and Caribbean community and that is manifested in the antisocial behavior of young people" (p. 48). Despite the infancy of family psychology, associated with the limited development of the science and profession of psychology in the region, the urgent need for family therapists capable of applying treatment approaches that are constructed on the extended family and communal traditions of the region is highlighted (Dudley-Grant, 2001; Ramkissoon et al., 2008). While acknowledging that there were striking differences between African Caribbean and African American experiences of chattel slavery, the soul wounding (Duran, Firehammer, & Gonzalez, 2008) was common as were some historical causes of the consequent disintegration of their families. Adaptations of multi-systems family therapy, which has enjoyed some success among African American families, especially in the southern United States, is proposed to hold good promise as a culturally-appropriate model of intervention in the Caribbean (Brondino et al., 1997; Dudley-Grant, 2001). This is an example of the adaptation of a treatment system that has been demonstrated to be useful in another context.

Cultural adaptations, such as this, are being encouraged as the field of counseling embraces evidence-based psychological practice (EBPP) (Morales & Norcross, 2010).

The relationship of potentially adaptable, evidence-based treatments to Caribbean people's history and culture must be carefully explored, however. There must be suspicious and careful adaptations given the fact that there is incontrovertible evidence that culture and context are in almost every aspect of the diagnostic and treatment process (Bernal, Jimenez-Chafey & Rodriguez, 2009). The notion of epistemological hybridity, or the ability to become "enmeshed in the cultural life-world of the person or community seeking [or needing] . . . help" (Duran, Firehammer, & Gonzalez, 2008, p. 291), emerges to be of grave importance as Caribbean psychologists complement their consideration of the best available research from more Eurocentric contexts with a more critical consideration of their client's characteristics, culture, and preferences (Morales & Norcross, 2010). One of the increasingly recognized limitations of the Eurocentric professional perspective is its relegation of spirituality beyond the reach of professional helpers.

Spirituality, Traditional Healing Practices, and Mental Health

The infusion of spirituality into our systems of conceptualization and intervention would likely augment their appropriateness and efficacy as well as their reach. The advocacy is mounting that spirituality should not merely be subsumed within mental health, one of the three pillars of biopsychosocial health. It has, in fact, been proposed that the World Health Organization's classic definition of health be expanded to explicitly include spirituality so that health is promulgated to be a state of complete physical, mental, spiritual, and social well-being and not merely the absence of disease or infirmity (Kwan, 2007). Indeed, some psychologists have emphasized the critical buffer that spirituality provides in contexts of historical trauma (Duran, Firehammer, & Gonzalez, 2008; Sutherland, 2011).

Comprehensive discussions of the types of spiritual practices extant in the Caribbean, including the ways in which they are or may be used to shore up health in the region, are quite timely. It has been suggested that traditional healers are an ever-present resource that Caribbean clients have always used in the absence of, and even in preference to, mental health professionals. The latter may only be an alternative treatment option, used as a first or last resort or in tandem with a native healer (Lefley, 1981; Maharajh & Parasram, 1999; Ramkissoon et al., 2008). Irrespective of the rates of utilization across the diversity of extant practices, that spirituality should be situated in efforts to indigenize a psychology for the Caribbean is clearly recommended (Hickling, 2007; Sutherland & Moodley, 2010).

Obviously, there will have to be much closer collaborations between the professional counseling community and religious practitioners if spiritual belief systems are to be incorporated into the efforts of professional counselors. Some collaborations are easier than others (Griffith, Mahy, & Young, 2008), but broad-based collaborations are, nonetheless, encouraged if counselors are to improve the efficacy of their treatment strategies (Sutherland & Moodley, 2010). It is the client's experience rather than the counselor's preference which should dictate the range and nature of collaborative efforts. Yet engaging a full range of spiritual practices introduces competing epistemological constructions and related tensions. Yeh, Hunter, Madan-Bahel, Chiang, and Arora (2004) argued that indigenous forms of healing follow a collective and holistic approach, which is largely absent in Western practices. They further note, "most Western helping practices remain within the mental and the physical boundaries of human experience. Often ignored in Western psychological thought and practice is that domain considered to transcend the mental and the physical . . . the realm of spirituality" (p. 414). The other significant difference is the linearity emphasized by the scientific method, associating human behavior with a "discrete cause-and-effect-framework" (Yeh et al., 2004, p. 414).

Developing or tolerating a more holistic concept of human health, with increasing attention to spiritual functions and a more multifactorial and interactive ecological understanding of cause and effect, can be challenging. However, greater tensions are encountered when different and largely incompatible notions about the Divine, and the nature of transcendental relations surrounding and including human beings, collide as counselors seek to incorporate alienating ideas about spiritual phenomena into their own frameworks. When counselors are generally contemptuous of, or indifferent to, spiritual beliefs, or hold a complacent ecumenicism or diunital flexibility (Dixon, 1976), collaborations are more easily established. However, professional counselors who hold personally-significant, crystallized cosmological convictions would find it much more difficult to develop what might be called cosmological hybridity. Nonetheless, when working with individuals and communities from cultural backgrounds with cosmological constructions that shape their perception of mental health in ways that are different from the perception of mainstream psychological counselors, pathways have to be found if effective efforts are to be launched.

Traditional healing practices, embedded within Caribbean cultural traditions, provide contextual meanings for understanding and addressing health concerns, including mental health problems, a fact that is finally influencing psychology-based helping professionals (Hickling & James, 2008; Ramkissoon et al., 2008). Indeed, even those counselors who place primacy on a sociogenic analysis of the etiology of psychological problems recognize the indispensable instrumentality of sharing the client's cultural construction of his or her experience. Despite an understanding that the sociostructural conditions in which people are sequestered, such as extreme poverty or lack of access to basic education and health care, rather than spiritual explanations, are the basis of their psychocultural stultification, required transformations will be elusive if clients' phenomenology cannot be accessed as the platform on which therapeutic relationships are constructed.

Collaboration and Integration

The delivery of culturally accessible health services requires that collaborative bridges are built between the traditional and the professional healer. This would be facilitated if each category of therapist becomes more informed about the other. Attempts have been made to organize traditional healers into different typologies to facilitate their demystification among psychotherapists (McKenzie, Tuck, & Noh, 2011; Vontress, 1991), and systems of comparisons have also been presented (Krippner, 1995; Wing, 1998). Among other steps that have been proposed are the acceptance by both parties of the value of each other's practices, the awareness of the limitations of their respective practices, the willingness to help those receiving services to understand the value of the interventions, and the willingness by both parties to share their philosophies, values, and beliefs as well as to recognize underlying similarities (Yeh et al., 2004). Ultimately, a cosmological and epistemological hybridity—an ability to become "enmeshed in the cultural life-world of the person or community seeking [or needing] . . . help"—is going to have to be developed (Duran, Firehammer, & Gonzalez, 2008, p. 291).

McKenzie, Tuck, and Noh (2011) suggested that there are three types of interfaces that can occur between professional psychotherapists and traditional healers: integrative, inclusive, and tolerant, while expressing a clear preference for the integrative approach. An approach that would qualify as merely inclusive is the provision of a shared space in which traditional healers offer their services side by side with professionally-trained providers. An example is provided in Suriname in which professional practitioners are housed in a clinic that is next door to a clinic in which shamanistic practitioners treat persons (O'Neill, Bartlett, & Mignone, 2006).

Wing (1998) argued for more integrative efforts by attempting to draw attention to many similarities between traditional and more contemporary healing concepts, while Nuñez-Molina (1996) expressed the view that "the healing process itself has generic properties which can be found in several therapeutic systems" (p. 227). Other ways of integrating the two systems of healing include training professional therapists from the same cultural background as potential clients so that they can synthesize cultural healing systems and the psychotherapeutic strategies with which they have become equally familiar (Martinez-Taboas, 2005). A critical step towards integration is the need for traditional healers, with access and influence in their communities, to be recruited to work on preventing conditions which threaten the health and longevity of community members. The penchant of traditional healers to wait to respond to illnesses limits their potential role in health promotion and disease prevention (Aarons, 1999; Archibald, 2011). Their influence as community elders, cultural brokers, and healers must be incorporated in the cultural struggle against the strident erosion of the communal fabric and the marching epidemic of diseases of lifestyle and privation (Sutherland, 2011).

Utilizing traditional healers and community leaders as informal helpers and sociocultural mediators is a way to bridge cultural and socioeconomic gaps that keep culturally-disenfranchised and economically disadvantaged individuals and communities from accessing professional or formal mental health services. These religious advisors, healers, and other elders and aficionados of social and cultural activities in their communities possess the charisma, leadership skills, and cultural knowledge to expand the reach of professional mental health providers in their communities.

Conclusion

The critical and growing need for a cadre of psychological counselors in the Caribbean region proportionately and paradigmatically adequate to meet the wide array of psychobehavioral challenges, including mental illnesses with some transcultural features, was discussed. Issues ranging from the prevention and control of chronic non-communicable diseases, particularly diabetes, hypertension, cancer, and obesity, requiring effective changes in behavior and habits of diet, physical activity, smoking, and alcohol use, to profound pathologies of identity and culture, including violence and gender-based maladaptations were elaborated. These issues were presented as protracted consequences of the region's history of violence and human degradation— a contemporary profile of arresting psychosocial patterns and a crying need for effective psychological responses to this assortment of behavioral, cultural, and social maladies. The argument was made that a Caribbean psychology, promising accurate analyses and effective interventions, requires foundational grounding in the people's history (beyond slavery and colonialism), culture, and social realities, including their spiritual reserves.

These matters were raised in the context of a discussion of the dire and unmet need for psychobehavioral service providers with a capacity to effectively respond to the region's population. The available human resources to tackle these conditions were presented as inadequate as are the ways in which services are conceptualized and made available when they exist. Selected elements and examples of a culturally-appropriate psychology were discussed to illustrate both the special needs of this population and efforts that have been recommended or tried to build or adapt promising systems of healing. Among the innovations recommended is the infusion of spirituality into counseling. Indeed, the reportedly ubiquitous nature of traditional spiritual practices across the region promises that significant numbers of persons seeking, or needing, interventions by professional counselors will present with backgrounds and beliefs that mandate their incorporation into efforts to be helpful. Professional helpers are being encouraged to establish ways in which their efforts may be augmented by practitioners who are more familiar with these practices. While illustrating some difficulties that may be encountered in the process of establishing these pathways, the chapter discussed certain ways through which these collaborations may be advanced.

References

Aarons, D. E. (1999). Medicine and its alternatives: Health care priorities in the Caribbean. *Hastings Center Report, 29*(4), 23–27.

Archibald, C. (2011). Cultural tailoring for an Afro-Caribbean community: A naturalistic approach. *Journal of Cultural Diversity, 18*(4), 114–118.

Bernal, G., Jimenez-Chafey, M. I., & Rodriguez, M. M. D. (2009). Cultural adaptation of treatments: A resource for considering culture in evidence-based practice. *Professional Psychology: Research and Practice, 40*(4), 361–368.

Brondino, M. J., Henggeler, S. W., Scott, W., Rowland, M. D., Pickrel, S. G., Cunningham, P. B., et al. (1997). Multisystemic therapy and the ethnic minority client: Culturally responsive and clinically effective. In D. K. Wilson, J. R. Rodrigue, & W. C. Taylor (Eds.), *Health-promoting and health compromising behaviors among minority adolescents: Application and practice in health psychology* (pp. 229–250). Washington, DC: American Psychological Association.

Bulhan, H. A. (1985). *Frantz Fanon and the psychology of oppression.* New York: Plenum Press.

Byrd, W. M., & Clayton, L. A. (2000). *An American health dilemma: A medical history of African Americans and the problem of race, beginnings to 1900.* New York: Routledge.

Dixon, V. J. (1976). Worldviews and research methodologies. In L. M. King, V. J. Dixon & W. W. Nobles (Eds.), *African philosophy: Assumption and paradigms for research on black persons* (pp. 51–102). Los Angeles, CA: A Fanon Center Publication.

Dudley-Grant, G. R. (2001). Eastern Caribbean family psychology with conduct-disordered adolescents from the Virgin Islands. *American Psychologist, 56*(1), 47–57.

Duran, E., Firehammer, J., & Gonzalez, J. (2008). Liberation psychology as the path toward healing cultural soul wounds. *Journal of Counseling & Development, 86*, 288–295.

Fanon, F. (1967a). *Toward the African revolution.* New York: Grove Press.

Fanon, F. (1967b). *Black skins, white masks.* New York: Grove Press.

Fanon, F. (1968). *The wretched of the earth.* New York: Grove Press.

Fouad, N., & Arredondo, P. (2007). *Becoming culturally oriented: Practical advice for psychologists and educators.* Washington, DC: American Psychological Association.

Freire, P. (1972). *Pedagogy of the oppressed.* New York: Penguin Books.

Gibson, R. C., Matthies, B. K., & Hickling, F. W. (2007). CARIMENSA's master's degree in cultural therapy. In F. W. Hickling (Ed.), *Dream a world: CARIMENSA and the development of cultural therapy in Jamaica* (pp. 23–26). Kingston: CARIMENSA.

Girvan, N. (2001). Reinterpreting the Caribbean. In F. Lindahl & B. Meeks (Eds.), *New Caribbean thought*. Kingston, Jamaica: UWI Press.

Griffith, E. E., Mahy, G. E., & Young, J. L. (2008). Barbados spiritual baptists: Social acceptance enhances opportunities for supporting public health. *Mental Health, Religion & Culture, 11*(7), 671–683.

Hickling, F. W. (2007). *Psychohistoriography: A post-colonial psychoanalytic and psychotherapeutic model.* Kingston: CARIMENSA, University of the West Indies.

Hickling, F. W., & James, C. (2008) Traditional mental health practices in Jamaica: On the phenomenology of red eye, bad-mind, and Obeah. In F. W. Hickling, B. K. Mathies, K. Morgan, & R. C. Gibson (Eds.), *Perspectives in Caribbean psychology* (pp. 465–486) . Mona: Caribbean Institute of Mental Health and Substance Abuse, University of the West Indies.

Hickling, F. W., & Paisley, V. (2011). Redefining personality disorder: A Jamaican perspective. *Revista Panamericana de Salud Publica, 30*(3), 255–261.

Hospedales, C. J., Samuels, T. A., Cummings, R., Gallop, G., & Greene, E. (2011). Raising the priority of chronic noncommunicable diseases in the Caribbean. *Revista Panamericana de Salud Publica, 30*(4), 393–400.

Hutchinson, G., & Hickling, F. W. (2005). Epidemiology of mental illness. In F. W. Hickling & E. Sorel (Eds.), *Images of psychiatry: The Caribbean* (pp. 121–136). Kingston: Department of Community Health and Psychiatry, University of the West Indies, Mona, Jamaica.

Krippner, S. (1995). A cross-cultural comparison of four healing models. *Alternative Therapies, 1*(1), 21–29.

Kwan, S. S. (2007). Clinical efficacy of ritual healing and pastoral ministry. *Pastoral Psychology, 55*, 741–749.

Lefley, H. P. (1981). Psychotherapy and cultural adaptation in the Caribbean. *International Journal of Group Tensions, 11*(1–4), 3–16.

Lewis, D., Joseph, S. C., & Roach, K. (2010). The implication of the current financial and economic crisis on integration: The Caribbean experience. *Global Development Studies Journal, 6*(1–2), 49–98.

Maass, J., Mella, C., & Risco, L. (2010). Current challenges and future perspectives of the role of governments in psychiatric/mental health systems of Latin America. *International Review of Psychiatry, 22*(4), 394–400.

Maharajh, H. D., & Parasram, R. (1999). The practice of psychiatry in Trinidad and Tobago. *International Review of Psychiatry, 11*, 173–183.

Maharajh, H. D., & Rampersad, P. (1999). The practice of psychiatry in Trinidad and Tobago. *International Review of Psychiatry, 11*, 173–183.

Martinez-Taboas, A. (2005). Psychogenic seizures in an *espiritismo* context: The role of culturally sensitive psychotherapy. *Psychotherapy: Theory, Research, Practice, Training, 42*(1), 6–13.

McKenzie, K., Tuck, A., & Noh, M. S. (2011). Moving traditional Caribbean medicine practices into healthcare in Canada. *Ethnicity and Inequalities in Health and Social Care, 4*(2), 60–70.

Morales, E., & Norcross, J. C. (2010). Evidence-based practices with ethnic minorities: Strange bedfellows no more. *Journal of Clinical Psychology, 66*(8), 821–829.

Morgan, K., & O'Garo, K.-G. N. (2008) Caribbean identity issues. In F. W. Hickling, B. K. Mathies, K. Morgan, & R. C. Gibson (Eds.), *Perspectives in Caribbean psychology* (pp. 3–31) . Mona: Caribbean Institute of Mental Health and Substance Abuse, University of the West Indies.

Murdoch, H. A. (2009). A legacy of trauma: Caribbean slavery, race, class and contemporary identity in Abeng. *Research in African Literatures, 40*(4), 65–88.

Núñez Molina, M. (1996). Archetypes and spirits: A Jungian analysis of Puerto Rican Espiritismo. *Journal of Analytical Psychology, 41*, 227–244.

O'Neill, J., Bartlett, J., & Mignone, J. (2006). *Best practices in intercultural health.* Washington, DC: Inter-American Bank.

Ramkissoon, M., Gopaul-McNichol, S.-A., Davidson, B., Matthies, B. K., & Brown Earle, O. (2008). Family life in the Caribbean: Assessment and counseling models. In F. W. Hickling, B. K. Mathies, K. Morgan, & R. C. Gibson (Eds.), *Perspectives in Caribbean psychology* (pp. 93–112). Mona: Caribbean Institute of Mental Health and Substance Abuse, University of the West Indies.

Samuels, T. A., & Fraser, H. (2010). Caribbean wellness day: Mobilizing a region for chronic noncommunicable disease prevention and control. *Revista Panamericana de Salud Publica, 28*(6), 472–479.

Sheridan, R. B. (1985). *Doctors and slaves: A medical and demographic history of slavery in the British West Indies, 1680–1834.* Cambridge: Cambridge University Press.

Sutherland, M. E. (2011). Toward a Caribbean psychology: An African-centered approach. *Journal of Black Studies, 42*(8), 1175–1194.

Sutherland, P., & Moodley, R. (2010). Reclaiming the spirit: Clemmont E. Vontress and the quest for spirituality and traditional healing in counseling. In R. Moodley & R. Walcott (Eds.), *Counseling across and beyond cultures: Exploring the work of Clemmont E. Vontress in clinical practice* (pp. 263–277). Toronto: University of Toronto Press.

Vontress, C. E. (1991). Traditional healing in Africa: Implications for cross-cultural healing. *Journal of Counseling and Development, 70*(1), 242–249.

Ward, T., & Hickling, F. (2004). Psychology in the English-speaking Caribbean. *The Psychologist, 17*(8), 442–444.

Wing, D. M. (1998). A comparison of traditional folk healing concepts with contemporary healing concepts. *Journal of Community Health Nursing, 15*(3), 143–154.

World Health Organization. (2011). *WHO-AIMS report on mental health systems in the Caribbean region.* Geneva: WHO.

Yeh, C. J., Hunter, C. D., Madan-Bahel, A., Chiang, L., & Arora, A. K. (2004). Indigenous and interdependent perspectives of healing: Implications for counseling and research. *Journal of Counseling and Development, 82*, 410–419.

18

PRACTICAL MAGIC IN THE US URBAN MILIEU

Botánicas and the Informal Networks of Healing

Anahí Viladrich

Introduction

The growing market of religious healing in the United States (US) has called attention to the role of religion in American society and to the multiplicity of coexisting healing systems, as a cultural epiphenomenon resulting from the country's ethnic and religious diversity. Folk healing practices have been blossoming in recent decades along with the holistic health movement (developed in the 1970s) and its successor, the New Age trend, followed by the newly-institutionalized field of complementary and alternative medicine (Baer, 2001; Baez & Hernandez, 2001). Nevertheless, there has been a paucity of research on the intertwining fields of religion, spirituality, and health, particularly pertaining to Caribbean healing traditions.

Contrary to the popularity of New Age and holistic therapies, folk healing practitioners have remained an understudied universe in the US. Conversely, while the safety net for health services has become more unraveled in recent years, the burden of health care has increasingly shifted to immigrant communities that mostly serve the poor and the undocumented (Viladrich, 2006a; 2007a). In this context, traditional healing systems, rather than being diluted by globalization and the ubiquitous presence of Western practices, have been blossoming more than ever before. Undoubtedly, the popularity of African and Caribbean traditions in the US has been prompted by an increasing international clientele searching for either traces of the Americas' indigenous cultural forms, or for innovative versions of transnational healing therapies (see Polk, 2004).

This chapter examines the presence of botánicas in New York City (NYC), which are ethnic-religious stores that provide a physical and social space for the reproduction of informal faith-healing networks on the basis of religious belonging (e.g., *Santería* and Spiritism). Botánicas are main healing outlets serving a pan-ethnic population of Latin American and Caribbean immigrants in urban milieus. Either in El Barrio of upper Manhattan or in "the United Nations of New York City" (as the borough of Queens is often called, see Tyree, 2005) or in the Hollywood outskirts of Los Angeles, botánicas' products and services unveil the overlapping fields of religious healing and community bonding in ways which, until recently, had mostly remained unexplored. Rather than opposing bio-medicine, the main argument of this chapter aims at underscoring botánicas' contribution to providing unique responses to their clients' needs on the basis of complementing what the former system of healing has to offer (see Moodley, Sutherland, & Oulanova, 2008; Viladrich, 2007b). It begins with an examination of the literature on the role of botánicas in promoting Caribbean and Latin American folk healing traditions in the US, and examines the social geography of healing expressed in botánicas' changing locations due to the ongoing gentrifi-cation taking place in main urban centers, such as NYC. This is followed by an analysis of informal healing networks that extend both within and beyond the botánicas' premises. Lastly, it highlights the need for developing conceptual models that incorporate indigenous etiologies, including reliance on spirituality and religiosity as holistic systems of healing.

Botánicas' Religious and Spiritual Realm

Botánicas, which literally means botany, are local dispensaries that offer spiritual and religious goods to mostly a Latino and Caribbean clientele (Murphy, 2010). While their origin can be retraced to the *droguerías* (pharmacies) that existed as early as in the 1900s, through time they evolved into becoming eclectic outlets that combine healing practices with religious traditions (Long, 2001). Botánicas are found almost anywhere in the Americas, and are named with a variety of terms including *hierberías, herbarias,* and *botanicos* in places such as Brazil, Colombia, and the French Caribbean. In fact, the presence of botánicas has become ubiquitous in many urban regions, where they combine an uncanny financial enterprise with a witty array of multicultural religious icons and products. In agreement with Romberg (2003), in her study on religious healing practices in Puerto Rico, rather than witnessing the birth of homogeneous healing trends as a product of globalization, botánicas represent myriad healing influences that are dynamically expressed (and transformed) into unique versions of religious faith.

Additionally, it is in the US where botánicas' eclectic nature achieves an ultimate multinational and wide-ranging concoction. This is concomitant with immigrants relying on culturally familiar healing practices (e.g., folk healers or *curanderos*) while they are literally "crossing borders" to get services in different countries (Byrd & Law, 2009; Loera, Muñoz, Nott, & Sandefur, 2009). In the US, botánicas can be found in most Latin American and Caribbean neighborhoods, where they represent the main selling outlets of religious and spiritual objects along with natural remedies (Anderson, McKee, Yukes, Alvarez, & Karasz, 2008; Dearfield & Pugh-Yi, 2011). Rather than being solely associated with one particular national or racial group, these stores have become multiethnic settings, since they are owned by (and serve) a variety of immigrant populations including Dominicans, Haitians, Cubans, Puerto Ricans, Mexicans, Colombians, Ecuadorians, and Guatemalans. With immigrant groups rising in numbers in the US' gateway cities, botánicas have begun to share their front doors with magic and fortune-teller services, while offering myriad products and services—from herbs to magical potions, and from tarot reading to marriage counseling (Jones, Polk, Flores-Peña, & Evanchuk, 2001; Reyes-Ortiz, Rodriguez, & Markides, 2009; Viladrich, 2007c).

Furthermore, botánicas combine a mosaic of ethno-religious practices that merge Afro-Caribbean religious beliefs and traditions such as *Santería*, Palo Monte, Voodoo, and Spiritism (see Gomez-Beloz & Chavez, 2001; Fernandez Olmos & Paravisini-Gebert, 2011; Gelb, 2005; Romberg, 2011; Trotter & Chavira, 1981). The transnational liaisons taking place between immigrants' country of origin and of destiny, as in the case of *Santería* practitioners in Puerto Rico and NYC, make of their "spiritual capital" (Romberg, 2011) a matter of ongoing religious and commercial exchanges across nation-states. Among botánicas' diverse products, one can find aromatic candles named after Latin American saints, who are well known for their healing powers, as well as herbs often imported from Puerto Rico and the Dominican Republic. Botánicas' staples also include oils, tinctures, and candles aimed at cleansing both the physical and the spiritual environment (see Reyes-Garcia, 2010).

As a result, most botánicas have become vivid representations of transnational faiths, as they offer every key charm revered and utilized in Afro-Caribbean spiritual traditions—from necklaces (or *Elekes de Santo*) to *caracoles* (cowry shells used for divination) and voodoo dolls for *trabajos* (used for spells and other magical works). These religious practices, which evolved in the Americas as part of a culture of resistance among African slaves, are expressed through a syncretic blend of Yoruba and Catholic beliefs, which find a common ground in the communication with and possession by an array of incorporeal spirits (McCarthy Brown, 1991; Murphy, 2010; Singer & Garcia, 1989).

The Changing Social Geography of Botánicas

Social geography is defined in this chapter as a multi-level layered map that interweaves physical location with the sociodemographic and cultural characteristics of Latin and Caribbean immigrants in urban milieus. In any big US city, it is easy to observe the large (and rising) number of botánicas, mostly located in neighborhoods where ethnic minority groups reside. Paradoxically, and despite their outstanding presence in key urban areas, these establishments seem to be catering to a diverse clientele in search for unique religious and healing products.

Being unique aesthetic places that feed on transnational liaisons, the social geography of botánicas in NYC are embedded in immigrants' grassroots settings in the *barrios* (Latino neighborhoods), where they coexist along with *bodegas* (Latino grocery stores), amid a variety of community organizations, including Latino churches and immigrant organizations (Solimar, 2007).

In tracing the botánicas' physical and social settings in NYC, Viladrich (2006a) found that the largest location of these establishments correlated with the highest percentage of Latinos per neighborhood. Furthermore, the higher the density of Latino residents, the bigger the number of botánicas—independent of residents' country of birth. Conversely, most geographical areas that register the lowest percentage of Latinos also have the least number of botánicas.[1] By all means, the presence of botánicas in NYC reflects both the current ethnic composition and the ongoing changes taking place in the city's urban fabric. Viladrich's study showed that the shifting patchwork of botánicas symbolizes the paradigmatic displacement of minority populations from NYC's gentrified neighborhoods, marked by their disappearance of ethnic stores from most upwardly mobile areas, vis-à-vis their slow (but steady) emergence in others.

For example, botánicas found in the Manhattan neighborhoods of Washington Heights and Inwood are mostly located within the Dominican enclave, while the ones in East Harlem reflect the vanishing Puerto Rican presence in that area as a product of ongoing gentrification. Finally, the botánicas scattered around Manhattan represent spotted vestiges of the former presence of Latinos, as it is the case with the neighborhoods of the Lower East side and Morningside Heights (Viladrich, 2006b). In sum, the distribution of botánicas in NYC is living proof of the demographic shifts that have lately taken place in many large cities in America.

Latin and Caribbean immigrants typically tend to have less access to health care because of their lack of health coverage, and due to the many barriers (e.g., financial, linguistic, and logistic) that deter them from seeking and obtaining adequate medical care in the US (Viladrich, 2007a). According to the Community Health Survey 2002 (New York Department of Health and Mental Hygiene, 2002), the density of botánicas does not change by insurance level, suggesting that their use is a matter of cultural affinity more than a surrogate for the unavailability of insurance. Furthermore, a strong correlation was found between the high presence of botánicas and the large percentage of Latinos reporting no personal doctor, which suggests that botánicas are more likely to be placed in areas where Latinos mostly lack a regular source of care.

Nevertheless, rather than using botánicas as the only point of entry, it seems that their customers combine services with those of allopathic medicine. Concomitantly with the literature on immigrants' healing practices, botánicas provide unique products that complement those offered by other local businesses including the selling of herbs and other botanical products (Menard et al., 2010; Vandebroek et al., 2010). Moreover, the fact that botánicas tend to share the front space with drugstores, pharmacies, and other health-related outlets located on main commercial avenues, further supports the idea that these diverse businesses coexist, rather than compete, with each other. For instance, studies on ethnobotany suggest that botánicas are key points of entry for immigrants' access to plants and herbal infusions for the treatment of specific health problems, as in the case of women's health conditions such as infertility and menstrual dysfunction (Balick et al., 2000; Menard et al, 2010; Reiff et al., 2003).

Therefore, it appears that the services provided by botánicas (including counselors working on site) are somehow surrogates for the personal doctor, particularly among those of lower socioeconomic status who lack health insurance and/or are undocumented. Finally, and in agreement with research on the nonmedical sources of prescription drugs (see Vissman et al., 2011), botánicas also sell allopathic medicines, particularly non-prescription drugs. In this vein, the literature usually defines botánicas as affordable and culturally competent "invisible pharmacies," where clients are treated by those speaking their language and sharing their cultural and religious beliefs (Balick & Lee, 2001; Gomez-Beloz & Chavez, 2001; Pignataro, 2009; Polk, 2004; Tafur, Crowe, & Torres, 2009).

Botánicas' Informal Healing Networks

Regardless of the specific products they offer, the success of botánicas greatly depends on the informal social webs held by those working in their premises on the one hand, and by those who regularly visit them as either providers or clients on the other. Although the owners and employees of botánicas do not usually call themselves "healers," they are actually key players in the informal economy of care (Viladrich, 2007c). Comparable to the figure of the *farmacista* (pharmacist) in many Latin American cultures, botánicas' employees are pivotal in helping their customers navigate a complex pharmacopoeia of herbs and natural ointments, along with the provision of referrals and the prescription of home remedies. As noted by Dearfield and Pugh-Yi (2011): "Botanico staff are a primary or influential source of medical advice for some clients, and therefore are an important potential referral source to clinical practice as well as potential educator for clinicians who want to reach their clientele"(p.21). In fact, botánicas and religious healers do not claim to be biomedical experts, and they usually refer their clients to conventional medical care when dealing with health conditions they cannot treat.

Botánicas' owners and folk healers are known by word of mouth; therefore they build their reputation at face value on the basis of the esteem and popularity of their clientele (see Reiff et al., 2003; Viladrich, 2006a; 2006b). As *immigrants treating immigrants* (Viladrich, 2006b) botánicas' employers are seen as cultural brokers par excellence that are acknowledged by the community they serve, including members of hidden populations (e.g., unauthorized immigrants) who are unlikely to be beneficiaries of the health system's safety net. From tarot readers to "lay injectionists" (Rahill, Dawkins, & De La Rosa, 2011), botánicas help their clients deal with specific health ailments, such as diabetes and high blood pressure as well as emotional and family issues (Caban & Walker, 2006; McNeill & Cervantes, 2008; Ransford, Carrillo, & Rivera, 2010).

Not only do botánicas offer a physical and a social space for the exchange of information and resources, but they also support informal faith-healing networks on the basis of religious belonging (Viladrich, 2006b). Botánicas' back rooms are typically turned into offices where healers regularly greet and treat clients seeking informal counseling and health advice. As participants of the same alternative model of cure, customers and providers are linked by social relationships that become alive in the many religious ceremonies that often take place at the botánicas' basements, waiting rooms, and adjacent spaces. In fact, the communal aspects of ritualistic healing is one of the most conspicuous elements of *Santería* and other Caribbean-religious systems, in which surrogate families of parents and godchildren remain tied to a spiritual house led by particular *Orishas* (e.g., deities such as Shango or Obatala).

Within healers' faith networks, reciprocity becomes a shared trait that rests on a system of redistribution in which key resources (material and symbolic) are exchanged between godparents and their followers. Overall, disease is understood as the result of the combined effect of the natural, social, and supernatural realms, which overlap in convivial liaisons toward creating a balance in the sufferer's life. Illnesses expressed through biological and organic symptoms are often diagnosed, treated, and cured through divine intervention—for example, via Yoruba protectors who have the ability to both harm and cure. In their study on religious healing in the Caribbean, Fernández Olmos and Paravisini-Gebert (2011) point out the following:

> Afro-Cuban religious practices focus on the relationship of devotees with the deities and the spirits. Those who require balance and harmony in their lives due to a physical or emotional illness or a life crisis seek out the help of a priest of Ocha who will undoubtedly consult the oracle to hear the spiritual solution proffered by the deities. The remedies can range from a spiritual cleansing, a *resguardo* or protective charm, to more advance initiatory steps.
>
> *(p. 59)*

One of these *Orishas*, Babaluú Ayé, embodies the *Santería* representation of the Catholic Saint *San Lázaro*. He is highly respected among religious healers as one who not only can cure but also cause illness—a duality found in many of the divinities composing the Afro-Caribbean pantheon. Pugliese (2010) notes that: "He is an Orisha that is respected but at the same time highly feared. These two extremes exist because as he cures he can simultaneously bring sickness and disease upon you" (pp. 4–5). Furthermore, rather that opposing biomedicine, *Orishas* (or *Santos*, saints in the Catholic faith) and other spiritual beings actually represent the ultimate biomedical allies, particularly by warning and protecting the living regarding organic ailments which, even if latent, may be waiting to arise. For example, surrounding envies may weaken the physical body by making a person more vulnerable to common diseases—from the common cold to chronic asthma or allergies. Finally, rather than being passive observers of their own maladies, patients turn into active participants in the healing process by following the *Santos'* prescriptions through offerings and cleansing ceremonies (Fernandez Olmos & Paravisini-Gebert, 2011; Viladrich & Abraido-Lanza, 2009).

Botánicas and Community Mental Health

Despite the findings presented above, not all voices are as optimistic when it comes to assessing botánicas' impact on the clients they serve. Botánicas have been labeled with offering products that have dubious curative powers (see Long, 2001) and that may even be dangerous, as in the case of their alleged selling of mercury for spiritual–religious purposes (Masur, 2011). The literature also questions the labeling of botánicas as "unlicensed clinics" vis-à-vis the unclear distinction between folk and complementary medicine (Holliday, 2008a; 2008b). Critical perspectives have also noted that botánicas' folk healing practices have been swept away from their authentic ethnic and cultural roots, at the expense of turning into samples of petty capitalist enterprises, or as new representations of hermeneutic practices (see Jacobs, 2001).

There is still much to be learned in terms of understanding the liaisons between religious faith and immigrants' physical and mental health, along with the efficacy of non-biomedical systems on health outcomes. Future work should shed light on the actual therapeutic effect claimed by botánicas' products and services, while promoting community-based strategies toward educating the public about the use of potentially dangerous substances. From a research perspective, religion and spirituality are often seen as frozen concepts that miss the dynamic fluxes of the healing experience along with the subjective meaning of transcendence (Viladrich & Abraido-Lanza, 2009). This speaks to the importance of developing conceptual models that incorporate the beneficial impact of indigenous etiologies of health and disease, including reliance on spirituality and religiosity as a holistic/integrative way of healing.

In many ways, the chasm between folk practices and Western medicine has dissociated the possibility of learning from indigenous healing forms, while minimizing the contributions of the latter to Western models of thought. Health researchers should consider the multidimensional and complex influence of religious practices on both physical and mental health, including the importance of collective healing (Broad, 2002; McKenzie, Tuck, & Noh, 2011). Among the positive therapeutic outcomes of these practices, the literature suggests the power of group support and the self-reliance in the positive help of others (Hoogasian & Lijmaer, 2010).

As it was sought in the past (see Koss, 1980; Koss-Chioino; 1992), health services that work with community-based organizations and folk practitioners could lead to forging bridges between formal and informal mental health services, while providing care in less structured contexts. Recent efforts in countries like the US and Canada (Broad, 2002; Hoogasian & Lijtmaer, 2010; McKenzie et al., 2011) stress the need to include traditional medicine into integrated health care systems. This body of research shows that service organizations are key in linking botánicas with both grassroots organizations and broader social institutions, including government agencies and biomedical services (Motta-Moss, 2008). On this line, the religious-healing practices that take place during ritualistic and collective ceremonies, often in botánicas' premises, have remained an unexplored area of research from a Western psychotherapeutic perspective. Future studies should provide an in-depth understanding of religious healing, including the influence (both positive and negative) of the social environment in promoting physical, mental, and spiritual health.

Conclusions

Botánicas constitute the visible entry to the concealed world of immigrant healers' practices in urban milieus. This is supported by studies that emphasize botánicas' role as a viable substitute of health care, given the financial and cultural barriers that minority populations face in the US. These establishments provide alternative sources of care by making their products highly visible in storefronts, which are run by their owners or employees, many of whom are healers themselves.

Despite the rising of international trade of spiritual and religious products, botánicas (and the healers associated with them) have remained loyal to their Latino and Caribbean clientele, which find in their premises unique answers to both their organic and spiritual ailments. Botánicas' customers are mostly drawn from disadvantaged populations that have little access to formal health care, and for whom religious healing offers an available outlet to both their physical and emotional needs. To a certain extent, these ethnic businesses have become an integral part of the city's informal networks of healing as they offer personalized attention to spiritual, mental, and organic conditions that would probably remain unattended otherwise.

As part of the urban fabric, botánicas function as informal hubs for the dissemination of information about community resources: from where to obtain a cheap second-hand piece of furniture to the newest treatment for children's *empacho* (indigestion). As discussed in this chapter, Latino and Caribbean folk healers, and their followers, tend to recreate familiar surroundings through communal practices that promote emotional bonding and interpersonal support, while building relational buffers against social stress, discrimination, and isolation in urban settings.

Botánicas found in cities such as NYC, Los Angeles, or Miami are mostly located in areas where Latino and Caribbean populations live, by offering products not typically available in other health stores and services. Nevertheless, slowly but steadily, botánicas have been moving away from places that have experienced deep ethnic and social transformations due to gentrification. As a result, they tend to be either concentrated in transitional areas or in neighborhoods where immigrants have increasingly become the majority (e.g., Jackson Heights in Queens).

Botánicas may continue changing their locations in years to come, but they are meant to stay as long as they keep offering unique products and therapies sought by a growing Latino and Caribbean clientele residing in urban milieus. The unsolved health and social problems of low-income immigrants, along with the importance of religiosity and spirituality in their lives, promise to keep botánicas thriving in most American cities in decades to come. In their pivotal role as main outlets for community bonding, botánicas are called to stay as long as they continue providing practical, emotional, and spiritual responses to their clients' unmet needs.

Note

1. The neighborhoods where the correlation between the high number of botánicas and the density of the Latino population was the strongest included: Washington Heights, Inwood, and East Harlem, in Manhattan; the middle and southern Bronx; Jackson Heights, Queens; and in East New York, East Williamsburg, Bushwick, and Sunset Park, Brooklyn.

References

Anderson, M. R., McKee, D., Yukes, J., Alvarez, A., & Karasz, A. (2008). An investigation of douching practices in botánicas in the Bronx. *Culture, Health & Sexuality, 10*, 1–11.

Baer, H. E. (2001). *Biomedicine and alternative healing in America: Issues of class, race, ethnicity, and gender.* Madison, WI: University of Wisconsin Press.

Baez, A., & Hernandez, D. (2001). Complementary spiritual beliefs in the Latino community: The interface with psychotherapy. *American Journal of Orthopsychiatry, 71*, 408–415.

Balick, M. J., Kronenberg, F., Ososki, A. L., Reiff, M., Fugh-Berman, A., O'Connor, B., Roble, M., Lohr, P., & Atha, D. (2000). Medicinal plants used by Latino healers for women's health conditions in New York City. *Economic Botany, 54*, 344–357.

Balick, M. J., & Lee, R. (2001). Looking within: Urban ethnomedicine and ethnobotany. *Alternative Therapies, 7*, 114–115.

Broad, L. (2002). Nurse practitioners and traditional healers: An alliance of mutual respect in the art and science of health practices. *Holistic Nursing Practice, 16*, 50–57.

Byrd, T. L., & Law, J. G. (2009). Cross-border utilization of health care services by United States residents living near the Mexican border. *Pan American Journal of Public Health, 26*, 95–100.

Caban, A., & Walker, E. A. (2006). A systematic review of research on culturally relevant issues for Hispanics with diabetes. *The Diabetes Educator, 32*, 584–595.

Dearfield, C. T., & Pugh-Yi, R. (2011). Neighborhood botanicos as a source of alternative medicine for Latino Americans: Implications for clinical management of HIV/AIDS. In G. A. Downer (Ed.), *HIV in communities of color: The compendium of culturally competent promising practices: The role of traditional healing in HIV clinical management* (pp. 21–26). Washington, DC: Howard University College of Medicine.

Fernández Olmos, M., & Paravisini-Gebert, L. (2011). *Creole religions of the Caribbean: An introduction from Vodou and Santería to Obeah and Espiritismo.* 2nd ed. New York: New York University Press.

Gelb, R .G. (2005). The magic of verbal art: Juanita's Santería initiation. In M. Farr (Ed.), *Latino language and literacy in ethnolinguistic Chicago* (pp. 323–349). Mahwah, NJ: Lawrence Erlbaum Associates Publishers.

Gomez-Beloz, A., & Chavez, N. (2001). The botánica as a culturally appropriate health care option for Latinos. *The Journal of Alternative and Complementary Medicine, 7,* 537–546.

Holliday, K. V. (2008a). "Folk" or "traditional" versus "complementary" and "alternative" medicine: Constructing Latino/a health and illness through biomedical labeling. *Latino Studies, 6,* 398–417.

Holliday, K. V. (2008b). La limpia de San Lazaro as individual and collective cleansing rite. In B. W. McNeill & J. M. Cervantes (Eds.), *Latina/o healing practices: Mestizo and indigenous perspectives* (pp. 175–193). New York: Routledge/Taylor & Francis Group.

Hoogasian, R., & Lijtmaer, R. (2010). Integrating curanderism into counseling and psychotherapy. *Counselling Psychology Quarterly, 23,* 297–307.

Jacobs, C. F. (2001). Folks for whom? Tourist guidebooks, local color and the spiritual churches of New Orleans. *Journal of American Folklore, 114,* 309–330.

Jones, M. O., & Polk, P. A. with Flores-Peña, Y. & Evanchuk, R. J. (2001) Invisible hospitals: Botánicas in ethnic health care. In E. Brady (Ed.), *Healing logics. Culture and medicine in modern health belief systems* (pp. 39–87). Logan, UT: Utah State University Press.

Koss, J. (1980). The therapist-spiritist training project in Puerto Rico: An experiment to relate the traditional healing system to the public health system. *Social Science and Medicine, 14,* 255–266.

Koss-Chioino, J. (1992). *Women as healers, women as patients: Mental health care and traditional healing in Puerto Rico.* New York: Westview Press.

Loera, S., Muñoz, L. M., Nott, E., & Sandefur, B. K. (2009). Call the *Curandero*: Improving mental health services for Mexican immigrants. *Praxis, 9,* 16–24.

Long, C. M. (2001). *Spiritual merchants.* Knoxville, TN: The University of Tennessee Press.

Masur, L. C. (2011). A review of the use of mercury in historic and current ritualistic and spiritual practices. *Alternative Medicine Review, 16,* 314–320.

McCarthy Brown, K. (1991). *Mama Lola: A Vodou priestess in Brooklyn.* Berkeley, CA: University of California Press.

McKenzie, K., Tuck, A., & Noh, M. S. (2011). Moving traditional Caribbean medicine practices in healthcare in Canada. *Ethnicity and Inequalities in Health and Social Care, 4,* 60–70.

McNeill, B., & Cervantes, J. M. (Ed.) (2008). *Latina/o healing practices: Mestizo and indigenous perspectives.* New York: Routledge.

Menard, J., Kobetz, E., Diem, J., Lifleur, M., Blanco, J., & Barton, B. (2010). The sociocultural context of gynecological health among Haitian immigrant women in Florida: Applying ethnographic methods to public health inquiry. *Ethnicity & Health, 15,* 253–267.

Moodley, R., Sutherland, P., & Oulanova, O. (2008). Traditional healing, the body and mind in psychotherapy. *Counselling Psychology Quarterly, 21,* 153–165.

Motta-Moss, A. (2008). The role of immigrant service organizations in the transformation of cultural capital. *Dissertation Abstracts International*, Section B: The Sciences and Engineering. *68*, 6391.

Murphy, J. M. (2010). Objects that speak Creole: Juxtapositions of shrine devotions at botánicas in Washington. *Material Religion, 6*, 86–108.

New York Department of Health and Mental Hygiene. (2002). *Community health survey.* Retrieved from http://www.nyc.gov/html/doh/html/survey/survey.shtml

Pignataro, M. E. (2009). Botánica Los Angeles: Latino popular religious art in the city of Angeles, book review. Polk, P. A. (Ed.), *Chasqui: Revista de literatura latinoamericana, 38*, 206–207.

Polk, P. A. (2004). *Botánica Los Angeles. Latino popular religious art in the city of Angels.* Los Angeles, CA: UCLA Fowler Museum of Cultural History.

Pugliese, A. (2010). *The inaccurate saint: Devotion to San Lázaro / Babalú Ayé in Cuban culture in Miami, Florida.* Miami, FL: Goizueta Foundation Undergraduate Fellowship.

Rahill, G. J., Dawkins, M. P., & De La Rosa, M. (2011). Haitian picuristes/injectionists as alternatives to conventional health care providers in South Florida. *Social Work in Public Health, 26*, 577–593.

Ransford, H. E., Carrillo, F. R., & Rivera, Y. (2010). Health care-seeking among Latino immigrants: Blocked access, use of traditional medicine and the role of religion. *Journal of Health Care for the Poor and Underserved, 21*, 862–867.

Reiff, M., O'Connor, B., Kronenberg, F., Balick, M., Lohr, P., Roble, M., Fugh-Berman, A., & Johnson, K. D. (2003). Ethnomedicine in the urban environment: Dominican healers in New York City. *Human Organization, 61*, 12–26.

Reyes-García, V. (2010). The relevance of traditional knowledge systems for ethnopharmacological research: Theoretical and methodological contributions. *Journal of Ethnobiology and Ethnomedicine, 6*. Retrieved from http://www.ncbi.nlm.nih.gov/pmc/articles/PMC2993655

Reyes-Ortiz, C., Rodriguez, M., & Markides, K. (2009). The role of spirituality healing with perceptions of the medical encounter among Latinos. *Journal of General Internal Medicine, Supplement 3, 24*, 542–547.

Romberg, R. (2003). *Witchcraft and welfare: Spiritual capital and the business of magic in modern Puerto Rico.* Austin, TX: University of Texas Press.

Romberg, R. (2011). Spiritual capital: On the materiality and immateriality of blessings in Puerto Rican brujería. *Research in Economic Anthropology, 31*, 123–156.

Singer, M., & Garcia, R. (1989). Becoming a Puerto Rican espiritista: Life history of a female healer. In C. Shepherd McClain. (Ed.), *Women as healers: Cross-cultural perspectives* (pp. 157–185). New Brunswick, NJ: Rutgers University Press.

Solimar, O. (2007). Barrio, bodega, and botánica Aesthetics. *Atlantic Studies, 4*, 173–194.

Tafur, M. M., Crowe, T. K., & Torres, E. (2009). A review of curanderism and healing practices among Mexicans and Mexican Americans. *Occupational Therapy International, 16*, 82–88.

Trotter, R. T., & Chavira, J. A. (1981). *Mexican American folk healing.* Athens, GA: University of Georgia Press.

Tyree, J. M. (2005). The United Nations of Queens: The undiscovered borough. *The Antioch Review, 63*, 646–665.

Vandebroek, I., Balick, M. J., Ososki, A., Kronenberg, F., Yukes, J., Wade, C., Jimenez, F., Peguero, B., & Castillo, D. (2010). The importance of botellas and other plant mixtures in Dominican traditional medicine. *Journal of Ethnopharmacology, 128*, 20–41.

Viladrich, A. (2006a). Botánicas in America's backyard: Uncovering the world of Latino immigrants' herb-healing practices. *Human Organization, 65*, 407–419.

Viladrich, A. (2006b). Beyond the supernatural: Latino healers treating Latino immigrants in New York City. *The Journal of Latino-Latin American Studies, 2*, 134–148.

Viladrich, A. (2007a). From shrinks to urban shamans: Argentine immigrants' therapeutic eclecticism in New York City. *Culture, Medicine and Psychiatry, 31*, 307–328.

Viladrich, A. (2007b). Between bellyaches and lucky charms: Revealing Latinos' plant-healing knowledge and practices in New York City. In A. Pieroni & I. Vandebroek (Eds.), *Traveling cultures and plants: The ethnobiology and ethnopharmacy of migrations* (pp. 64–85). New York & Oxford: Berghahn Books.

Viladrich, A. (2007c) Welcome to el Barrio: An afternoon in the company of Doña Josefa. *Latino Studies, 5*, 364–373.

Viladrich, A., & Abraido-Lanza, A. (2009). Religion and mental health among immigrants and minorities in the US. In S. Loue & M. Sajatovic (Eds.), *Determinants of minority mental health and wellness* (pp. 149–174). New York: Springer.

Vissman A. T., Bloom F. R., Leichliter, J. S., Bachmann, L. H., Montaño, J., Topmiller M., & Rhodes, S. D. (2011). Exploring the use of nonmedical sources of prescription drugs among immigrant Latinos in the rural Southereastern USA. *The Journal of Rural Health, 27*, 159–167.

19

CARIBBEAN TRADITIONAL HEALING IN THE DIASPORA

Roy Moodley and Michel'e Bertrand

Introduction

Caribbean traditional healing has been a part of the social, cultural, and geopolitical landscape of the West since the time of slavery, a process that has taken several decades to evolve and develop to the degree that many are now regarded as part of the mainstream in the Caribbean and rapidly becoming accessible in the diaspora. Religious and healing practices such as Voodoo, Shango, Spiritual Baptist, *Santería*, *Espiritismo* and others that are a unique blend of African Animism, Christianity, and the healing modalities of the Amerindians have been reconceptualized in ways that are relevant to modern metropolitan urban living in the West. As a result these healing practices have become deeply engraved into the psyche as something that is frightening, dangerous, and grotesque, and reinforced through its Eurocentric representations in literature, art, popular culture, and film, particularly in Hollywood's depiction of some of these practices (e.g., voodoo) as immoral, violent, and evil. The fear and trepidation of Caribbean healing practices illustrates the complex relationship between the Caribbean and the West. For example, the history of slavery, the struggles for liberation and independence, and the current neocolonial relations between the West and the Caribbean are riddled with numerous signifiers that construct Caribbean people as inferior and uncivilized despite the rise of liberal humanism within a postcolonial, multicultural, and diverse environment.

The post-World War II period saw an increase in immigrants from several Caribbean islands to rescue North America and Europe from economic depression through cheap labour in various sectors of industry, transport, social, and health care services. Amongst these new Caribbean immigrants were many traditional healers whose healing practices offered hope and wellness in an environment where they felt alienated and disavowed, resulting in stress, psychological distress, and psychosomatic responses to racism. The limitations of conventional medicine became apparent not for want of trying but a consequence of hegemonic meanings embedded in colonialism. The research and literature demonstrating racist and oppressive practices in psychiatry, psychotherapy, and counseling are explicit about the dehumanizing ways in which Caribbean and other black people are treated in Western mental care (see, for example, Fernando, 1988; 2010; Moodley, 2011; Moodley & Palmer, 2005).

Indeed, the lack of awareness of Caribbean culture and wellness practices by health and mental health practitioners led many new Caribbean immigrants to seek help from traditional healers in their midst. The traditional healers were forced as a result to practice deep in the heart of the inner city and out of visual gaze of mainstream culture; indeed, while remaining "underground" these practices were responding to the sociocultural and political reality of the time alongside other cultural healing practices undergoing similar challenges, amongst them the Aboriginal communities (see, Poonwassie & Charter, 2005), the new immigrant communities from the Asia continent (Laungani, 2005), Africa (Vontress, 2005; Bojuwoye & Sodi, 2010), and South America (Hoogasian & Lijtmaer, 2010). Individuals and groups from mainstream dominant cultures too were seeking alternative and complementary health and healing strategies outside the framework of conventional medicine. Acupuncture, yoga, meditation, Ayurveda, qigong, Chinese traditional medicine and many others were in vogue and becoming acceptable as treatments for health and mental health care (see Moodley & West, 2005). Consequently, research and training evolved and developed, indicating that traditional healers and their healing practices appeared to have a proven, and even superior, efficacy with some patient groups (Wessels, 1985). Moreover, traditional healers and their healing practices were becoming critical spaces within which larger questions of social justice, anti-racism and anti-oppression were being interrogated. In addition, the role of the healers and their healing practices were shifting the discourse of an essentialist and positivistic Western medical science.

Moreover, the traditional healing practices are a way of keeping indigenous traditions alive; by recording psychosocial and illness experiences of the community, and through healing individual's bodies, a dictionary of illness, health, and wellness for Caribbean people in the diaspora is established. In this way traditional healing tends to become the oral and embodied historical archive of a culture/ethnicity (race) undergoing transformation. Traditional healers and healing by becoming the carriers of culture and Caribbean theology and by acting as guardians of indigenous sociocultural, economic, and political spaces against the onslaught of colonialism, oppression, racism, and capitalism constructs a significance in the diaspora that appears to be greater than the one that it played in the Caribbean.

In this chapter, we discuss how the Caribbean traditional healers and healing practices are configured and reconfigured in the diaspora. We explore the underlying philosophical and psychological constructs that underpin these changes, and how it has changed our illness representations and perceptions as a result. We discuss the role of traditional healers as conduits of the spirit world and protectors of the "divine," and how traditional rituals and ceremonies converge upon shared ontological and epistemological trajectories of cures within which Caribbean people in the diaspora can fulfill their desire for health, wellness, and spiritual healing.

Caribbean Philosophy of Healing in the Diaspora

For many who were transported to the Caribbean during slavery and indentureship, and for those people indigenous to Caribbean lands, the philosophy of health and healing evolved during the course of slavery, the resistance to oppression, and the fight to gain freedom for oneself and the community. In a time when the body and mind were shackled through Western cultural, socioeconomic, and political ideologies, Caribbean people were able to understand and heal themselves through their own construction of health and wellness. From the very beginning the concept of health meant freedom from oppression and slavery, resisting the representations of the body and mind as inferior by pseudo-scientific ideologies, and engaging the spiritual in ways that were culturally specific to Caribbean experiences. In combining Western religions and African gods they developed spiritual and healing institutions that required them to speak simultaneously in multiple opposed tongues, worshipping at the feet of statues of Christian saints, and emotionally eulogizing the spirits of African deities while at the same time planning to escape oppression and captivity. Indeed, this created the possibilities of accommodating several cognitive and emotional schemas with much dissonance in their psyches. They lived on the edge of hyperconsciousness; it is no wonder that Frantz Fanon (1952) argued that the black man has no time to make experience unconscious.

The capacity to code, mask, and integrate various indigenous worldviews with an increasingly Westernized approach came to define how Caribbean people determined and treated physical, psychological, and spiritual problems. While the Cartesian body–mind determinism constructed the way in which Caribbean people were perceived historically, with a racist emphasis of the (working, or exotic/erotic) black body and an inferior mind, the Caribbean people themselves were less interested in what the "whites" thought of them but rather concerned with their relationship with the African, Asian, and indigenous gods. However, for Caribbean communities this polarized body–mind discourse was the place of tension and illness, while the place of spirit provided an avenue for solitude and an integration of the self. The notion of spirituality then becomes a strong foundational construct for Caribbean communities to assert and validate their presence, health, and well-being in the West. The idea of the spirit is embodied and enacted through membership of spiritual communities, such as the charismatic

Christian churches, the Voodoo health centers, and community mental health groups. A philosophy emerges with spirit as its center point that ontologically configures the self and other. An ensuing spiritual worldview then evolves to replace the body–mind division and its racist constructions.

In evolving a philosophy of spirit, Caribbean healing traditions conceptualize an understanding of spirit that involves spirit as a larger, undifferentiated realm, as well as a differentiated and localized spirit that is specific to an individual. For the Pentecostal and Spiritual Baptist healers of the "Spirits of a drum beat: African Caribbean traditional healers and their healing practices in Toronto" research (Moodley & Bertrand, 2011), spirit is the primordial presence of God, or the divine spirit, whom we sometimes know and experience as the holy spirit. Alongside this, spirit can manifest in other ways. The Pentecostal healers encounter spirits in demonic possessions into which they intervene. Psychoanalytically, it seems that the racisms, tensions, and oppressions of day to day living in the West are embodied in the possession and exorcised through a Pentecostal healer's intervention.

The Spiritual Baptist healer encounters spirits as spiritual (spirit-form) mothers and fathers who help train and guide them in the practice of healing. The spirit is then the center of the healing process. For example, a Spiritual Baptist healer would treat high blood pressure with medical advice, exercise, keeping the head wrapped to restore balance in the head, as well as with the body, heart, and spirit, alongside prayer and meditation as channels of direct access to spirit (Moodley & Bertrand, 2011). For the *Santería* healer, spirit is a pantheon or collectivity of Orishas or Yoruba deities, to whom one can appeal individually and in turn, using one's own spiritual power. These powers of course differ for each traditional healing tradition. For some it's direct ancestry or being claimed by a spirit, between innateness itself and receiving a calling later in life, and between families of biological origin and chosen families; some converge and others are divergent from each other, but for the healers the ontological dialectic is between the spirit and the self as a manifestation of being human. This in turn outlines the contours of a particular philosophy of medicine, health, and illness.

Where spirit also refers to the spirits of people who have passed, "spirits of the dead" including ancestral spirits, this concept then becomes the guiding philosophy of Caribbean traditional healing. Acquiring the ability to read and access spirit involves intensive learning, often over several years, and a lifetime commitment to maintenance and renewal of the spirit, through intergenerational mentoring and accountability. This process is dedicated to developing the spirit(s) within, and, through them, the ability to attain insight directly or indirectly from spirit (Moodley & Bertrand, 2011). No doubt these constructions are a response to the ways in which Caribbean people are attempting to answer ontological and existential questions in the West. It seems that healing and transformation are facilitated by the transmission of supernatural powers from the spirits of the ancestors to humans to help them "to come into harmony with problem-causing spirits, to forgive them, and in so doing regulate emotions, lifestyles, physical complaints and destiny" (Moodley & Sutherland, 2009, p. 18).

The concept of "being" is derived from spirit as a universal configuration which manifests itself in the situated spirit enacting through the various dimensions of the individual: spiritual, emotional, mental, and physical. The state of equilibrium of the self is manifested through the condition of alignment or relationship with spirit; disequilibrium results in health problems and healing occurs when the spirit is restored to its harmonious and aligned place within the individual and the universe. In this way, traditional healing practices for singular health complaints are often multi-axial within a dimension, across dimensions, and in terms of realigning with spirit, involving a cultural and indigenous rituals, herbs, prayer, meditation, sacrifices, spirit dances, and on occasions even a referral to a Western health care professional. The *Santería/Lucumi* practitioner channels direct connections with an Orisha to prescribe a pathway for action in life, and also prescribes herbal cleanses to prepare and maintain openness to that connection along the intersecting axes of body, mind, and spirit. Multi-axial treatment may involve more than one practitioner working on the same, seemingly singular health complaint (Moodley & Bertrand, 2011).

Reconfiguring Traditional Healing Practices in the Diaspora

Caribbean traditional healing practices have been undergoing a metamorphosis since arriving in the West, responding to sociocultural and political events that confronted them as new immigrants, as well as the varied ways in which Caribbean people represented and presented their illnesses and psychological distresses. Throughout this period cultural and traditional healing practices have reconfigured, "reconstituted and modified to suit current contexts" (Moodley, 2011, p. 74), for example, Voodoo healing has been a direct response to slavery and racism (Chireau, 2003), while Maat, an Afrocentric healing method, empowers individuals and groups to resist the racial discrimination and cultural marginalization in the inner cities (see Graham, 2005, for discussion).

In any engagement in reconfiguring healing philosophies in the diaspora, the protagonists of these traditions were invariably pitted against each other; transformations were undertaken in an environment in which there were competing, contesting, and complex interests, motivations, and ideologies at play. For example, the Caribbean Christian charismatic churches portrayed non- Christian healers and healing traditions as evil, uncivilized, and illegal, clearly a reflection of a colonial mentality. The enduring strategy for these non-Christian healing traditions was to go underground. For example, Voodoo, *Santería*, and many others were the enterprise of many subversive healing communities in the larger metropolitan inner cities. Others of course flourished. For example, the Charismatic, Pentecostal, and other denominations of black churches with the unique blend of existential theologies and survival strategies in the face of racism in the US,

England, and Canada are still the central places of healing and worship. Yet, others, such as the Caribbean Islamic and Hindu healing traditions while not quite underground appear to be invisible or silenced by the new immigrant healing traditions from the Middle East or South India.

Clearly, the diasporic space presents each healing tradition with challenges and opportunities for transformations and reconfigurations in a new world, and indeed continues to do so in relation to the changing contexts within which their particular communities find themselves in. During the process of reconfigurations of traditional healing from slavery days to the diaspora many of these practices took on a more Eurocentric version in their enactments. For example, a Voodoo healer may work out of a modern office (a room in her or his apartment), schedule timely sessions, and make referrals to Western health care practitioners where appropriate. Voodoo healers themselves could be in full-time employment (e.g., a school teacher) during the day and see patients at night and on weekends. While these modern enactments of an age-old traditional ceremony and ritual give the impression that they have undergone a postmodern change, not much has changed at some levels since their evolution in the Caribbean. For example, Voodoo which evolved as a spiritual healing tradition combines Catholic practice and African spiritual traditions and still maintains at its core this integration and belief system even after coming to the West where Christian traditions are strong and are strongly opposed to Voodoo. However, since Voodoo is an integrated system concerning human activities between the natural world and the supernatural, fusing African animism with Western Christianity, it bridges the body/mind/spirit complex. The healing for many patients is through the rituals of dancing, offering gifts, ancestor worship, deification of material artifacts, and inebriation from herbs and plants; ritualized and sacred drumming and dancing, and animal sacrifice are also an important part of the healing practice, particularly when animal sacrifice to appease the spirits and gods is performed (see Courlander, Bastien, & Schader, 1966; Fernandez-Olmos & Paravisini-Gebert, 2003; Gomez-Beloz & Chavez, 2005; Moodley & Bertrand, 2011).

Undertaking some of these rituals, such as animal sacrifice, in the West is always problematic and may lead to contravening metropolitan city health and environment bylaws; moreover, mainstream cultures not familiar with these rituals can and do object to these practices being performed in their neighborhood, meaning that ritual animal sacrifices need to be toned down, modified, or even removed from some healing practices. These modifications take place to then appease the mainstream culture at the expense of tradition and possibly one's own healing. Clearly, as the newer forms of healing emerge they intersect, converge, collide, and/or compete with the older forms, they invariably change the way in which we represent and present health, illness, and wellness (Moodley, 2011).

While these processes and practices are continually changing and transforming according to the dynamic cultural, geopolitical, and socioeconomic terrain of the Caribbean and the diaspora, the function and purpose of the spiritual, religious, and healing practices remain the same, i.e., to connect people with the "divine", more so in the diaspora against competing healing discourses within Western multiculturalism. The importance, relevance, and revival of Caribbean healing practices have been gaining ground not only amongst Caribbean people but amongst other cultural and ethnic communities as well (see Moodley, 2011).

Caribbean Healing and Western Health Care in the Diaspora

The fact that Afrocentric religious practices remain relevant despite the hegemonic influence of centuries of sustained colonization is a testament to the strength of the intergenerational transmission of traditional healing practices (Gibson, Morgado, Brosyle, Mesa, & Sanchez, 2010). Alongside this, Caribbean communities deem their traditional healing practices to be outside the framework of conventional Western medicine and mental health care. In addition, many see the current Western health care practices as culturally insensitive, discriminatory, and even racist (see Moodley & West, 2005).

A core asymmetry exists where Caribbean healers and people who seek them would also turn to Western practitioners for complementary points of entry into the same problems, but on the whole receive less recognition and referrals from them even where these are vital. In "Spirits of a drum beat" (see Moodley & Bertrand, 2011), for example, healers often recommended clients to seek Western medical assessments and treatments when and where it was necessary, including when the assessments and/or treatments required were beyond the scope of their own practice and training. The healers were especially open to referring their clients to Western health care professionals who either shared or respected the healers' beliefs and practices, and received referrals from these professionals when the client's concern was believed to have a spiritual dimension. In the larger framework, however, this was often not the case. In the healers' perspectives, one of the key recurring reasons for this is the dissonance between the beliefs of Western medical science, on the one hand, and spirituality, on the other. This dissonance plays out in differences between Western medical approaches and spirituality-based approaches to understanding client psychological difficulties. Western professionals might not recognize the spiritual aspects of a client's concern; a client's treatment might be limited because the appropriate spiritual healing interventions might not be undertaken, or referrals to spiritual healers might not take place.

On the surface, the conflict between Western medical sciences and the spirit-based epistemologies of Caribbean traditional healing might seem impossible to bridge. Yet, through the intersectionality of the physical, emotional, mental, and spiritual, spirit-based epistemologies offer healers numerous ways to be open to scientific ways of knowing, and to integrate them into their own conceptions of health and healing. Notwithstanding this, collaborating and networking with Western health care practitioners continues to involve various obstacles, barriers, and skepticisms, as well as perceived illegitimacy of their specific faiths, cultural beliefs, and healing practices. For example, where Voodoo health is acceptable amongst many African and Caribbean communities, it remains suspect to many non-African Caribbean communities, including Western medical practitioners. Additionally, there are current structural limitations that need to be addressed, such as the legislation that forbids and creates systemic barriers to the referral systems, the recognition of traditional herbs or plants as part of indigenous pharmacy, and the need for health care institutions to include traditional healers in patients' treatment choice in the same way that health care practitioners are increasingly doing in some countries, such as China, Brazil, India, and South Africa. With these barriers in place, the holistic address of Caribbean healing systems comes to be ruptured: interventions that are primarily spirit-based or those that cognitively and psychosomatically perform are engaged with while physical challenges are, of necessity, referred to a regulated health professional in the Western system. In this way, the split of the Cartesian complex comes to be embodied through assimilation and integration, within which cultural healing practices situate themselves (Moodley & Bertrand, 2011).

There is still a long way to go in achieving respectful collaboration and integration. The beliefs and practices of traditional healing and of Western health care practices need to be acknowledged, accommodated, and understood by all practitioners within a framework of cross-cultural epistemological and epidemiological differences. The move towards getting more and more Western health care practitioners to become more familiar and acquainted with indigenous, traditional, and cultural practices is gaining ground (see Moodley & Sutherland, 2009; Moodley & West, 2005). However, there still lingers the pervasive issues of expropriation and commercialization of indigenous and traditional healing practices in the West. This raises key questions as to future trajectories for Caribbean healing practices in the diaspora. If there are possibilities for these practices to be recognized by and implemented within Western health professions, they bear much risk. Conscious of the ways that other traditional knowledge—such as mindfulness and yoga—have been taken up in Western health care industries, Caribbean healers in the diaspora have raised concerns that their own practices could be reformulated and repackaged without reference to their ancestral, cultural and spiritual base, and that the healers themselves would be replaced (Moodley & Bertrand, 2011). The uncertainty about the relationship between these traditions and Western health professions bears the colonial echo of rupture and recursive non-belonging.

Conclusion

For mainstream culture, as long as Caribbean traditional healing practices do not threaten Western religious, cultural, and health care ideas and ideologies, they are left alone for the Caribbean people to indulge in. For Caribbean people the engagement with traditional healing was and still is a very complex and confusing process, positioning them at the interface of African spirituality, and the diaspora experience of acculturation, integration, and assimilation. Many would seek the services of a "witchdoctor" or Voodoo healer at night in "borrowed robes" to avoid the European colonial gaze, professional peers, and even family members.

For Caribbean people in the diaspora, the syncretism of African or Asian or Islamic spiritual and religious practices and the colonial gods and belief systems continues to enable a tentative, shifting expression of indigeneity and ancestral knowing that ruptures a contained and containing subject of the new world. This process is geared to accommodate the ongoing condition in which ancestral origins and ultimate destinations are psychically and physically withheld. At the same time, it forestalls the kinds of densely rooted cultural self-articulations and self-assertions that are necessary to resist fragmentation, expropriation, and erasure by dominant discourses and structures, including those of health care, in the West. Caribbean systems of thought need to be sufficiently theorized to discursively re-indigenize Caribbean processes and projects of being, but sufficiently un-theorized so as to allow Caribbean people to genuinely be able to recognize, imagine, and reinvent themselves.

References

Bojuwoye, O., & Sodi, T. (2010). Challenges and opportunities to integrating traditional healing into counselling and psychotherapy. *Counselling Psychology Quarterly, 23*(3), 283–296.

Chireau, P. Y. (2003). *Black magic: Religion and the African American conjuring tradition.* Berkeley, CA: University of California Press.

Courlander, H., Bastien, R., & Schader, R. P. (1966). *Religion and politics in Haiti.* Washington, DC: Institute for Cross-Cultural Research.

Fanon, F. (1952) *Black skins, white masks.* London: Grove Press (1967).

Fernandez-Olmos, M., & Paravisini-Gebert, L. (2003). *Creole religions of the Caribbean: An introduction from Vodu and Santeria to Obeah and Espiritismo.* New York: New York University Press.

Fernando, S. (1988). *Race and culture in psychiatry.* London: Croom Helm.

Fernando, S. (2010). *Mental health, race and culture.* Basingstoke: Palgrave Macmillan.

Gibson, R. C., Morgado, A. J., Brosyle, A. C., Mesa, E. H., & Sanchez, C. H. (2010). Afro-centric religious consultations as treatment for psychotic disorders among day hospital patients in Santiago de Cuba. *Mental Health, Religion, & Culture, 1*(1), 1–11.

Gomez-Beloz, A., & Chavez, N. (2005). The botanica as a culturally appropriate health care option for Latinos. *The Journal of Alternative and Complementary Medicine, 7*(5), 537–546.

Graham, M. (2005). Maat: An African-centered paradigm for psychological and spiritual healing. In R. Moodley & W. West (Eds.), *Integrating traditional healing practices into counseling and psychotherapy.* Thousand Oaks, CA: Sage

Hoogasian, R., & Lijtmaer, R. (2010). Integrating Curanderismo into counselling and psychotherapy. *Counselling Psychology Quarterly, 23*(3), 297–307.

Laungani, P. (2005). Hindu spirituality and healing practices. In R. Moodley & W. West (Eds.), *Integrating traditional healing practices into counseling and psychotherapy*. Thousand Oaks, CA: Sage.

Moodley, R. (2011). *Outside the sentence: Readings in critical multicultural counselling and psychotherapy*. Toronto: CDCP.

Moodley, R., & Bertrand, M. (2011). Spirits of a drum beat: African Caribbean traditional healers and their healing practices in Toronto. *International Journal of Health Promotion and Education, 49*(3), 79–89.

Moodley, R., & Palmer, S. (Eds.) (2005). *Race, culture and psychotherapy. Critical perspectives in multicultural practice*. London: Routledge.

Moodley, R., & Sutherland, P. (2009). Traditional and cultural healers and healing: Dual interventions in counseling and psychotherapy. *Counselling and Spirituality, 28*(1), 11–31.

Moodley, R., & West, W. (Eds.) (2005). *Integrating traditional healing practices into counseling and psychotherapy*. Thousand Oaks, CA: Sage.

Poonwassie, A., & Charter, A. (2005). Aboriginal worldview of healing: Inclusion, blending, and bridging. In R. Moodley & W. West (Eds.), *Integrating traditional healing practices into counseling and psychotherapy*. Thousand Oaks, CA: Sage.

Vontress, C. E. (2005). Animism: Foundation of traditional healing in Sub-Saharan Africa. In R. Moodley & W. West (Eds.), *Integrating traditional healing practices into counseling and psychotherapy*. Thousand Oaks, CA: Sage.

Wessels, W. H. (1985). The traditional healer and psychiatry. *Australian and New Zealand Journal of Psychiatry, 19*, 283–286.

GLOSSARY

Chapter 3 Traditional Medicine

caul. A person born with the placenta over the face (born with the veil/caul) is considered to have special powers that allow him or her to be clairvoyant and see into the spirit world.

etiology. Cause of disease.

fallen angels. Evil spirits; duppies.

Chapter 4 Herbal Medicine—Scientific and Common Plant Names

Each plant is shown firstly by its botanical name and is then followed by its common names.

Abelmoschus moschatus: gumbo musque, musk mallow, musk okra, ambrette seeds

Achyranthes aspera: devil's horsewhip, prickly chaff-flower

Agave sp.: lechuguilla, century plant

Ageratum conyzoides: Mexican agcratum, z'herbe á femme, caringa de bode

Allium cepa: onion, zechalot, cebollin

Allium sativum: garlic, áil, ajo

Aloe vera: aloes, sâbila

Ambrosia cumanensis: perennial ragweed, western ragweed, cumin ragweed

Ambrosia hispida: coastal ragweed

Anacardium occidentalis: cashew, cashew apple, pomme cujou

Annona muricata: soursop, custard apple, guanabana

Annona reticulata: custard apple, sugar apple, bullock's heart

Argemone mexicana: Mexican prickly poppy, goatweed, bird-in-the-bush
Aristolochia rugosa: matroot, anico
Aristolochia trilobata: Dutchman's pipe, pipevine, birthwort
Artocarpus altilis: breadfruit, breadnut
Bambusa vulgaris: bamboo
Beta vulgaris: beetroot, beet, remolacha
Bidens pilosa: Spanish needles, begger's tick, amor seco
Bignonia longissima: French oak, Jamaican oak, mastwood
Bixa orellana: roucou, lipstick tree, anhiote
Borreria verticillata: botón blanco, shrubby false buttonweed, cardio de frade
Cannabis sativa: marijuana, ganja, weed
Casearia ilicifolia: holly-like-leaf, castor, casearia
Cassia fistula: Golden shower, Indian laburum, purging cassia
Cassia fruticosa: Christmas bush, drooping cassia
Catharanthus roseus: Madagascar periwinkle, guajaca
Chamaesyce hirta: malomay
Chaptalia nutans: dandelion, costa branca, bretonica
Chenopodium ambrosioides: worm grass, worm seed, bitter weed
Chiococca alba: West Indian milkberry, snakeroot
Chromolaena odorata: bitterbush, Jack-in-the-bush, agonoi
Cinnamomum verum: cinnamon, canela
Cissus sicyoides: possum grapevine, cow-itch vine, marine ivy
Citharexylum spinosum: spiny fiddlewood, fiddlewood
Citrus aurantifolia: limón, lime, citron
Citrus sinensis: sweet orange naranja dulce, oranj
Cocus nucifera: coconut, coco-tree, cocotero
Cola nitida: obie seed
Costus speciosus: crepe ginger, malay ginger, cane reed
Crescentia cujete: calabash tree, gourd
Cucurbita maxima: pumpkin
Curcuma domestica: tumeric, hardi
Cymbopogon citrates: lemongrass, fevergrass, molojillo criollo
Datura stramonium: datura, jimson seed, thorn-apple
Eleusine indica: Indian goose-grass, crows' foot-grass, silver crab-grass
Eleutherine bulbosa: dragon's blood, lagrimas de la virgen
Eryngium foetidum: spiritweed, shadon beni, fitweed, bhandania
Erythoxylum havanense: barberry, bracelet, tea bush
Eupatorium macrophyllum: z'herbe chatte
Eupatorium triplinerve: white snakeroot, yapana, pool root
Gomphrena globosa: bachelor button
Gossypium barbadense: sea island cotton, Creole cotton, long staple cotton
Jatropha gossypifolia: belly ache bush, physic nut, African coffee
Kalanchoe gastonis-bonnieri: leaf of life, donkey ears, good luck leaf

Lantana camara: red sage, kayakeet, lantana, graterwood

Leonotis nepetifolia: shandileer, Christmas candlestick, lion's ears

Mangifera indica: Mango, mangot, mamuang, manguier

Mintha viridis: spearmint, peppermint, garden mint

Momordica charantia L.: cerasee, bitter gourd, bitter melon

Myristica fragrans: nutmeg, neuz moscada

Neurolaena lobata Syn. *Pluchea symphytifolia*: Jackass bitters, zeb-a-pique, cure-for-all

Ocimum basilicum: sweet basil, basilik, fon bazin

Ocimum gratissimum: wild basil, vane van

Panax ginseng: ginseng

Parinari campestris: bois bandé

Paspalum conjugatum: buffalo grass, sour grass

Peperomia pellucida: shiny bush, silver bush, man-to-man

Persea Americana: avocado, zaboka, aguacate

Phyllanthus urinaria: shatter stone, chanca piedra, meniran

Pimenta racemosa: bay rum, wild cinnamon, bwaden

Piper auritum: bull hoof, root beer plant, hoja de Santa Maria

Piper marginatum: anesi wiwiri, marigold pepper, hinojo

Portulaca oleraceae: little hogweed, pigweed, pourpier

Pouteria sapota: mammee sapote, sapote

Rhoeo spathacea: oyster plant, Moses-in-the-cradle, wandering Jew plant

Richeria grandis: bois bandé, mang blanc, bwa bandé

Rolandra fruticosa: yerba de plata, herbe argentee, tete negresse

Roystonea regia Syn. *Roystonea reglia*: royal palm, palmier royal

Saccharum officinarum: sugar cane, canne à sucre

Scoparia dulcis: sweet broom, broom weed, bitter broom

Sechium edula: chayote, christophene, Madeira marrow

Senna occidentalis: coffee senna, septic weed, bruca

Serenoa serrulata: saw palmetto, dwarf palmetto, pan plant

Solanum torvum: prickly solanum, devil's fig, turkey berry

Stachytarpheta cayennensis: verbena, blue snakeweed, Brazilian tea

Stachytarpheta jamaicensis: vervine, blue snakeweed, worry vine

Stemodia durantifolia: white wooly stemodia, white wooly twintip

Swietenia mahogoni: mahogany, West Indian mahogany

Tagetes patula: marigold, tall marigold, French marigold

Tamarindus indica: tamarind, tangal asam, celagi

Thevetia peruviana: lucky nut, yellow oleander, cabalonga

Vismia macrophylla: wild plantain leaf, carachero, shittin cloud

Xylopia frutescens: malagueto, blister wood, malagueto chico

Zingiber officinale: ginger, jengibre

Chapter 6 Haitian Vodou

dyab. Monster believed to eat people in the Haitian culture.

Erzuli. Spirit of love, beauty, purity, and romance; wife of Damballa, Agwe, and Ogou.

giyon. Equivalent of depression; clients with *giyon* present with a high level of anxiety and also report sensations of weakness and vulnerability.

hunfo. Vodou temple; vodou clinic where healing takes place.

lwa. A vodou spirit.

les invisibles. The spirits; those we cannot see.

lwa kenbe. Retaliation from the spirits for unperformed duties or broken promises.

manbo. A vodou priestess.

mèt tèt. Master of the head; Principal protective spirit. Big guardian angel; consciousness or personality.

pase leson. First step of vodou healing where the vodou priest or priestess diagnoses the nature of a problem or illness.

Peristil/hunfo. Vodou temple; vodou clinic where healing takes place.

pitit fèy. Little leaf; vodou priests (ess) call their clients *pitit fèy;* a vodou follower.

Chapter 8 Santería

Sp. = Spanish Yor.= Yoruban (many of the Yoruban words here are reproduced in their Spanish translation/format.

Abakuá. A secret society of Ekpe origin (Nigeria), open only to men. *Abakuá* has been present in Cuba since the 1830s.

abiku (Yor.). "Born to die"; usually refers to children/spirits who are born on earth only to return within a short time to *orun* (heaven).

aché (Yor.). Spiritual power/energy; life force.

Ángel de Guardia (Sp.). Guardian angel; in *La Regla de Ocha* refers to the guardian spirit of ones' head.

apertura (Sp.). Refers to the era of political and cultural opening that occurred in Cuba in the 1990s (the Special Period).

babalawo (Yor.) a priest of *Ifá*, in Cuba a position held only by males.

babalochas (Yor.). A male priest of *oricha*; "father of the *orichas.*"

Babalú-Ayé (Yor.). *Oricha* of smallpox, infectious diseases, and leprosy; syncretized in *La Regla de Ocha* with the Catholic saint San Lázaro.

brujería (Sp.). Witchcraft.

collares (Sp.). Necklaces; in *La Regla de Ocha* refers to the beaded necklaces (each representing a specific *oricha*) given as a first initiatory step in the religion.

diloggun (Yor.). A Cuban adaptation of a Yoruban divinatory system using 16 cowrie shells. The highset form of divination done by *Oloricha*.

dueño (Sp.). Lord, ruler.

ebbo (Yor.). Offering or sacrifice designed to influence *oricha*, *eggun*, or other spiritual entities. A fundamental part of *La Regla de Ocha* practice.

egun (Yor.). Ancestors by blood.

eleda (Yor.). Head, inner being, spirit that resides in one's head.

espiritismo (Sp.). A branch of spiritual practice that is based on the teachings of 19ᵗʰ century French educator Allan Kardec, who wrote several books on mediumship. A central belief of *espiritismo* is that spirits need light and prayer to elevate them spiritually. *Espiritismo* became very popular with the middle classes of Latin America and the Hispanic Caribbean around the turn of the century. In Cuba, *espiritismo* mixed with *La Regla de Ocha* so that today the two are intertwined. Evidently, *espiritismo* replaced important *egun* rituals and worship which did not survive African slavery.

espiritista (Sp.). One who practices *espiritismo*.

Guerreros (Sp.). Warriors; refers to the quartet of warrior *orichas Elleguá, Ogun, Ochossi,* and *Osun,* who are generally received together as a secondary step (after receiving *collares*) as an initiatory step in the religion.

Ifá (Yor.). Corpus of 16 major *odu,* which are further developed into 256 lesser *odu* which is the central body of wisdom Yoruban origin. Priests of *Ifá* are known as *babalawos.*

ikin (Yor.). Nuts of the oil palm; used by *babalawos* in divination.

ile (Yor.). House; spiritual family joined by initiatory lineage (godparents and godchildren).

iré (Yor.). Good luck, blessing.

iré ariku (Yor.). Blessing of long life and victory over death.

iyalocha (Yor.). Priestess of the *orichas;* "mother of the *orichas*"; equivalent to *santera.*

letra (Sp.). Letter; refers to the *odu* that falls in a divination.

limpieza (Sp.). Cleansing; in *La Regla de Ocha limpiezas* may involve baths, flowers, fruits, and vegetables, animals, grains, alcohol, tobacco, etc.

Lukumí (Yor.). Another name for Yoruban that was adopted in Cuba and became the common name for Africans of that ethnic group as well as another name for *La Regla de Ocha.*

maldiciones (Sp.). Curses.

malojo (Sp.). Evil eye.

malpensimientos (Sp.). Bad thoughts of others; the sending of negative energy.

misa (Sp.). Spiritual mass for the spirits of the dead.

nervios (Sp.). Anxiety/mental illness.

Obatalá (Yor.). *Oricha* of white cloth, wisdom, coolness; rules the head, bones, nerves; punishments are insanity, blindness, paralysis.

odu (Yor.). One of 16 bodies of knowledge contained in the entire corpus of *Ifá,* a compilation of verse and wisdom developed in the oral culture of the Yorubans centuries ago. Each *odu* contains a wealth of allegories, parables, advice, examples of correct conduct, *patakis* or moral fables, and remedies.

Olofin (Yor.) Supreme God (of a trinity with *Oludumare* and *Olorun*).

Oloricha (Yor.). Collective name for both *babalochas* and *iyalochas.*

Olorun (Yor.) Supreme God (of a trinity with *Oludumare* and *Olofin*).

Oludumare (Yor.). Supreme God (of a trinity with *Olofin* and *Olorun*).

omi tutu (Yor.). Cool water.

opele (Yor.). A chain with eight coconut shell pieces which is used by *babalawos* to divine *odu*.

Ori (Yor.). *Oricha* of one's head; one's personal *oricha*.

oricha (Yor.). A deity of the Yoruban pantheon; the most well known in *La Regla de Ocha* include *Elleguá*, *Ogún*, *Ochossi*, *Obatalá*, *Changó*, *Ochún*, *Yemayá*, *Oyá*.

osogbo (Yor.). Bad luck; evil.

palero (Sp.). A practitioner of *Palo Monte*.

Palo Monte (Sp.). Afro-Cuban religion of Bantu/Congo origin.

patakis (Yor.). The stories/moral fables found in the *odu*.

resolver (Sp.). An expression used frequently by Cubans to refer to the day-to-day struggle to meet the basic needs of life—food, clothing, water, work, money.

Santería (Sp.). Literally "worship of the saints"; another name for *La Regla de Ocha*.

santero/santera (Sp.). Spanish name for *bablocha/iyalocha*.

Vodou (Kreyol). Religion of Haitian origin which is a syncretism of African and Catholic influences; also found in the eastern part of Cuba.

voudouisants (Kreyol). Devotees of vodou.

Chapter 9 *Espiritismo*

dis-obsession Therapy. A psycho-spiritual therapeutic technique that disrupts the influence of an obsessed spirit over an incarnated person.

medium. A person (incarnated spirit) through whom spirits are able to communicate.

obsession. A pervasive, persistent, and intrusive spiritual entity who influences an incarnated or disincarnated spirit entity.

radical empathy. Personal and spiritual identification between healer and supplicant that fully bonds both within a realm of confidence, understanding, and support.

spirit guide. Spiritual entity that protects or guides those with whom it is identified.

Chapter 10 Revival

angels. Spirits that Revivalists "work" within Jamaica; mostly Biblical figures.

balmyard. A place of spiritual healing in Jamaica, generally operated by a Revivalist.

bush. Herbal medicines used in Jamaica.

duppy. A Jamaican term for the spirit of a deceased person.

Kumina. A Jamaican religious tradition found principally in the parish of St. Thomas that is associated particularly with funeral rites and has a strong African component.

modda. A revered woman in Jamaica who is leader of a Revival group or a healer with a balmyard.

Myalism. A spiritual tradition in Jamaica that developed from Obeah in the 18th century and is associated with a dance, healing, spirit possession ("myal"), and opposition to "witchcraft."

Native Baptists. An indigenous religious tradition of 18th century Jamaica that imbued Baptist missionary Christianity with Myalist practices such as visions, dreams, and spirit possession.

Obeah. The practice of magic in Jamaica and the British West Indies.

Obeah doctor or Obeah man. Individuals with the power to intercede with spirits, to practical ends: healing the sick, protecting crops from thieves, finding lost of stolen property, gaining revenge, predicting the future, casting spells, and offering protection from spells.

Obia. Spiritual knowledge brought from Africa to Jamaica and other parts of the African diaspora.

Pocomania. A religious tradition indigenous to Jamaica, also known as Pukkumina. A derisive term used to refer to indigenous, particularly African, spiritualism in Jamaica.

reading. A diagnostic exam performed on a client or patient by a Revival healer, using spiritual techniques or divination.

Revival. A religious tradition indigenous to Jamaica, emerging in response to the Great Revival of 1860–1861. Also known as Zion or Zion Revival.

science. A modern term for Obeah in Jamaica, particularly when it involves de Laurence.

seal. A sacred shrine that attracts spirits in Jamaican Revival religion. The term also refers to

sigils. Distinctive occult signs or drawings representing the spirits to be invoked. A shrine must contain a sigil-seal, but a sigil-seal can be used without a shrine.

Chapter 11 Shango

doption. Vigorous dancing trance session that allows one to travel quickly to the spiritual lands, normally done in groups in a church meeting.

jumbie. An evil spirit.

lock up. Soul loss, the belief that one's soul is outside of one's body, the symptoms of which correspond to depression.

maljo. Harming someone supernaturally through envy, corresponding to many cultures' ideas of the evil eye.

meditation. Trance session consisting of quietly closing one's eyes and travelling in the spiritual world.

mother. A female leader among the Spiritual Baptists, often a female pointer.

mourning. Long trance sessions while blindfolded.

Obeah. Black magic.

Orisha. A Yoruba-derived religion originating in Trinidad, "orisha" being the Yoruba term for a god.

pointer. The head of a Spiritual Baptist congregation who has the ability to guide one in mourning (to point the way to the spiritual lands).

Shango. Aan older term for Orisha, now often considered derogatory. Shango is one of the chief orishas.

Chapter 13 Rastafarl

Babylon. Name given to objects of Western society; represented by the police, governmental organizations.

ganja. Cultivated Indian hemp from the female plant; also called marijuana (of Mexican-Spanish roots) collie weed, grass, weed, hemp (Indian hemp origin).

Rastafari scholar E. E. Cashmore:

> I and I is an expression to totalize the concept of oneness, the oneness of two persons. So God is within all of us and we're one people in fact. The bond of Ras

> Tafari is the bond of God, of man. But man itself needs a head and the head of man is His Imperial Majesty Haile Selassie I (always pronounced as the letter 'I,' never as the number one or 'the first') of Ethiopia.

The term is often used in place of "you and I" or "we" among Rastafari, implying that both persons are united under the love of Jah.

irations. Creation; reasoning.

livity. Natural way of life or totality of one's being in the world.

ones. People in general.

overstanding. *Overstanding* (also "innerstanding") replaces "understanding," referring to enlightenment that raises one's consciousness.

Chapter 15 Islam

The list below is in the main either Urdu or Hindi terms but are not here identified as such. They are familiar to both Muslims and Hindus who are the 19th to mid-20th century diaspora from the Indian subcontinent, a familiarity that is suggestive of the cultural fluidity discussed in the essay.

'Aashura. The 10th day of Muharram. For Shi'as it is day of mourning. For Sunnis, it is a day of rejoicing for the glorious events with cosmic significance that happened on that day.

Awliya' Allah. Friends of God, pious ones, interceding for divine assistance.

ayat. A verse of the Qur'an, the holy text of Islam.

babu. An older Hindu person, term used as a form of respect.

baqarah. Meaning cow, the name for a chapter of the *Qur'an*—Surah al Baqara.

bhuts. Evil spirits in Hindi.

bucra. Used in mockery to refer to oppressors, white sugar planters.

dam. Breath, air, life, scent, and stewing over a slow fire.

damiidan. To blow or breathe, and is associated with the Arabic "*dam*/blood."

dam karna. To do the blowing after making the supplication or recitation of passages from the *Qur'an* that for adherents is a life-giving or affirming book.

dhikr. Remembrance of God, through repetition of his name as a way of purifying the heart.

didi. Aunt, used as a term of respect.

du`ā'. Humble supplication to God or prayer using Qur'anic verses.

imam. Leader of Friday worship in the mosque, and a spiritual leader of the Muslim community.

iman. Faith or belief.

jhadu. Magic involving the idea of waving a wand or stick to expel evil spirit.

jharay. Hindi word for healing practice that drives out evil sprits.

karamaat. Charisma, blessed by being a friend of Allah, close to God.

karna. The act of doing

maangna. To ask or beg as in knocking from door to door for alms.

maangna du`ā'. An Urdu expression meaning "supplication," but often rendered as prayer, and used here as such, humbly asking or begging God.

maiya ji. An older and respected person, a term for the imam.

mamu. Uncle in Hindi, used as a form of respect to an older person.

nazar. An evil eye or gaze cast on a child.

sadhu. A Hindu revered or holy person, used in showing respect.

salāt. Prayer done five times daily in Islam, a pillar of Islam.

shaykh. Head of a larger family, and term used to show respect to the head.

Surah – chapter of the Qur'an.

Surah al Baqara. The name for a chapter in the Qur'an meaning "cow."

tabeej. Amulet.

tadjha. A bamboo made frame decorated with colored paper to represent the tomb of Prophet Mohammed's martyred grandsons at Karbala; a gathering commemorating the martyrdom and occurring on '*Aashura*, that is the 10th day of Muharram, first month in the Islamic calendar, that in Guyana became festive and riotous , and is known as the Hosay festival in Trinidad.

taqwah. God-fearing Muslim; one watchful over oneself morally and spiritually so as not to stray away from God.

ta'ziya. Mourning or consolation.

INDEX